PRAISE FOR
The Arm

"This is the most important baseball book in years, not just for major league pitchers like me who had Tommy John surgery but for every parent who wants a child with a healthy arm. This is an epidemic that can be fixed, and *The Arm* is a great first step."

—John Smoltz, Cy Young Award winner

"A timely and comprehensive look at all aspects of a baseball problem that in recent years appears to approach a crisis."

—Bob Costas

"This is a stunning exposé of the hidden story behind the most frequent operation performed on the most important players in this most important game in our country."

—Ken Burns

"*The Arm* makes it official—Jeff Passan is the best young baseball writer in America. This searing, meticulously reported account of the orthopedic revolution that began with Tommy John is must reading for every manager, general manager, pitcher and, most especially, every parent whose child has 100-mph dreams."

—Jane Leavy, *New York Times* bestselling author of *The Last Boy: Mickey Mantle and the End of America's Childhood*

"Passan varies his approach to his subject like an ace mixing his speeds, leaving the reader happily guessing at what's coming next."

—*New York Times Book Review*

"Passan has written an important book. For arms, if there is Tommy John surgery, maybe we now also have Jeff Passan education."

—Frank Deford, *Washington Post*

"The best baseball book of the year. . . . Jeff Passan spent several years in clubhouses and operating rooms to report *The Arm*. It's a close, exceptionally well-written look into the game's epidemic of ruptured elbow ligaments, and the hard fact that medical science still has no real answers for it."

—*Boston Globe*

"One of the more important books on baseball of the decade, a superbly researched and detailed look at the current 'epidemic' of arm injuries in the sport."

—*Publisher's Weekly* (starred review)

"Passan makes you care deeply about pitching arms and the boys and men attached to them. In doing so, he transforms medical jargon and inside-baseball minutiae back into flesh and blood. You sweat every second of the journey."

—Jonah Keri, *Wall Street Journal*

"A must-read for any sports dad or anxious Mets fan. Grade: A."

—*Entertainment Weekly*

"Jeff Passan's *The Arm* is the real deal—a book that's both readable as hell and that has something meaningful to say about the way the game works. . . . This human element lends the book its propulsive quality, but every part is fascinating."

—*BookPage*

The Arm

The
Arm

Inside the
Billion-Dollar Mystery
of the Most Valuable
Commodity in Sports

Jeff Passan

HARPER

NEW YORK • LONDON • TORONTO • SYDNEY

A hardcover edition of this book was published in 2016 by Harper, an imprint of HarperCollins Publishers.

HarperCollins books may be purchased for educational, business, or sales pro-motional use. For information, please e-mail the Special Markets Department at SPsales@harpercollins.com.

FIRST HARPER PAPERBACK EDITION PUBLISHED 2017.

Designed by William Ruoto

Library of Congress Cataloging-in-Publication Data has been applied for.

ISBN 978-0-06-240037-6 (pbk.)

17 18 19 20 21   OV/LSC   10 9 8 7 6 5 4 3 2 1

FOR DUK, HE WHO'LL NEVER AGAIN
BE FORGOTTEN.

CONTENTS

VIII / Contents

The Arm

For 130 years, pitchers have thrown a baseball overhand, and for 130 years, doing so has hurt them. Starter or reliever, left-handed or right-handed, short or tall, skinny or fat, soft-tossing or hard-throwing, old or young—it matters not who you are, what color your skin is, what country you're from. The ulnar collateral ligament (UCL), a stretchy, triangular band in the elbow that holds together the upper and lower arms, plays no favorites. If you throw a baseball, it can ruin you.

When the UCL breaks, only one fix exists: Tommy John surgery. Over the past decade, the procedure became a frequently uttered curse word as pitcher after pitcher felt the pain of a torn ligament, huffed anesthesia a few days later, and woke up an hour after that with a fresh scar and an exasperating rehabilitation schedule. Some of the biggest names in Major League Baseball needed Tommy John. Even more kids, some barely teenagers, blew out their elbows and underwent surgery. At the highest levels of the game, a panic swelled. Not only were the arms of current pitchers failing, elite players from the next generation were going down before they could sign their first professional contract.

The culture of baseball seemed backward to me. The more I thought about the pervasiveness of Tommy John, the more I understood it needed demystifying. I heard stories of kids getting Tommy John surgery at fourteen years old. (They were true.) And of kids who underwent Tommy John even when they weren't hurt, because they thought it would help them throw harder. (Neither the stories nor the implication was true.)

Mostly, I wanted to understand this for my son. He was five years old. He loved baseball. He wanted to play catch every day. He was hooked, like his dad. And the more I heard stories from other parents—of their sons getting hurt or boys they know quitting baseball because their arms no longer worked—the more I needed to figure out what was happening to the arm.

So I spent three years traveling the world to find out. I saw a mad scientist in rural Florida who believes he can fix the arm and a couple of geniuses in Chicago who saw fit to spend more than $150 million on one. I went to Seattle to watch a human being throw a baseball almost 106 miles per hour and to Kansas City to see a teenager flirt with 100. I flew to Arizona to get Sandy Koufax's opinion on the greatest sports orthopedist ever, asked that orthopedist how he came up with Tommy John surgery in the first place, and learned from Tommy John himself how he once worried that his hand was going to be permanently clawed because of it. I sat in laboratories, saw doctors tend to bodies living and dead, went halfway across the globe to a place where the problem is even greater, read medical studies, and scavenged through data, all to answer two vital questions:

How did baseball fail the pitching arm, and what can be done to save it?

Eventually, I found two pitchers who allowed me to infiltrate their lives at their nadir so I could fully understand what happens when an arm—and a career—blows up. Daniel Hudson was twenty-five when his UCL burst. He threw differently from most, his arm slot a low three-quarters, his release almost like a slingshot, each pitch stoking the cauldron's fire. Even so, the Arizona Diamondbacks had never bothered tinkering with his mechanics. A pitcher is fine until he isn't. The other pitcher, Todd Coffey, was a right-handed reliever with a personality as big as the scar on his elbow. He needed two Tommy John surgeries, the first when he was nineteen, the next at thirty-one. A study on two-time Tommy John patients showed that the ligament from Coffey's first surgery lasted the longest of any pitcher who needed another surgery. This didn't guarantee his return from the second. Nothing can.

I marveled at Hudson's and Coffey's daily existence, which toggled between triumph and failure. They balanced loneliness and tedium with excitement and redemption. Optimism got into daily head-on collisions with reality. These two men are the faces of every arm. And yet before I tell their stories, it's important to understand the arm's place in the rest of the baseball world and what's at stake beyond billions of dollars and World Series titles.

The problem is not going away. The sport's foremost doctors believe it's worsening. The current generation of pitchers is lost, the product of a broken system, their arms ticking time bombs. If that doesn't change, today's kids will be the next casualties. They throw more and harder at younger ages than ever. Do the same thing again and again and again, and no matter how natural—like many things about the arm, the idea that throwing is an unnatural motion is a complete myth—it will break.

I don't want that to be my son. I don't want that to be your son. Baseball knows it needs top-to-bottom change. The $1.5 billion Major League Baseball spends annually on pitchers' salaries is five times more than the combined cost of every starting quarterback in the NFL. It exceeds the top two hundred NBA salaries put together. When I call the pitching arm the most valuable commodity in sports, it is not an exaggeration. And yet the most overanalyzed sport in the world, with an industry of bright minds studying its intricacies, loses half a billion dollars a year to injuries. More than 50 percent of pitchers end up on the disabled list every season, on average for two months–plus, and one-quarter of major league pitchers today wear a zipper scar from Tommy John surgery along their elbows.

People in the sport call arm injuries an epidemic. Solutions do exist. They aren't easy, and they'll take the sort of overhaul baseball seems loath to implement, but they can happen. Because one thing I now know is that for all of its travails, all the heartache it can cause, all the frustration left in its wake, the arm is capable of wondrous things.

CHAPTER 1

A Dead Man's Tendon

HE DIDN'T WANT A PIECE of the dead guy holding his elbow together. That's all he asked.

Todd Coffey had resigned himself to spending the next year learning how to throw a baseball again. He had accepted the mind-numbing rehabilitation process after tearing his ulnar collateral ligament, the two-inch elastic band that had prevented the upper and lower bones of his right arm from flying apart when he pitched. He simply couldn't stomach the new ligament coming from someplace other than his own body. "I think about it as a used car that has 40,000 miles on it," Coffey said. "You don't know what the previous 40,000 miles were like. I don't know what it's been through."

He had spent his entire adulthood in baseball. Got married, had kids, fought his way to the major leagues, made his first million and a few more, played the hero and the goat. Now his elbow had popped, and it was fix it or be done. He was used to binary outcomes after spending nearly half his life as a relief pitcher. Ball or strike. Win or loss. Save the game or blow it. He knew nothing else. He didn't want to know anything else. And here he was, at thirty-one, with that career, that life, at risk, and the doctor wanted to reconstruct his elbow with a dead man's tissue because Coffey's own body didn't have any to spare.

On July 17, 2012, Coffey slid into an MRI tube at the Kerlan-Jobe Orthopaedic Clinic in Los Angeles. The next day he was scheduled to undergo Tommy John surgery, the procedure that revolutionized baseball in 1974, when Dr. Frank Jobe used a tendon from the wrist of John, a left-handed pitcher, to replace his torn elbow ligament. At the time, Jobe said it had a 1 percent chance of success. In the forty years since, the procedure has saved nearly one thousand professional players' careers, including that of Todd Coffey. It had given Coffey everything, and now it was threatening to take it away. Coffey was a well-traveled reliever, having bounced from Cincinnati to Milwaukee to Washington to Los Angeles, and now to Dr. Neal ElAttrache's operating room.

Nobody needs a pitcher with arm problems, not when there are kids in the minor leagues who throw harder and come cheaper. While Coffey wanted again to be among the 80 percent whose careers Tommy John surgery saves, a second procedure poses far more risks. Revisions, as they're called, aren't nearly as successful. Compound that with the possibility of foreign tissue mending Coffey's elbow and a ripped tendon in his forearm that required repair, too, and even ElAttrache warned this was no typical sew and go.

"This," he said, "is the toughest Tommy John I've ever done."

Were it up to ElAttrache, he would've skipped the MRI and gone straight to an allograft, the technical name for a tissue transplant from a cadaver. Coffey insisted, so the MRI machine growled and confirmed what ElAttrache had thought: maybe, just maybe, there would be sufficient tendon in his left leg for a graft. It probably wasn't twelve centimeters, the minimal length needed, and the scar tissue from the previous surgery might have compromised its integrity. Discouraged, Coffey asked ElAttrache to cut into his leg and poke around for something better anyway. Coffey would know only when he awoke from the anesthesia whether he might join the short list of major leaguers striking out batters with an elbow not entirely his.

On the morning of the surgery, Coffey was supposed to arrive at seven thirty. He showed up a half hour early at Kerlan-Jobe with his wife, Jennifer, and his mother-in-law, Cathy Singer. Palm trees swayed in front of the five-story building plopped in the middle of West LA. Celebrities and athletes and every-day people mingle daily in the third-floor waiting room, burying their heads in magazines and smartphones before appointments with ElAttrache. Coffey plopped into an old chair and started to fill out paperwork. The signatures seemed endless. Coffey didn't bother reading the documents. His eyes drooped. He hadn't slept very well. Stan Conte, a trainer for Coffey's team, the Los Angeles Dodgers, slipped into the room and pulled Jennifer aside.

"How is Todd?" Conte asked.

"He kept saying he didn't want to have surgery," she said.

Coffey didn't know what to feel. His livelihood mocked him. It wasn't just the allograft. Jennifer, his second wife, was five months pregnant with their first child, and Coffey wanted to come back in twelve months whereas the doctors said it was going to take eighteen, and, God, was the rehab brutal, and what if the surgery didn't go well and kept him from even trying to come back, which didn't happen much, but maybe it would happen to him. And the dead guy. Please, Doc, not the dead guy.

He buried his head in the papers, looped his signature, tried not to listen.

"Time to go," a nurse said.

Coffey leaned over and gave Jennifer a kiss. She told him everything would be OK, and he wanted to believe her.

"I love you," he said.

The nurse whisked him through a door and back to an operating room, where ElAttrache soon would join them. Todd Coffey's career was not dying, not there, not then. Neal ElAttrache promised he'd save it.

THE FIRST TIME TODD COFFEY'S UCL blew, the surgeon tried to harvest the palmaris longus, a tendon in his right wrist, to tie the elbow back together. The tendon was too thin to stabilize the joint. He sliced open the other wrist. Same problem. So he went to Coffey's left leg and removed the gracilis, a hamstring tendon. It broke as the doctor tried to loop it through Coffey's elbow. One more cut yielded a fresh gracilis. Mercifully, it worked. Coffey made history on May 11, 2000: He was the first—and still the only—patient in the history of UCL reconstruction to go in for a surgery that entailed two cuts and leave with five scars.

Over his fourteen years in the game, Coffey had left behind an almost-unparalleled trail of apocryphal stories that were actually true. Like the time he asked the Arizona Diamondbacks' visiting clubhouse manager to make him a snack. He wanted peanut butter on one side, jelly on the other, two Reese's Peanut Butter Cups in the middle, all griddle-fried with butter. To this day, visiting players at Chase Field still can order the Todd Coffey Sandwich. His new teammates always wondered about the extra piece of luggage he hauled from city to city. The hard-shelled suitcase carried just one item: Coffey's baseball glove.

Justin Todd Coffey was born September 9, 1980, in Shelby, North Carolina. He stands six feet four, weighs approximately three hundred pounds, and has a shock of red hair with a beard to match. Fans know him best for his exuberant sprints from the bullpen to the pitcher's mound, during which many of those three hundred pounds gyrate in manners only physicists can explain, and which tens of thousands of YouTube viewers have enjoyed. For seven years, he clawed through the minor leagues: the twelve-hour bus trips and fast-food dinners in bunk-ass towns for nothing pay and even less hope. Eventually, he found a role as a bullpen piece for the Cincinnati Reds, where he became a cult favorite. Although he is smarter than his goofy persona might suggest, Coffey fits the stereotype of a man playing a kids' game: he still drinks whole milk, watches *Star Trek*, and obsesses over Blood Bowl, a football-rugby hybrid dice game that involves painting figurines and having them disfigure one another.

Coffey's career had been far better than most, even if instability defined it. His career earnings totaled nearly $7 million as an average reliever for eight years. Cincinnati had released him on his birthday in 2008, and the Milwaukee Brewers and Washington Nationals subsequently let him walk via free agency, and his current Dodgers contract would expire at the end of 2012, leaving him jobless for the first time since a Reds executive tried to talk him out of signing as a seventeen-year-old. It was another of Coffey's odd stories. After Cincinnati chose him in the forty-first round of the 1998 draft, the team wanted to watch him pitch in junior college for a season and, if he looked good, sign him for a far more significant bonus before the next draft. To show their best intentions, the Reds asked area scout Steve Kring to pay Coffey a visit after the draft.

"I sent the scout into the house to go ahead and offer him a thousand dollars," said DeJon Watson, the Reds' scouting director at the time. "There was no bonus. It was just the minor league contract. And he fucking accepted it! The scout's calling me from the house, freaking out. I said, 'Did you explain to him we want him to go to college and give him more money later on?' And he said, 'Yeah. He doesn't care.'"

Watson had already spent every dollar budgeted for the draft by his skinflint owner, Marge Schott, and did not want to draw her ire for dropping even a thousand dollars on a forty-first-round pick from North Carolina who threw 88 miles per hour. He started screaming at Kring.

"D," Kring said, "Todd wants to talk to you on the phone."

Watson figured he could convince Coffey to go to college. He sweet-talked his way into deals. Surely he could sweet-talk his way out of one. Watson told Coffey he was excited to have him in the Reds family and that everyone wanted to see him grow as a pitcher—in college. To which Coffey replied that he'd rather sign. Watson thought Coffey didn't understand. He did. He understood clearly. He just refused to listen. Coffey was signing his contract.

"And I promise you," he said, "I'm gonna pitch in the big leagues."

He reported to Billings, Montana, one of eight future major leaguers on the Reds' rookie-ball team. He didn't throw hard, not yet. He was awkward, Watson said, "like a big Baby Huey at the time. They teased the shit out of him. I felt so bad. Everybody rode him so hard." Coffey stomached the jokes, kept improving, gaining velocity, fighting through his first Tommy John recovery, not just making it but staying. "It was something special about him," said Watson, who later helped bring Coffey to Los Angeles, where he was an assistant general manager. "He said he was gonna pitch in the big leagues. And he kept his end of the bargain."

Coffey loved pitching for the Dodgers. They had spent most of the first three months that season in first place. Dodger Stadium was paradise for pitchers. The sale of the team to a Magic Johnson–backed consortium invigorated the city. When Coffey came into the game in relief in the top of the eighth inning against Cincinnati with his team down 3–1 on July 2, 2012, he figured it would be just like his previous 460 appearances in the big leagues: throw sinkers and sliders, get ground-ball outs, head home. On Coffey's fifth pitch, a slider that plunked his former teammate Jay Bruce on the foot, he felt a twinge in his elbow. He shook his arm and thought little of it. Coffey bounced his next pitch in the dirt. His catcher, A. J. Ellis, visited the mound.

"Something doesn't look right," he said.

"It feels fine," Coffey said.

"You're not extending," Ellis said.

"I will, I will," Coffey said.

Three pitches later, Dodgers outfielder Elian Herrera mis-played a Todd Frazier hit into a triple. Manager Don Mattingly headed to the mound with the team's head trainer. Coffey threw a couple of warm-up pitches, and even though he shook his arm after each, he swore he was good, and they believed him.

Coffey struck out the next two hitters. He still has no idea how.

"Maybe adrenaline?" he said. "My elbow was done. And the tough thing is, in my case, it didn't hurt. I didn't have any pain. There's no swelling. It just felt like normal inflammation. My body is telling me: You can pitch."

He gave up a hit on his next pitch, and Mattingly yanked him and sent him into the clubhouse so ElAttrache, the Dodgers' team physician, could examine him. Coffey is almost certain his elbow blew when he hit Bruce, meaning he fired sixteen pitches, most up around 92 miles per hour, with a UCL shredded for the second time.

An MRI the next day confirmed the tear. The misery of Tommy John surgery had struck Coffey again, as it would strike at least twenty more pitchers through the end of 2012. Even if his career in Los Angeles was done, Coffey promised to follow the Dodgers the rest of the season. He swore he would not forget them, no matter where he was or what he was doing.

Coffey needed just one favor before he left and went on to the rest of his career. He asked for Mitch Poole, the home clubhouse attendant, to wrap up his spikes. He wasn't going to waste a perfectly good pair of shoes, not when he planned on using them again.

THERE WAS BLOOD ON THE floor of the stark-white Operating Room 2 at Kerlan-Jobe, and the surgery hadn't even started.

Coffey, who hated needles, had warned the staff about his elusive veins. "I've always been a hard stick," he said. "My veins hide." On the first attempt at inserting an IV in Coffey's arm, the vein blew and spurted crimson. It took three more tries before an IV worked.

Coffey breathed deeply. At least he wouldn't have to watch the rest. The nurse warned him he would feel some burning. Propofol, the creamy white sedative doctors call "milk of amnesia," started to course through Coffey's body.

The door opened and ElAttrache walked in.

"Doc," Coffey said. "This is some good shit."

"We're going to get you taken care of," ElAttrache said.

"Well, good luck," Coffey said, drifting off to sleep. Once he was out, the medical team covered everything except his right arm with a sheet. ElAttrache first needed to assess the havoc. Years of damage can leave a pitcher's elbow looking like a grenade went off inside. ElAttrache started the scalpel above Coffey's first Tommy John scar on his upper arm, sliced over the elbow and ended beneath the bottom of the old scar—about twelve inches total, four inches longer than with a first-time UCL patient. He split the muscles around the elbow and used retractors to expose the UCL area—an inscrutable mess of red muscles blending into ligaments mingling with tendons camouflaging bones. ElAttrache needed to navigate the mess, and the first task called for someone even more specialized than him.

Dr. Steve Shin worked as a hand surgeon at Kerlan-Jobe, and ElAttrache needed his precision. Shin looked into the exposed elbow and prepared his one assignment: move an eight-inch portion of Coffey's ulnar nerve, a tube of fibers that originates at the spine, snakes down the arm, and controls fine-motor movement in the hand. The ulnar nerve allows you to pinch, make a fist, type. A hand is a hand, and not a claw, because of it. Even the slightest bit of irritation to the nerve can have a profound effect; since Coffey's first surgery, the numbness in his ring finger and pinky hadn't abated. Not only could mishandling of the nerve set back his rehab schedule, it could leave him with permanent damage barely five minutes into the surgery.

Shin wore a pair of jeweler's loupes in order to distinguish the nerve and its tiny branches from the surrounding scar tissue. During Coffey's first operation, the surgeon, Dr. Timothy Kremchek, had brought the ulnar nerve to the front of the elbow, laying it over the reconstructed ligament, a procedure that in the dozen years since had fallen out of favor. Shin, a kind of neural cat burglar, carefully lifted the nerve away from the disarray inside Coffey's arm and fastened it temporarily to his skin with three sterile rubber loops weighted down by clamps. The ulnar nerve would rest there, a spectator to the rest of the operation, which at ten a.m. was barely under way.

Now ElAttrache could gauge the true damage, and it was grim. An MRI provides a working theory on an arm's condition, though it rarely tells the entire truth. In 2012, Minnesota Twins pitcher Scott Baker went in for surgery on the flexor-pronator mass, a bundle of muscles in the forearm, and went out with a new ulnar collateral ligament, too. ElAttrache feared Coffey's flexor mass had ripped away from the bone and torn his flexor tendon, and his suspicion was correct. Now an already trying surgery would prove a test of ElAttrache's patience and stamina as much as his technical know-how.

"Stan, look at this," ElAttrache said, calling over the Dodgers' trainer, who had scrubbed in. The last twelve years of pitches had turned Coffey's elbow into spaghetti, and the flexor tendon tore because of what Stan Conte calls "shearing force"—the minute stresses that, when repeated thousands upon thousands of times, can cause ligaments and tendons to fray and, eventually, to snap.

ElAttrache wasn't exaggerating when he called this his toughest surgery. Hundreds of Tommy John operations have earned him the title of the fastest gun in elbow reconstruction, powering through some UCL repairs in as little as sixty minutes. His preferred technique requires drilling holes to create new pathways in the humerus (upper arm) and ulna (one of the lower-arm bones) through which he can slide the tendon until perfectly taut. Over the next two years, the new tissue slowly undergoes a process called ligamentization, in which tendon cells called tenocytes modify their function and how they secrete the regenerative protein collagen, and, after about two years, change their entire form. In adapting to its new role holding the upper and lower arms together, the tendon actually morphs into a ligament, connecting bone to bone.

ElAttrache went to work, asking for pickups—medical tweezers—and a scalpel. The last track of a Counting Crows song strained through a subwoofer and two cube speakers. Conte stepped away from the table. He had sat in on plenty of surgeries, and he never tired of what they represented: a miracle of modern medicine that could give injured pitchers a new lease on a baseball career. Even with Tommy John's success rate, he didn't shrug it off as some routine procedure—"almost like a root canal," as former Atlanta Braves manager Fredi González once called it.

"A lot of people talk about Tommy John, how you're back in twelve months," Conte said. "It's not that easy. There are complications. There are issues. There are a ton of decisions to be made in the OR that can change things. It's like we're walking up to the tee right now and the hole is five hundred yards away. This is our tee shot.

"And I hope nobody shanks it."

EVERYBODY IN THE ROOM STOOD except for Neal ElAttrache. He sat in blue scrubs on a swiveling stool, a green surgical mask over his mouth. Although Todd Coffey's arm was flayed open, all eyes were on ElAttrache, who happens to have movie-star looks and a clientele to match. Earlier in 2012, a picture of Arnold Schwarzenegger and Sylvester Stallone resting in adjacent hospital beds had gone viral. ElAttrache had done their surgeries back-to-back. Schwarzenegger went to him on the recommendation of ElAttrache's brother-in-law: Stallone. He is married to the model Jennifer Flavin, and ElAttrache to her sister Tricia, a nurse he met on his first day at Kerlan-Jobe twenty-five years ago. Tricia doesn't see much of him, nor do their three daughters. He misses parent-teacher conferences and lets mom handle boy trouble. Sleep is a luxury for ElAttrache, golf a rarity. He is fifty-four, in the prime of his career, the prime of his life, and he spends most of his time tending to other people's problems. When Los Angeles Lakers star Kobe Bryant blew an Achilles, ElAttrache fixed it. When Los Angeles Dodgers ace Zack Greinke fractured a collarbone, ElAttrache mended it. He performed both of those surgeries the same April day in 2013. Hundreds of millions of dollars ride on his scalpel.

"I always have to take care of my patients and do surgery and do that well. That trumps everything else," ElAttrache said, "That level of intimacy, that relationship you make with a patient, celebrity or athlete or not, is almost like a sacred thing. I tell the guys we're training: if that privilege doesn't strike you right in the chest, to have that given to you, you're missing the most beautiful thing about what we do. It doesn't matter how famous they are. It's that you can really be involved in someone's life."

Orthopedics called him, as it did his father, Selim, who attended Jesuit school in Lebanon as a kid, studied medicine in France, and came to Chicago in the mid-1950s to complete his residency at Northwestern University. He didn't know much English, so he learned by joining a local YMCA for three months. He met a nurse named Vera, got married, graduated, moved to Utah, started a family, and relocated to Pittsburgh, where he took care of the United Mine Workers. Three of his children would grow up to be doctors. Neal was the famous one. When he gave lectures around the country, his father sometimes showed up unannounced and snuck into the back row for a listen.

"My first day in medical school, my first class in anatomy, I knew I had been blessed to find maybe the only thing I'm any good at in my life," ElAttrache said. "I feel very, very fortunate to have been able to find it. I immediately knew I was home."

More than an hour into the surgery, ElAttrache laced sutures through the holes he had drilled in Coffey's humerus and ulna to help guide the graft and, ultimately, hold it in place. The ends of the sutures stuck out like guitar strings that hadn't been clipped.

ElAttrache conducts his team like he's leading an orchestra, his hand movements signaling exactly where the other half-dozen people should be and what they should be doing. When he opens his hand, his scrub tech, Ken Newmark, knows what instrument ElAttrache needs. When he releases a tourniquet, Leslie Quinn, his nurse, is standing over the wound with a suction instrument. When he readies to drill into a limb, his equipment tech, John Hale, hands him a tool loaded with the proper bit. The movement of the team is balletic.

At 10:44 a.m., with the ulnar nerve resting safely to the side and the preliminary holes drilled and the sutures strung, ElAttrache started spelunking for whatever piece of the gracilis might be left. He ran his scalpel along Coffey's thigh. Tourniquets allowed the flesh inside to remain a pearly white. ElAttrache wasted no time in jamming his index finger into the hole. As he rooted around, ElAttrache pushed the skin of Coffey's leg out from the inside. "It's all feel," Conte likes to say. ElAttrache wasn't feeling much and asked for help. Shin and a surgical fellow each pulled back one side of Coffey's leg to give ElAttrache a better look. When doctors need something, they will MacGyver it. And if it meant Coffey's leg was going to hurt like mad when he woke up because two grown men were playing tug-of-war with it, well, he's the one who rejected the dead man's tendon, and that's what pain meds are for, anyway.

The extra leverage proved no help; no matter how much ElAttrache searched, he couldn't find what he was looking for.

"I shouldn't have to dig this out," ElAttrache said.

"It's melted down," Conte said.

Quinn, the nurse, knew what that meant. She went over to a workstation near the operating table and came back with two eight-and-a-half-by-eleven sheets of paper and showed them to ElAttrache.

"There are two choices here," she said. "You like any one better?"

She held one piece of paper in her left hand and the other in her right. ElAttrache scanned the left first, then went to the right.

"Give me that one," he said, pointing to Quinn's left hand.

As Quinn left the room, ElAttrache dug back into Coffey's leg. It was 10:56. He had already spent twelve minutes fishing. He wanted to search one more time so he could tell Coffey he made every effort. Quinn walked back in, holding a blue bedpan filled with warm water and a plastic bag with a long, white strand inside.

"You want it open?" she asked ElAttrache.

"Not yet."

A minute later, he found what he was looking for: the last remnant of Coffey's left gracilis. ElAttrache slung his fingers behind it and pulled the tendon out of the wound to show the onlookers.

"I can see through it," ElAttrache said.

"That's not great tissue," Conte said.

"This would be the weakest link of our operation if we went with that," ElAttrache said.

Nothing is as critical during Tommy John surgery as the length and diameter of the graft. Having a good piece of tissue emboldens a doctor. Had ElAttrache used Coffey's remaining gracilis, it may not have been enough to tie even a single loop, let alone the double-stranded approach ElAttrache prefers. He gestured toward the bedpan and said to Quinn: "Open it."

At 10:58 a.m., she sliced through the bag and pulled out Todd Coffey's new elbow ligament. Quinn dipped it in the water and let it continue to thaw as ElAttrache stitched together Coffey's leg and laid a few Steri-Strips over the sutures. Six minutes after its water bath began, the allograft was ready.

If Todd Coffey wanted to pitch again, it would be with the semitendinosus tendon of Donor ID 101079556, a twenty-four-year-old male who'd died in a car accident. Nobody in the room knew his name. Coffey's new tendon (cost: three thousand dollars) had arrived vacuum sealed from RTI Biologics in Gainesville, Florida, packed in dry ice inside a cooler stuffed into corrugated cardboard, just another brown box among the many dropped off at Kerlan-Jobe, a frozen miracle to undo what years of pitching had wrought.

The tool kit for ElAttrache's standard UCL replacement includes sutures made of collagen-coated, polyester-wrapped plastic polymer, stainless-steel alloy drill bits manufactured to eat through bone without burning it, chamfers to round off sharp edges of bone that could slice the fresh tendon, and the battery-powered Arthrex 600 drill. ElAttrache stood above Coffey, ready to begin the most delicate phase of the surgery: drilling two holes in the ulna that intersect like a V in the middle of the bone. The graft would come in one side and out the other. Then both ends would slide into a 5.0-millimeter tunnel on the bottom of the humerus, where two smaller drill holes on the top of the bone would create separate paths for the two ends, which would be yanked taut by the sutures ElAttrache laid earlier. Once the tension was correct, ElAttrache would knot the sutures together on the outside of the bone, stabilizing the new UCL.

The tiniest error could end Coffey's career. During Coffey's first Tommy John, this was a ho-hum portion of the proceedings, but in a revision—particularly one lasting this long—maintaining bone integrity presented the greatest danger. Forget baseball being a game of inches. Surgery dabbles in fractions of millimeters. The drill holes from Coffey's first surgery left his ulna in danger of cracking. ElAttrache needed holes small enough to ensure the bone's stability and large enough to accept the thick graft. Already he had shaved down the semitendinosus to accommodate it. He took a deep breath, sucking in his mask, and leaned in toward the ulna, ready to fix Coffey's elbow using the docking method, a variation on Jobe's original surgery.

As he depressed the drill's trigger, ElAttrache used a guide to stop the bit from plunging too far. "I have to be careful on the ulnar side," he had explained earlier. "I don't want to break the bridge." The bridge is the area between the two holes. The bigger the bridge, the less likely the bone is to crack. If the bone did fail, ElAttrache could attach the UCL with a metal button or screw, an inferior solution. Broken bone meant no more baseball.

Immediately ElAttrache knew the 3.5-millimeter holes in the ulna were too small. He took away the guide and free-handed one hole to a 3.6-millimeter width. He tried to pull the graft through. Not even close. He didn't want to thin it any more, either. Most blowouts leave most of the original UCL in place; the surgeon can tie the new tendon on top of it, using the native ligament's collagen to help in the healing process. Coffey's had practically vaporized, the remaining pieces infinitesimal.

ElAttrache asked for a 4.0-millimeter bit. As Hale prepared the drill, ElAttrache debrided tissue from the bone. Shin, the hand doctor, suctioned away the refuse. ElAttrache wanted a closer look. The bridge was getting smaller by the moment, the peril growing larger.

"I'm ready," ElAttrache said. He widened the holes to 4.0 millimeters and tried to pass the graft again. It wouldn't budge. He was getting pissed. In a normal surgery, he could drill the ulnar tunnel with his eyes closed. He asked for a 4.5-millimeter guide but kept the 4.0-millimeter bit. The slightest mistake meant total failure, and ElAttrache was inviting it by free-handing the drill to expand the tunnel's opening by that fraction of a millimeter.

"That's high-tech art right there," Conte whispered. "Notice how quiet it got? Everyone knows this is technically difficult."

The drill buzzed and emerged with a bloodied bit. It was 11:31. A normal Tommy John surgery takes seventy-five minutes. This had already gone twice as long, and it wasn't close to done. Dustin Volkmer, a surgical fellow at Kerlan-Jobe, continued filming the procedure and snapping pictures with an iPhone. ElAttrache couldn't remember another revision with a blown flexor mass, so he wanted to document it for future such cases, rare though they may be.

"Graft," ElAttrache called. Quinn retrieved it from the bean-shaped pan. ElAttrache tugged at it. Still nothing. "Fat part of the graft," he said.

Then, finally, movement.

"Here it goes," ElAttrache said. "Here it goes."

The room perked up.

"A little oil?" he said. "I do not want to break this thing."

Quinn, the nurse, squirted a dab of mineral oil where graft met tunnel. The tendon started to slide.

"Whew!" ElAttrache said.

Sutures pulled the graft through the ulna and out the second hole. ElAttrache looped it into the humeral tunnel and used two more sutures to guide them down their respective paths. He measured where he needed to trim the tendon so it would fit perfectly, detached both ends from the suture sherpas, and removed it from Coffey's elbow.

No longer was the allograft white. Blood covered it as ElAttrache began trimming it to size. He admired the finished product. "I love the length," he said. After using the titanium chamfer to smooth the ulnar tunnel, ElAttrache once again slinked the tendon through, this time for good. He knotted the sutures strong and true.

The hard part was over. At 12:12, just as the Dodgers were about to take the field a few miles away, ElAttrache tied the final three knots. He lifted Coffey's limp arm in the air with the help of two others. He bent it at the elbow and rotated it in and out, like Coffey does on every pitch. If the graft slacked, ElAttrache would need to start over.

"OK," he said, "feel that."

"Whoo!" Shin said. "That's tight!"

ElAttrache sutured the new UCL to the remaining shreds of the old one. A suction tube drained away a river of blood. Every few minutes, Quinn cleared blood clots and tossed them into a biohazard wastebasket nearly filled to the brim. ElAttrache moved down to the flexor mass, the muscles that connect the elbow to the wrist, and began to fix their torn tendon and reattach them. The dried blood on his gloves was almost black. He took a deep breath and groaned. "My ass is numb," ElAttrache groused.

He had been parked in the same swivel chair for three hours. ElAttrache gently carried the ulnar nerve to its new location, away from the bone and protected by subcutaneous fat, a precaution to keep it away from bone chips that could develop, sever the nerve, and leave the hand useless.

ElAttrache hooked the first stitch to close Coffey's wound at 12:48. He cinched the final one six minutes later. After nearly four hours, Todd Coffey had a new arm.

JENNIFER COFFEY SAT IN THE chair closest to the waiting-room door, glancing at it every few minutes, hoping ElAttrache would walk through and assure her everything had gone well. She played a slot-machine app on her iPad to pass the time. Her whole morning felt like a game of chance.

She was a newly minted baseball wife, five months pregnant but barely showing. She felt that awful cocktail of nerves and fatigue. Coffey had kept her up most of the previous night, asking rhetorical questions, catastrophizing—the dead guy and what comes next and life without baseball and on and on and on.

"You think one thing," Jennifer said, "and your mind takes you further and further into the future. Not just now, but once he starts playing again. How many years does he have left to play? He has to be precise and particular and so careful. One more thing goes wrong and he's done. I don't know if anyone has had a third Tommy John. I think the more it happens, the less likely you are to return."

It wasn't just his career causing her the agita. Where would they have the baby? Pasadena, where they moved for the summer? Phoenix, where Coffey would rehab? Milwaukee, where she grew up? Rural North Carolina, their offseason home? Their wedding gifts were in Wisconsin still, and she wasn't going to be able to travel soon, and—she stopped midsentence. The door into the waiting room opened. ElAttrache and Stan Conte appeared.

"He did great," ElAttrache said.

She sighed.

"He has a very big graft," ElAttrache said. "The only issue was I wasn't able to use his own tissue. It was precariously short. And I could see through it. It was a little bitty thing. This was much better tissue."

"On my son, in that circumstance, I would've used the allograft," Conte said. "I think that's the best chance for him to get back. It really is."

"The allograft—is his body going to accept it?" Jennifer said.

"When you transplant his own tendon, there are still some living cells that emit chemical signals to attract blood vessels and things like that," ElAttrache said. "The same thing is going to happen on this, in the environment it's in, because it's a very vascular environment. That process may be a little slower. We don't know that clinically, but we think it's correct. It's definitely safe tissue to use. And it works."

"So," Jennifer said, "when will he be back?"

"I don't see this being a twelve-month return to competition," ElAttrache said. "And based on the time of the year, the chances of him making it back for next season aren't good. He just needs more time."

Jennifer would deal with their onerous year ahead soon enough. After nearly five hours, she just wanted to see her husband. She thanked ElAttrache and Conte and headed back to the recovery area, where Coffey, supine on a bed, was regaining consciousness. He wore a hospital gown and booties on his feet. He would leave two hours later with pain meds to be taken every four hours. Best of all, his fingers weren't at all numb from the handling of the ulnar nerve.

The first question Coffey asked Jennifer wasn't about the dead guy. He knew it had been likely, and he'd get used to it. Nor was it about the rehab. His relentless optimism told him he would be back in twelve months, and so he'd aim for twelve months. And it wasn't about the baby, or how Jennifer was feeling, or where they would move, or anything of that ilk. Like Neal ElAttrache, Todd Coffey was a man who kept his promises. And the day his elbow failed, he had made a promise to his teammates that he'd never forget them. Not even Propofol could break it.

He looked at Jennifer, smiled, and asked: "What's the score?"

CHAPTER 2

Dummyball

Doctors consider Tommy John surgery one of the most successful medical procedures ever because it solved a problem. When an elbow ligament tore, it could be fixed. Baseball rejoiced. "We thought elbows were solved," former Red Sox general manager Ben Cherington said. "So we stopped thinking about them."

Because an answer for elbow issues existed, the sport never bothered to concern itself with the root cause of such injuries. Maybe it was mechanics, the way a player throws the ball and its effect on his body. Perhaps it was usage, the volume of pitches or innings in a single game, over a whole season, or even longer. Certainly a player's genetic makeup could factor in, too, or how hard he threw, or what pitches he preferred, or his between-start workouts, or his diet, or any other sort of measurable factor.

Tommy John surgery, it turned out, was a paradox, the procedure that worked too well. It lulled baseball into a false sense of security, and by the time the sport realized what had happened, an epidemic was on its hands. Elbows are breaking more than ever and younger than ever. And while the rash of Tommy John surgeries that spread across Major League Baseball over the last five years took out some of the game's finest pitchers, children ages fifteen to nineteen make up a disproportionately high number of patients. Baseball is thus left scrambling to figure out how to keep its million-dollar arms healthy while fixing a feeder system that keeps sending damaged goods to major league teams.

"It's a huge issue," said Rob Manfred, Major League Baseball's commissioner. "You know why it's a huge issue? Because that's a competitive space, and the single biggest competitive advantage baseball has in that space is the fact that it may be the safest sport your kid can play. It still doesn't mean that we don't have a responsibility to make the play of the game as safe as possible for kids. And we do. We take that seriously."

Over the last two decades, baseball's youth apparatus has been filched and privatized, and the single-sport-specialization craze has transformed the game. The best players spend most weekends year-round traveling to tournaments across the country. They participate in so-called showcase events, in which maximum-effort throws and pitch velocities that light up radar guns separate the elite from the rest.

In hindsight, the results were predictable. Stephen Strasburg, the right-hander with a 102-mph fastball who shattered signing-bonus records out of college, blew out his arm twelve games into his rookie season with the Nationals. More big names followed: New York Mets ace Matt Harvey, Texas Rangers star Yu Darvish, and the late José Fernández, a Miami Marlins wunderkind who died in a boating accident in 2016.

Latin American countries, where the best kids spend their early teen years playing baseball for a living so they can cash in with bonuses at sixteen, were hardly spared: Iván Nova and Danny Salazar from the Dominican Republic, Martín Pérez and Carlos Carrasco from Venezuela, even José Contreras, the forty-year-old

Cuban. Every day, it seemed, another went down. During one two-week span early in the 2014 season, nine players underwent Tommy John.

The number one pick in the draft two months later, Brady Aiken, didn't sign with the Houston Astros because of an abnormality in his elbow and eventually needed Tommy John. Two more first-round picks in 2014, Jeff Hoffman and Erick Fedde, were chosen despite their blown-out elbows, and potential number one picks in 2015 (Michael Matuella) and 2016 (Cal Quantrill) underwent Tommy John while still in college. "It's almost like it's a sci-fi film where they're going to take the best and the brightest with a light ray coming down," Oakland Athletics GM Billy Beane said. "The ligaments remaining are the ones you don't necessarily want pitching for you."

Arm injuries are nothing new. In the days of three hundred–and four hundred–inning seasons, plenty of pitchers were injured. Sports medicine, in its nascent stages, had next to no understanding of how the arm worked. Salaries were minuscule, and the cost of losing a player was negligible. Today, the science for progress exists. It's lunacy to call arm injuries the cost of doing business when the business loses hundreds of millions of dollars as a result of them annually. Baseball nevertheless has fostered an environment in which all thirty teams treat pitchers' health as proprietary information instead of banding together to solve the sport's greatest mystery. "Teams are hesitant to invest because they think they're going to seed the money and then everyone is going to share in the information," New York Yankees president Randy Levine said. Competition gets in the way of the greater good, greed in the way of greater health, and any advances that could rejigger the system at lower levels stay in-house. "This is one where you need the it-takes-a-village approach," Beane said. "We've got to stop pretending we know the answers. Because whatever we're doing doesn't seem to be working."

As injuries piled up, teams panicked and started treating their best young players with kid gloves. In 2012, the Toronto Blue Jays sent their three top pitching prospects—Noah Syndergaard, Aaron Sanchez, and Justin Nicolino—to Class A Lansing. Syndergaard looked like a Nordic god, six feet six and 240 pounds, all muscle and blond hair. Sanchez was a six-foot-four twig with lightning in his right arm. Nicolino typified the command-and-control left-hander who kills batters softly.

For their first five starts of the season, each was limited to three innings pitched. This seemed senseless. No studies showed that unusually short outings keep pitchers healthier long-term. The restrictions felt similar to the thinking that limits most current major league starters to around one hundred pitches: a guess. I emailed then–Blue Jays general manager Alex Anthopoulos and asked why the team was handling young arms with restraint bordering on alarm.

"Overall, there's not much science to what we do," he wrote. "Just being overly cautious with our young arms. We have no evidence that shows it's the right way to go but we prefer to err on the side of caution."

Never before had I heard Anthopoulos, a studious sort whose analytical bent helped him land his job, admit to making a choice about vital pieces of his franchise's future with "no evidence." He personified a game spending a billion and a half dollars a year on something it didn't understand.

Baseball is a constantly evolving sport, challenging itself and its entrenched beliefs with rigorous self-examination. The current trend toward defensive shifts stemmed from a simple, epistemological question: What is a position? No boundaries define it, so why confine players to certain areas when the numbers show hitters deposit balls in certain pockets more often than others? The game struggles more with macro questions. It's why baseball has now settled on the reductive strategy for handling pitchers: throw them less. The fallacy of treating something as unique as a pitcher's arm collectively may be the acme of baseball senselessness.

Here's the truth: they're scared. And maybe they should be. A new generation of kids raised in travel-ball and showcase culture is throwing harder than ever, and the results are troublesome. "UCL reconstruction is becoming a victim of its own success," wrote Brandon J. Erickson, an orthopedic surgeon, for the *American Journal of Orthopedics*, "as younger and younger athletes who will likely never play at the major league level are undergoing this procedure at an alarming rate."

For a 2015 paper, Erickson used a supercomputer to access a private medical database that cataloged five years' worth of injuries. He typed in code 24346—UCL reconstruction with a tendon graft—and found 56.8 percent of cases were performed on teenagers. Surely some suffered from delusions of grandeur, others from overeager surgeons, but the reality of the numbers frighten those in baseball who understand what's happening.

This problem is only getting worse.

AT A YOUTH-BASEBALL COMPLEX SOUTHEAST of Phoenix, a ten-year-old boy named Harley Harrington stood on top of a mound and twirled pitch after gorgeous pitch. Harley's motion was a study in biomechanical beauty, his legs driving efficiently, his hips swiveling at just the right time, his non-throwing arm tugging down and pulling through his torso, and his right arm unfurling so smoothly it looked machine-taught. His peers chucked the ball; Harley delivered it.

He came here in March 2015 from San Diego with a traveling baseball team called the Show, which recruited some of the best ten-and-under kids in Southern California to compete in high-level tournaments like this one, the Spring Championship Super NIT in Gilbert, Arizona. Hundreds of other teams in all age groups, some as young as seven years old, came from around the country to feed the excesses of American youth baseball personified by the Big League Dreams complex. Built near a farm, it reeked of cow dung. Local politicians still kick themselves for spending more than $40 million to develop the campus for the private company that runs ten more such facilities across the West Coast.

Four fields, each built in the scaled-down image of a famous major league stadium, surrounded a central hub of video games, flat-screen TVs, bad food, and, most important, copious beer. The taps started flowing around eight a.m., when some fathers lubed themselves to forget they'd been conned into traveling hundreds of miles for games that just as easily could've taken place ten minutes from their houses. The youth baseball–industrial complex can hypnotize even the most mindful.

Nicola and Martin Harrington never expected to find themselves in a facility like this. Nicola once was a pop star in England whose band, the Simon Cowell–backed Girl Thing, fizzled amid great hype. Much of the drama involved Nicola's secret relationship with Martin, a music producer. They married, had Harley, left England, and ended up in Los Angeles, where a friend of Martin's told him that now that his boy was American, he needed a baseball glove. Harley fell in love with the game and showed enough aptitude that he craved better competition.

All Martin knew about the United States' travel-sports industry—whose estimated revenues now range from $7 billion to far more—was that it seemed crazy. Not just the cost of hotels or the time away from work, all so a kid could play at a novelty stadium or win a cheap championship ring, but the children on other teams who cowered in fear of criticism from their parents.

Three former number one overall picks in Major League Baseball's draft had played for the Show: National League MVP outfielder Bryce Harper and two pitchers, Stephen Strasburg and Brady Aiken, both of whom bear scars on their elbows. While Harley started as an outfielder, his coaches quickly recognized the fluidity with which he threw a ball. Pitchers spend a lifetime trying to look as natural pitching as Harley did the first time he stepped on a mound.

"Having been around some really good players in our program, sometimes we single out kids who remind us of others," said Hector Lorenzana, one of the Show's longtime coaches. "We had the privilege of having Bryce Harper since he was eight and a half, nine years old. We see flashes in things kids do at certain ages. And it reminds you of other players who have come through. Harley is one of those."

At the Spring Championship Super NIT, whose champion qualifies for an even bigger tournament later in the year at Disney World, the Show ran roughshod through its bracket to reach the semifinals, where it unleashed Harley. He mixed fastballs and off-speed offerings, all from the same release point, each pitch faster and crisper than his peers'. Harley exited in the fourth inning after fifty-two pitches, well short of the tournament limit of eight innings with no maximum pitch count. Martin always kept track of how many Harley had thrown, and when the Show squeaked out a victory to get into the finals, he approached Lorenzana about Harley's availability for the next game.

"Going in the same day back-to-back," Lorenzana said, "is a huge no-no for us."

And yet Martin Harrington, conscientious enough to download an app to track his son's usage, a voracious enough reader to realize that the rash of Tommy John surgeries points back to excessive and unnecessary throwing by children, wanted his son to pitch in the final game, if need be.

"It's not like it was the morning and there was a four- or five-hour gap," Martin said. "To me it was about two hours, and he'd thrown fifty pitches. I thought it wasn't a problem to throw twenty more. Honestly, I don't think the Show is going to abuse a kid to win a medal. That's not how they're going to do it. But he had more left in him. Harley is one of those kids where he has unfinished business. He doesn't need to show them he's the best. But I think he felt shortchanged in the semifinals. I knew he wanted to go out there and finish it off."

Another coach lobbied Lorenzana, too, pointing to Harley's parents. "Look at the mom! Look at the dad!" he said. Both were pictures of fitness. Also working in Harley's favor was that unlike almost every top travel-ball player, he actually took time away from baseball, spending his summers in England or playing club soccer. The single-sport-specialization malady that affected kids across the US landscape did not apply.

Still, nobody knew. Not Lorenzana, not Nicola or Martin Harrington, not the doctors urging coaches and parents to pump the brakes on excessive use. Nobody could say whether putting Harley in for a second time would cause damage years down the road. Every kid and every arm is different.

At 4:15 p.m., in the fifth inning of a blowout game the Show led, about two and a half hours after he had last pitched, Harley Harrington went back out to win a tournament for a group of ten-year-olds.

"If it was anyone other than Harley, we'd have shied away from it," Lorenzana said. "There are some horses you're going to ride a little longer. There's no science. There's no process. You just don't know."

INCREASINGLY, RESEARCHERS ARE LOOKING BEYOND the major leagues and down to kids like Harley Harrington and how they're being handled. Grave concern exists among those studying the arm that because of tournaments like the Super NIT, which lack pitch counts, the current generation of injured arms will look positively healthy compared with the kids' coming up.

The American Sports Medicine Institute (ASMI), the baseball industry's foremost think tank, followed nearly five hundred youth-league pitchers for a decade starting in 1999 and found that kids who pitched more than one hundred innings in a calendar year were three and a half times likelier to get injured than those who didn't. In 1997, Dr. James Andrews, the famous orthopedic surgeon who had founded ASMI in Birmingham, Alabama, was performing Tommy John surgery on one or two high school kids per year. Today, he estimates he does eighty or ninety a year. "Hell, I've got four to do tomorrow," Andrews said during an April 2015 conversation. He fears that even worse news is coming at the major league level. "If they don't get involved in it from a prevention standpoint at the youth level," he said, "they're not going to have anybody to draft out of high school or college who hasn't had their elbow operated on."

The future generation of baseball pitchers lives in a system that takes undeveloped and underdeveloped arms and pressures them to show off for the radar guns they're taught will determine their future. The easiest way to build velocity is through year-round throwing—and year-round throwing, according to the ASMI study, is the single highest predictor of future injuries among kids. Risk factors are highest for kids like Harley, whose arms are especially fragile at ten years old and, in many cases, remain so through the end of high school and beyond. Some surgeons have performed Tommy John on kids as young as thirteen years old, even as doctors at the top of the field warn against cutting still-growing arms. Children who regularly pitched with arm fatigue are thirty-six times likelier to undergo elbow or shoulder surgery, another study by Andrews and his peers at ASMI found. The same study said that kids who pitch in games more than eight months of the year need surgery five times as often. And another study, published in the *American Journal of Sports Medicine*, reported that children like Harrington who play travel ball are five times likelier to suffer from elbow pain.

"I have this conversation with every Tommy John patient," said Dr. Orr Limpisvasti, a surgeon at Kerlan-Jobe in Los Angeles. "Just so you know, I'm going to fix your arm so you can destroy it again. And this lightbulb goes off. Here's what we know: Throwing is bad for your arm. You're good at it and love doing it. And you tore your God-given UCL, probably the best one you'll ever have by a long shot, and if we put a new one in, you're refurbishing it so you can do the exact same thing that you did before."

UCL reconstruction is far from foolproof, too. The procedure involves cutting through skin and muscle, drilling into bone, and tying the elbow together. It is major surgery that calls for a brutal, monotonous rehabilitation. And while the return rate is around 80 percent, a study from Jon Roegele at the *Hardball Times* looked at the return of every pitcher who underwent Tommy John surgery from 2000 to 2009 and found the median threw just sixty games and one hundred innings for the rest of his career. The data also showed that pitchers on fourteen-to-sixteen- and seventeen-to-twenty-month timetables had performed better than those who rushed back, an indictment against a baseball culture intent on returning pitchers in a year.

There is nothing glamorous about Tommy John surgery. The urban legend of doctors performing it pre-emptively and prophylactically is unfounded. Forget another myth, too: the problem stems from kids throwing curveballs too young. Another ASMI study showed that curveballs cause less strain on the arm than the simple, humble fastball, whose greater velocity taxes pitchers more. In 2003, the average fastball in the major leagues didn't crack 90 miles per hour. Today, it's over 92, jumping annually for eight consecutive years and placing not just a physical burden on every kid who dreams of being a big leaguer but also a mental one: throw hard or your chances are grim.

So they travel like Harley Harrington, using pitch-all-you-want tournaments to ready themselves for the grind of their teenage years, when scouts will converge on showcase events to see kids who have been reared to do everything bigger, faster, harder.

"Travel baseball is completely different than it was twenty years ago," said Paul DePodesta, now the chief strategy officer for the NFL's Cleveland Browns after spending two decades in baseball front offices. "With all the showcases and these guys pitching, it's not just when they're seventeen. It's when they're fourteen and fifteen." DePodesta has four kids, three boys. His second son, Evan, played on an all-star team that was invited to a regional tournament in 2014. He got to stay in a hotel and wanted to keep doing that with a travel team. Sure, his dad said, except he might have to give up football and soccer and basketball.

"I don't think I'm ready to choose," Evan said.

"Well, you shouldn't," DePodesta said, "because you're six."

THE ULNAR COLLATERAL LIGAMENT IS a finicky little bastard, ill-equipped to stand up long-term to the single fastest movement the body can generate: the throwing motion. The arm moves thirty times faster than an eyeblink when it's firing a baseball. It's the final cog of a mechanism that steals energy from the legs, builds on it through the hips and butt, transfers it up the back and to the shoulder, and releases it with a whip of muscles and ligaments and tendons and bones that launch a round projectile at speeds of up to 105 miles per hour. It is beautifully chaotic and chaotically beautiful. It is different in every arm, from Harley Harrington's emergent one to that of Greg Maddux, the Hall of Fame pitcher who never did break over a twenty-three-year, five-thousand-inning career. All the gurus of biomechanics—the science, as the pioneering biomechanist James G. Hay once said, of "internal and external forces acting on a human body and the effects produced by these forces"—concur that Maddux's delivery was perfect, though one could argue that perfect mechanics are more than a series of proper motions. Perfection is the ability of a pitcher to find a delivery that keeps him productive and healthy.

Pitching consists of six generally accepted phases: windup, stride, arm cocking, acceleration, deceleration, and follow-through. Throwing a baseball differs from all other athletic tasks. Footballs are about ten ounces heavier and require slightly dissimilar mechanics. Tennis serves and volleyball spikes come more over the top than most pitchers' high three-quarters deliveries.

Windmilling softball pitchers rarely need Tommy John surgery, because the force generated simply isn't enough to rip the elbow apart.

Overhand throwing isn't in and of itself the villain or culprit. "When you grow up, that's what we do. We throw," said Chris Carpenter, the former St. Louis Cardinals ace. "It doesn't have to be a ball. It can be a toy, a Cheerio. You grow up, you chuck shit around. That's what I did anyway." Throwing is eminently natural, positively symphonic, an inevitable result of human evolution. What's unnatural is throwing a five-and-a-quarter-ounce sphere ninety-plus miles per hour one hundred times every five days.

The traditional pitching motion starts with a leg lift into a stride. This activates what's commonly known as the kinetic chain—a simplistic way of describing the sequential transfer of energy from body parts farther from the ball to ones closer. Something as simple as a leg lift starts building elastic energy, a type of potential energy that comes from the stretching of ligaments and tendons before it's stored in muscles. When the stride foot lands, the muscles in the butt clench—scouts look for pitchers with big asses for a reason: they're biomechanically advantageous—and start rotating the hips. Shortly thereafter, the muscles in the back activate, too, sending rapid signals from the brain to the muscles. Those nerve impulses open up calcium channels in the muscle. As calcium is released, muscles contract. The powerful contractions begin cascading up the chain to the torso. Good hip-to-shoulder separation—the opening of the hips while the torso stays in line with the plate, which creates even more elastic energy because hip rotation stretches its ligaments and tendons—is common in the hardest-throwing pitchers.

Front foot down, hips rotated, torso starting to twist, pitchers cock their arms and prepare for twenty to thirty milliseconds of wonder. What happens next is difficult to see with the naked eye. The shoulder externally rotates, bringing the elbow forward, the hand behind the body, and the forearm almost parallel to the ground. All of the elastic energy rushes into the shoulder, loading the muscles and ligaments and tendons and bones, like a coiled spring pushed flat. The UCL is screaming for mercy, particularly in players whose weak shoulder muscles cannot withstand the onslaught of energy and spill it down to an already-loaded elbow. The UCL is triangular, and the energy affects each side differently; the posterior and transverse bundles, biomechanists believe, endure less stress, while the anterior—the side that in almost every injury is torn—is burdened to the cusp of failure.

When the ligaments and tendons tell the shoulder it cannot rotate further, the elastic energy turns into kinetic energy, and the shoulder sends it down the arm by rotating internally at up to 8,000 degrees per second. No movement in the body matches the internal rotation of the shoulder, and along with the extension of the elbow, it propels the arm forward.

"If you're one-thirtieth of a second late or early, you're basically, over time, doing damage," said Brent Strom, the Houston Astros' pitching coach. "And that's how fine this thing is. It's like hitting a golf ball. You've got to be right on time. Those that can maintain that timing can stay healthiest the longest."

The UCL breathes a sigh of relief as the energy travels down the arm and through the ball. Shoulder muscles contract to help the arm decelerate safely, and the follow-through dissipates the remaining energy. And, if all goes well, pitchers do it ninety-nine more times that day.

Baseball has seen its share of anomalies who could throw 150 pitches without any arm soreness or regularly top 100 miles per hour without incident. R. A. Dickey, the Toronto Blue Jays' right-handed knuckleball pitcher, a thirteen-year major league veteran, throws a baseball for a living without a UCL, which is not supposed to be possible. He does not know if he was born without one or it just vaporized at some point during all the innings he tossed in high school. He is not sure if the muscles in his arm learned how to contract to keep it stable. Dickey simply knows he is a freak. And freaks are confusing. They defy explanation. And they challenge the modern theories of the pitching arm, which hold it to be a delicate flower never to be mistreated.

"I believe it's miraculous," Dickey said.

Dickey isn't wrong. Long before he mastered the knuckleball, he was a regular fastball pitcher, able to run it over 90 miles per hour. His arm's ability to function without a UCL is extraordinary; though, for that matter, every arm is a little miracle. It doesn't take an outlier to appreciate the arm's ability to survive the rigors of baseball.

"Every time I throw, it's a train wreck," then–Philadelphia Phillies starter Cole Hamels said on May 25, 2012. "I'm sore as heck. I don't even want to know what's going on inside me."

Two months to the day after Hamels said that to me, the Phillies signed him to a six-year, $144 million contract extension.

HARLEY HARRINGTON IS A LOT like a boy who grew up in San Diego a quarter century ago and later inspired hosannas to the beauty of his pitching. Even when Mark Prior spent afternoons in the backyard playing catch with his grandmother, his talent was obvious. He grew up to be the Vitruvian pitcher, ideal in every way until he wasn't.

"I tried to tell people: 'My mechanics are not perfect,'" Prior said. Nobody wanted to listen, of course, because baseball people are stubborn and Prior looked the part. He was six feet five, his 225 pounds perfectly distributed from his tapered torso to his strong legs. His delivery looked symmetrical, with an upright trunk, easy pace, and soft landing, all so his right arm could ride a rounded pathway to his release of the ball. Prior was supposed to be the Chicago Cubs' savior. He threw his last major league pitch when he was twenty-five, kicked around in the minor leagues after shoulder surgery, flopped in a few comeback attempts, and wound up in a front-office job. Today, he's responsible for helping keep the San Diego Padres' minor leaguers healthy.

Was it his delivery? Too much throwing as a kid? Bad genes? The unnecessarily high pitch counts he ran up as a Cubs rookie? A combination of all four? Something else that no one can name? Prior is the baseball horror story that frightens Nicola and Martin Harrington and every parent whose kid braves the pitcher's mound. Even if the unicorn that is a mechanically ideal delivery exists—one that spares the elbow in a motion that inherently stresses the elbow—so many other factors can derail it.

Harrington's teammates saved him from a stressful second outing by launching hits, including a mercy-rule-inducing home run to win the Super NIT. "The Harley thing could've easily blown up on us," said Lorenzana. Instead, another coach picked up Harley and swung him around while the rest of the team danced in their blue-and-orange uniforms. At the ceremony for their championship rings, a tournament organizer prattled on, ending with a prophecy for a group of ten-year-olds he'd never met: "I know these guys are destined for greatness."

The Harringtons drove back to San Diego that night. Harley took a week off from baseball. Martin wondered whether he had done the right thing, rationalizing that never had Harley thrown even seventy pitches before, and that he never would consider leaving him in a full game and pitching him a day or two later. "It's one of those situations where if you feel like your kid is being abused for one reason or another, we wouldn't stand for that," Martin said. "If our kid isn't on the field playing, he's depressed. To us, it makes sense. To Harley, it's terrible. 'How can you not put me on the field?'"

Dr. James Andrews hears different versions of that same story almost every day, and he worries about the youth system's half-hearted effort to clean itself up. Tommy John surgery is not a panacea. It requires time to rehab kids don't have, training they may not be prepared to handle, and maturity they almost certainly don't possess without parents and coaches emphasizing the importance of arm care.

"What twelve-year-old is going to say? 'Excuse me, coach, I'm feeling a little soreness in my elbow. I think it would be most prudent if I stopped now,'" said Dr. Glenn Fleisig, the research director at ASMI. "We have a kid who's on a travel team and is a good pitcher. He enjoys being a good pitcher. His parents enjoy it. And they have nothing but the best intentions. Same with the coach. They all enjoy it. So here's this kid. He's pitching on a Saturday afternoon, and he's spent. And his mom and dad are rooting for him. And so is this girl. And they're winning four to two. So of course he's going to keep pitching."

Doctors believe almost every UCL tear is an accumulation injury—a ligament worn down over time that finally relents. Kids play today more than ever, and while the correlation with the spike in UCL injuries is obvious, many in the sport see the relationship as causative, too. "There are so many misrepresentations of our game and how it should be taught and how kids should play it," said Tony Clark, the executive director of the MLB Players Association. "I shudder at the thought of being told at thirteen years old to choose a sport because that would be my only chance to make it."

If there's any good news, it's that the elbow's loss has been the shoulder's gain. Shoulder injuries used to be the bane of baseball, ending careers far more often than elbows and causing nearly seven thousand disabled-list days as recently as 2008, according to research by Jeff Zimmerman of the *Hardball Times*. By 2014, the number dipped to fewer than three thousand, thanks in large part to innovative exercise programs that strengthened shoulder muscles. Unfortunately, ligaments cannot be strengthened, which leaves the UCL to fend for itself against the onslaught of more throws and maximum-effort deliveries and pitches like the sinker, cutter, split-fingered fastball, and changeup that all call for some sort of hand manipulation.

"Medicine and science have come so far," Washington Nationals pitching coach Mike Maddux said. "A hundred years ago, a couple guys in North Carolina said let's fly this thing called an airplane, and people said these guys are smoking some hashish, man. As far as we've come in science and medicine, we still haven't come to the human element of a pitcher's arm. No matter how smart we get, all the advancements we've made, nature always will take its course."

I'm not sure that's true.

The arm is not a dead end. Obstructionism around baseball exists, and those in power need to take bold steps to fix a culture that has existed far too long for its own good. Over the three years I spent exploring the pitching arm's past, present, and future, I found brilliant people dedicating their life's work to saving it. They had ideas and technologies and strategies to help. Ingenuity still lives in the game. All it takes is one brilliant mind to change the culture. About forty years ago, baseball witnessed it firsthand.

CHAPTER 3

The Men Who Changed Baseball History

THE PITCH WAS SUPPOSED TO be a sinker, 82 or 83 miles per hour, effective in spite of its velocity and because of its dishonesty. In spin and look, it masqueraded as a fastball, only to dive to the dirt about ten feet in front of the plate. Hitters were aware of its charms and unable to resist them anyway. This particular sinker bore no such malice. It floated high and outside. Hal Breeden, who stood in the batter's box at Dodger Stadium in the third inning on July 17, 1974, took the last pitch Tommy John threw before he changed baseball forever.

Almost immediately, John ambled off the mound and toward the dugout. "Tommy John was a tough sumbitch," Breeden said. "When he walks off like that, something's bad." This wasn't pain; it was agony. John was thirty-one years old, a major leaguer for a dozen seasons already, and he knew soreness like every pitcher knows soreness. This was more acute, concentrated in his left elbow joint, distressing enough that he scuttled right past future Hall of Fame manager Walter Alston and into the dugout, where his message for Los Angeles Dodgers trainer Bill Buhler was succinct: "Get Dr. Jobe."

Frank Jobe left his box seat and wound his way to the trainer's room, a fifty-by-twenty-foot antechamber into which large men shoehorned themselves to receive treatment for sore muscles and other common ailments. Jobe, considered by many the best orthopedic surgeon in America, was also the Dodgers' team physician, on duty for a moment like this, when the pitcher with the fourth-best ERA in baseball winced and needed to know why his arm felt like someone had left it in a pizza oven.

Jobe steadied John's upper arm while moving his forearm, read his face for discomfort, and told him to head home, ice it, and visit the next afternoon. Medicine worked on a different timetable then, immediacy an impossibility, because the right technology didn't exist. It had been only five months since the United States issued its first patent on what would become the magnetic resonance imaging (MRI) machine. Jobe would rely on X-rays of John's elbow, and before he drew any conclusions, he wanted John to visit Dr. Herbert Stark, a hand surgeon whose patients included Sandy Koufax and Wilt Chamberlain. Stark manipulated John's arm in and out, same as Jobe. The meeting didn't last long.

"Boy, you sure did a job on it, didn't you?" Stark said.

"I guess," John said.

"Go on back to Dr. Jobe," Stark said.

By five o'clock, when John returned to Jobe's office, the X-rays were clear enough to confirm Jobe's fear: a torn ulnar collateral ligament. John didn't know what a UCL was. Few pitchers did. Players spent so much time dreading shoulder injuries that the elbow, such a simple, effective joint, not encumbered by sheaths of muscle braided together, was almost an afterthought. Elbow pain meant bone chips, or maybe a torn flexor-pronator mass, which John knew well; Jobe had sliced open his forearm to re-attach the forearm muscles following the 1972 season. The UCL was enough of a mystery that Jobe prescribed three or four weeks of rest to let it heal before trying to throw again. Twenty-six days later, before a game at Shea Stadium against the Mets, John tried to throw batting practice. After twenty pitches, his arm felt lifeless.

Without a working left arm, he tried to jerry-rig one. John asked Buhler, the trainer, to treat his elbow as he would a sprained ankle. Buhler mummified the arm in athletic tape, weaving a figure eight as John held his elbow at 90 degrees. Considering he couldn't straighten his arm, John threw rather respectably, though nowhere near well enough to get major league hitters out. His options were dwindling, his time fading, and on September 11, John called Jobe from San Francisco and lamented the lack of progress. Jobe told him to fly into Los Angeles the next morning, where he delivered a diagnosis: "It's not going to heal."

Jobe was the kind of doctor who gave the bad news first, hoping the good news to follow would act as an analgesic. John didn't need surgery. He would live a totally normal life without a UCL. His first child, a girl, was due in two weeks, and he would walk her down the aisle just fine. He could do anything except pitch in the big leagues.

"We just told him to go home," Jobe remembered. "He was through playing baseball."

He could go to Terre Haute, Indiana, where he was born, and sell cars. Or partner up with a friend in San Francisco who owned a jewelry business. The name Tommy John meant something. He could've parlayed it into success outside baseball if he weren't so much like his father. Thomas Edward John had worked for Public Service Indiana as a power-line serviceman, tacking himself to utility poles, climbing, hanging only by a belt and the grace of God. He did this for decades, until he was sixty-three years old. Nobody would take him away from the lines.

John refused to accept that his baseball career had ended on a garbage sinker to Hal Breeden. He prodded Jobe, asking for an alternative. None existed. Jobe said that the only possibility was theoretical. For years, doctors had used a tendon in the wrist, the palmaris longus, to strengthen the ankles of polio patients at Rancho Los Amigos National Rehabilitation Center. Hand doctors rebuilt finger joints with it. The success of those surgeries emboldened Jobe to consider extrapolating the technique: he would use the palmaris longus to rebuild the elbow, something he told John might have a 1 percent chance of success. "Tommy likes to tell the story that he was a math major and knew that one in one hundred is better than zero in one hundred," Jobe said. "But I thought it had a ninety percent chance to work."

Jobe sandbagged so as not to give John false hope. He wanted to wait two weeks and assemble a strong support team to help with the experimental surgery. He didn't know whether the tendon would turn into a ligament or fail in the elbow joint and require more surgery. He worried about the sensitivity of the ulnar nerve, the lack of a concrete rehabilitation plan, the speculative nature of the entire operation.

"Tommy," Jobe said, "I don't know what I'm doing."

More than anything, those words convinced John this was exactly what he wanted. Before Todd Coffey—before Stephen Strasburg and Matt Harvey and José Fernández and minor leaguers you haven't heard of and college kids who never made it and high school kids suckered by delusions of majestic major league careers—there was only Tommy John the ballplayer, not the brand name of a surgical procedure. The greatest triumph in the history of sports medicine exists because Jobe and John shared a feeling to which neither was accustomed: vulnerability. "I knew he wasn't bullshitting me," John said. "He's a friend first, a doctor second. But when a doctor admits he's not a god, a deity, and he can fuck up, that sold me."

John stared at Jobe and said three words that forever would wed them: "Let's do it."

Some doctor would have dreamt up the surgery at some point, but Jobe earned his reputation as the best. Take the procedure's name, because that more than anything captures his essence. Other doctors asked him what he wanted to call his new surgery. "The way you should say it," Jobe told me almost forty years later, "is 'reconstruction of the ulnar collateral ligament using the palmaris longus tendon.' It's not catchy enough." The convention was for doctors to name the procedure after themselves. Every skin cancer patient knows Mohs surgery. Salk and Sabin both developed eponymous polio vaccines. Even body parts sometimes carried doctors' names; the transverse bundle of the UCL is also known as Cooper's ligament. "Jobe surgery" didn't sound right, not to Jobe's ears. He believed he was little more than a man with a scalpel, a drill, and an idea. The courage and gumption were Tommy John's. If this worked—if it actually became something that could save baseball players' careers—John deserved the recognition.

Jobe had learned quick thinking as a medic for the 101st Airborne. He braved the Battle of the Bulge, slept in the snow, dodged machine-gun fire, and sent letters to his mother back in North Carolina that no mother should have to read. "I consider myself the luckiest guy in the world," Jobe said. "I've been lucky all my life. I was in World War II and didn't get killed." When Jobe returned from the war, he left his family's fifteen-acre farm for California, where the GI Bill funded his undergraduate degree, and his battlefield experience made medical school a natural step. After getting his MD from Loma Linda University, Jobe ran a family practice for three years to pay off twenty thousand dollars in student loans. Debt-free, he landed an orthopedics residency and met the no-nonsense midwesterner Dr. Robert Kerlan, another sports-medicine pioneer, who took a shine to him and invited the genteel southerner to partner up.

Jobe's first patient was Johnny Podres, a Dodgers left-hander with a bone chip floating in his elbow. Even before the advent of the arthroscope, removing bone chips was a relatively quick procedure, nothing like traversing the twenty-one muscles of the shoulder, which resemble a highway interchange. Digging deeper into the elbow wasn't an option, either, even though cursory research had shown the significance of the UCL.

In 1941, Dr. George Bennett, an orthopedist dubbed the "mender of immortals" by *Sports Illustrated*, studied arm injuries in pitchers. His resulting article in the *Journal of the American Medical Association* mentioned an elbow lesion "not seen in other occupations"—a torn UCL, though Bennett didn't call it by name. Five years later, a journal in Europe introduced UCL injuries through the prism of javelin throwers, whose technique is strikingly similar to pitchers' when viewed in slow motion. The stride, the external rotation of the shoulder, the deceleration during follow-through—everything was there, and javelin throwers blew out their arms frequently. For the next thirty years, the medical literature more or less ignored UCL tears, which Dr. James Andrews of the American Sports Medicine Institute later blamed on the difficulty of diagnosing the injury with X-rays.

Though far less frequently than today, torn UCLs did end pitchers' careers. Tired of telling pitchers the same sad two-word phrase—"You're done"—Jobe vowed to devise a work-around. Rather than get lost in fixing all three sides of the UCL, Jobe homed in on the anterior bundle, the most vital piece of the triangular ligament because it absorbs most of the energy that travels to the elbow. His choice of the palmaris longus was particularly intuitive, too, despite its success in other, unrelated surgeries. Its size was perfect, between 3.5 and 4.5 millimeters wide, almost an exact match of the anterior bundle. It was long enough to allow Jobe to drill tunnels in the humerus and ulna and wrap the tendon in a figure-eight pattern. The best part: the palmaris longus is altogether useless, anatomically inert, the appendix of the arm. Patients function no differently after its extraction than before. Doctors estimate 15 to 20 percent of people don't even have one. But when John touched his thumb to his pinky and flexed his hand, a palmaris longus popped up in the middle of his wrist.

"God put it there," Dodgers trainer Stan Conte said, "so Frank Jobe could do this surgery."

In between starts, when his elbow ballooned to cartoonish sizes because the damage in it invited fluid to congregate near the joint, Sandy Koufax would visit Dr. Robert Kerlan and brace himself. Relief came in the form of a needle that Kerlan jabbed into the swollen area. Red-tinged liquid oozed into an empty syringe. No matter how many visits to Kerlan it took, Koufax was not going to let his degenerative elbow stop him from throwing a baseball.

For the last three years of his career, Koufax, the Los Angeles Dodgers' ace, subjected himself to the treatment with regularity. His arm refused to cooperate otherwise. X-rays showed that three or four spurs hooked off the bones of his elbow. Nobody knew the full extent of the tumult inside, though the accumulation of fluid indicated that the body recognized trouble and was trying to protect it from further wreckage. On the day before, the day of, and the day after his starts, Koufax ate a white-and-orange capsule of Butazolidin, a brand of phenylbutazone, an anti-inflammatory originally intended for horses and today considered unsafe for human consumption. He eased the pain with a codeine-cut aspirin. Then, before Koufax pitched, the Dodgers' training staff snapped on rubber gloves, scooped a glob of Capsolin, a clear, pungent balm, and applied it to Koufax's elbow, shoulder, and back. Capsolin wasn't a salve so much as a declaration of war; it consisted of 3 percent pure capsaicin, the active ingredient in chili peppers, along with turpentine, camphor oil, and other elements that punished the body with heat. Nerve endings stood no match. They wilted and died from Capsolin overdoses. Koufax needed it to manage his misery.

Today, Koufax looks about two decades younger than his eighty years, fit and tan, a man who could star in a pharmaceutical commercial that features happy octogenarians taking a walk or tilling the garden. A half century after he walked away from baseball in his prime, Koufax remains one of the finest pitchers the game has ever seen. His friendship with Jobe blossomed in retirement, and Jobe has often said that if he'd conceived of UCL reconstruction a decade earlier it would be called Sandy Koufax surgery.

Koufax grants one-on-one interviews as frequently as a total solar eclipse. When I asked through an intermediary if he would talk about Jobe, Koufax was happy to make an exception, inviting me to Dodgers spring training to visit and reminisce.

"He was a very gentle man, but he was also very strong," Koufax said. "Great bedside manner, but wouldn't take any crap." Jobe never treated Koufax during his Hall of Fame career, probably because it ended almost as quickly as it began. When the pain in his elbow first materialized in April 1964, Koufax was twenty-eight years old. He couldn't straighten his arm. Injuries shelved him for one-third of his scheduled starts. Kerlan diagnosed him with traumatic arthritis, declared there was no cure, and suggested he pitch once a week. During spring training in 1965, Koufax woke up one morning to find the majority of his left arm black and blue. Undeterred, he pitched every fourth day, twirled a perfect game, and won the National League Cy Young Award. In the offseason, Kerlan suggested he quit. Koufax wanted one more year, needles and drugs and fear of permanent disability be damned.

His arm held up until the middle of the summer in 1966. On July 23, against the New York Mets, Koufax threw a 168-pitch complete game, which followed a ten-day stretch during which he had pitched in four games and tossed twenty-four innings. His manager, Walter Alston, thought he left Koufax in for 200 pitches. "I worried that maybe I should get him out of there,"

Alston told reporters. "I know he's not right, and I'm half-afraid of hurting him. But with a doubleheader coming up, I didn't particularly want to use the bullpen."

Koufax saw its effects instantaneously. Fluid gathered in his elbow, more than usual. Kerlan drained it and injected it with cortisone, the top-shelf numbing agent of the time. Four days after he threw 168 pitches, Koufax struck out sixteen in an eleven-inning complete game. He didn't miss a start the rest of that season and finished with more than three hundred innings pitched for the third time in four years.

Sandy Koufax retired after the 1966 season, done in by baseball's ignorance and sports medicine's primitiveness. He was thirty years old, at the peak of his greatness. Koufax was worried that his ravaged elbow would keep him from golfing or washing his face or shaving, and he refused to trade another year of throwing a baseball for a lifetime of disability. No doctor saved him, because no doctor knew how. "In those days, they believed if you opened an arthritic joint it got worse," Koufax said. "Medicine changed."

Koufax was never diagnosed with a damaged UCL. He doesn't think he tore it, either, though with all the trickery used to enliven his arm, he can't say for certain. He just believes its expiration date was thirty, and whether it was the spurs or the bursa sac or the ligament, his arm was too far gone for medicine at the time to remedy it.

"I was hoping I would live longer after baseball than before," he told me. "And I've made it. In those days there was the question of are you going to have full use of your arm, are you going to do this or that. . . . Because the draining, the eating Butazolidin, everything you can to get through—I thought when the doctor tells me it's time to stop, it's time to stop."

The arm in baseball has had two eras: Before Tommy John and After Tommy John. Koufax was perhaps the closest to that bridge. When Koufax joined the Dodgers organization, more than six hundred players came to spring training, an exercise in

Darwinism. Dozens developed arm injuries—either arm fatigue or tendinitis or dead arm or some other vague complaint—and never returned. The survivors were major leaguers.

In the final week of the 1954 season, the Dodgers summoned from Triple-A a twenty-three-year-old left-hander named Karl Spooner to start two games. In his first, against the New York Giants, the eventual World Series champions, Spooner threw a three-hit shutout and struck out fifteen. He followed with a four-hit shutout and twelve more strikeouts against the Pittsburgh Pirates. "He was as good as anybody you've ever seen," Koufax said. During spring training in 1955, after Dodgers starter Johnny Podres—later Jobe's patient—got pounded in an exhibition game, Spooner came in without sufficient time to warm up. His left shoulder barked. He exited the game and started treatment. The pain didn't ebb. He tried to rehab it. Nothing worked. Doctors went medieval.

"They pulled his teeth," Koufax said. "They thought poison was coming down into his shoulder." He was not exaggerating. With all medical options exhausted, doctors yanked teeth out of fear they were emitting harmful toxins into the bloodstream. Karl Spooner threw his final major league pitch when he was twenty-four. His shoulder never stopped hurting.

THE ARM NEEDED A SAVIOR, and even if he couldn't remedy the shoulder, Frank Jobe resolved to rescue the elbow. The surgery existed only in theory, in Jobe's mind, and still he went into it with a confident and fully supportive team. "The nurses in the operating room said, 'Your dad has a certain way of setting his jaw,'" said Dr. Chris Jobe, one of Jobe's sons and himself an orthopedic surgeon who today performs Tommy John surgeries. "It seems like the operating room is ten degrees colder all of a sudden. He didn't have to get mad. He was sensitive to you, and you became sensitive to him."

On September 25, 1974, eight years after Koufax retired from baseball, Jobe scrubbed in with Robert Kerlan, Herbert Stark, a doctor on fellowship named Stephen Lombardo, and a gang of support staff at Centinela Hospital Medical Center. In order to reach the UCL, Jobe detached the flexor-pronator muscles from their connection in the upper arm. Holes drilled, palmaris longus harvested, he wove it into position and tied it tight. Jobe transposed the ulnar nerve, tucking it beneath the muscles and securing it before closing John's elbow. The procedure took four hours, some of which consisted of Stark good-naturedly bugging Jobe for Lakers tickets.

"The most impressive thing to me as a rookie doctor was that technically he did the surgery like he'd done it a thousand times," Lombardo said. "It would be like you and me opening a door and walking into a room. It wasn't just a random thing that was done. It was very well thought out.

"He was a gifted surgeon. Most orthopedic surgeons are well trained. But he had a style and smoothness to his surgical technique that was many standard deviations above the rest. I knew it was special. He had a good patient, too. You can't win a dance contest unless you have a good partner, and Tommy John was a great dancer."

History glosses over an important part of the original Tommy John surgery: for almost three months, it looked like a complete failure. After the procedure, John's left hand curled into a claw, his pinky and ring fingers numb bordering on frozen, the other three suffering from varying levels of discomfort depending on the day. The tendon in John's elbow was assimilating fine, the pain dwindling, but his hand looked gnarled.

Jobe's fear had come true: damage to the ulnar nerve. It's why nearly forty years later Neal ElAttrache treated Coffey's with such care. The slightest mishandling can doom the recovery. In mid-December 1974, Jobe reopened John's arm, moved the nerve back to its original location, and hoped that rest for the remainder of the offseason would prepare him for spring training.

Everything was a guess. No protocol yet existed for the rehabilitation, leaving John to experiment. Jobe did offer John one nugget of advice: "Follow your body." A month after the removal of the cast that immobilized his arm, John joined his teammates at Dodgertown in Vero Beach, Florida, for conditioning activities. When they went to the pitching mounds, he sidled over to a concrete partition at the facility and taught himself to throw again. To fight the lingering numbness, John used athletic tape to bind his left pinky to his ring finger. He picked up a ball with his right hand, jammed it into his slowly cooperating clawed hand, and fired against the closest thing he'd seen to a batter in months: a wall.

Every Monday, the routine started again. "My reasoning," John said, "was if God took Sunday off, Tommy John can, too." John's arm felt the worst when he threw the day after his day off. The other six days he worked, him and the wall, him and his wife, him and anyone who wouldn't laugh when he threw a ball. Stamina built over time, particularly as the nerve surgery worked its magic, unfurled his claw, and allowed him to squeeze Silly Putty and complement his shoulder exercises with forearm-muscle building. Ten or fifteen minutes of throwing grew into sessions two and three times as long. It bore no resemblance to the manicured rehab protocols today, most of which mirror one another with slight variations. Tommy John simply embraced the conventional wisdom of the time, as imparted by his old pitching coach, Johnny Sain: the more you throw, the healthier you get. Little empirical evidence exists today to back that claim, though John continues to believe it. The return of his arm—the real return—was enough for him.

It happened on July 8, 1975, in Pittsburgh, with the temperature and humidity both in the eighties. John went to the bullpen with catcher Mark Cresse and settled into his typical rhythm: pitch, catch, pitch, catch, pitch, catch, metronomic in its efficiency. The heat loosened up his arm, and Cresse started to push

John. "Add a little more speed," he said. So John did. For more than forty minutes, John threw Cresse sinkers. They resembled the ones he had thrown all those years leading up to the Breeden at bat. "I finally felt good," John said. "I was following Dr. Jobe. My body was telling me what I needed."

He threw for forty minutes again the next day. "I was very tentative starting out," John said. "I'm throwing, and the more I throw, the more I sweat, and the better my arm feels, and [Cresse] says tonight was better than last night." He followed with another forty minutes on the team's last day in Pittsburgh, and a few days later, on the Sunday before the All-Star break in St. Louis, John asked his manager, Walter Alston, to let him throw batting practice. John looked good, good enough that he scrapped his plan in case the surgery didn't work: asking his old teammate Hoyt Wilhelm to teach him the knuckleball. The initial failure was evolving into a success story, though John never deluded himself into thinking he was safe. He was a lab rat, and lab rats weren't expected to survive.

At the end of the season, the Dodgers sent John to the fall instructional league, usually the domain of young prospects. On September 26, one year and one day after Jobe opened up his arm and did something no man ever had done before, Tommy John was back on a mound facing batters. The first was Danny Goodwin, the only player ever chosen number one overall in two drafts. On his third pitch, John dropped a curveball in for his first strike in over a year. He cruised through three innings on just thirty-six more pitches. Over the next twenty-eight days, John started seven games and threw thirty-seven innings. The rat lived.

The Dodgers asked John to go to the Dominican Republic and play winter ball, but Jobe refused to let him. Months of throwing six days a week had taxed John's arm, and Jobe didn't want to overwork it any more, especially after instructional-league games in which John had thrown with maximum effort.

Nothing guided Jobe's choices other than instinct. In a sense, Jobe had even more riding on John's recovery than John himself. Jobe knew UCL reconstruction was a legitimate solution for fixing a catastrophic injury, and he didn't want to jeopardize its future.

Following a lockout of the players during spring training in 1976, John reported to Dodgers camp, ready to rejoin the rotation. He was turning thirty-three in May. Only eight pitchers in baseball were older than thirty-four, the eldest of whom was spitballer Gaylord Perry, at thirty-seven. Even if the surgery proved successful, John figured he had only a few good years left.

Tommy John returned to the major leagues on April 16, 1976, for the 319th start of his career. He never missed another. There would be 382 postsurgery starts in all, more than twice as many as anyone who underwent UCL replacement at the age of thirty-one or older since. John threw nearly three hundred more innings with his new UCL than he did with his original. He retired at forty-six with 288 wins, the seventh-highest total among left-handers in major league history, a career ERA of 3.34, and almost five thousand innings pitched. He was a walking billboard for the power of medical innovation, the genius of Frank Jobe.

More than forty years later, the original Tommy John surgery remains the best. It saved the arm from what was millions of years in the making.

CHAPTER 4

Chimps, Quacks, and Freaks

Around two million years ago, long after they had split off from their chimpanzee ancestors and benefited from bipedalism, developed brains, lengthened legs, and expanded waists, the species that eventually evolved into human beings underwent a lesser-known adaptation involving the shoulder. The shrugged posture of earlier primates disappeared and grew to resemble our shoulders of today, with the glenoid cavity—the socket of the shoulder's ball-and-socket joint—no longer angled upward but pointed out and into the humeral head.

The slight difference changed humanity—and would eventually make Tommy John surgery necessary. No longer was *Homo erectus* bound by the physiological limitations of chimpanzees. Sandy Koufax himself couldn't teach a chimp to throw a ball much more than 20 miles per hour. Slightly lowering the junction of the shoulder in early humans opened up their range-of-motion treasure chest. The new shoulder allowed *H. erectus* to throw spears, rocks, and other hunting implements, which allowed them to expand beyond the vegetarian diet of their forebears, which facilitated moves across desert landscapes where no plants grew, which led to the dispersal of people worldwide. All because humans can throw things.

To understand the arm, I needed to understand its origins and what it went through to get where it is today. So I called Dr. Neil Roach, a biological anthropologist who specializes in human evolution. Roach had just published a paper in which he studied college-aged pitchers and tied modern man's superior throwing ability to the new body of *H. erectus* storing elastic energy in the muscles, tendons, and ligaments of the shoulder.

Today's shoulder can flex straight in front and extend directly back. It flares out to the side and moves up (abduction) or down (adduction). No movement in the entire human body can match its maximum speed at internal rotation. And this was the missing link Roach could explain: not how we got from Koufax to today but how we grew into overhand-throwing marvels in the first place.

"We had a hypothesis that elastic energy was being used for improved performance," Roach said. "I was surprised at how effective this mechanism could be. These are tiny little ligaments and tendons, and yet they're accounting for more than fifty percent of the energy used for these rapid motions."

While the expansion of the waist and similar vital changes occurred in other species, *H. erectus* first reaped the benefits of the shoulder's emergence about two million years ago, presumably ushering in the hunter-gatherer form of society. The first throwers were pragmatists. They just wanted to eat. The blather about throwing being an unnatural motion could not be further from the truth. It is nature personified.

Bows and arrows, traps, and guns eventually rendered spears, rocks, and blunt objects obsolete, turning the throwing arm into an antiquated device. Though we use our arms every day and would struggle to function without them, the ability to internally rotate the shoulder at 8,000 degrees per second serves no purpose in the modern world outside of athletic pursuits. Roach's study of twenty top-flight athletes, most of them college pitchers, affirmed his theory about the modern shoulder acting as a clearinghouse for energy generated mostly in the hips and glutes. Mankind didn't die in part because evolution in the shoulder helped it survive.

What it didn't do was give us an infallible joint. The shoulder can absorb a few full-power throws at prey, maybe a few more close-range rock assaults. Only the rarest are made for one hundred pitches. Shoulder problems, elbow problems—they're all the same, all the function of men pushing themselves to do something the body never intended it to do.

"Unfortunately, the ligaments and tendons in the human shoulder and elbow are not well adapted to withstanding such repeated stretching from the high torques generated by throwing, and frequently suffer from laxity and tearing," Roach wrote in the final paragraph of the paper, which was published in *Nature*. "While humans' unique ability to power high-speed throws using elastic energy may have been critical in enabling early hunting, repeated overuse of this motion can result in serious injuries in modern throwers."

Nearly one hundred years passed before anyone in baseball recognized that.

Baseball in the 1800s wasn't baseball, not as we know it today. It existed for scamps and scalawags, a sport governed by its utter lack of governance. It couldn't get the easy stuff right. Though baseball's first official game came in 1846, no strike zone existed until more than forty years later. The mound's sixty-foot, six-inch distance was not established until 1893. Expecting even a whit of care when it came to protecting pitchers' arms was like asking Old Hoss Radbourn to stay sober during the 1884 season.

Much as Frank Bancroft, the manager of the National League's Providence Grays, tried to keep his ace away from booze, Charles Radbourn found a sip here, a nip there, every last drop used as an analgesic to dull the pain in his arm. He refused to let his teammates pitch, and Bancroft knew better than to argue with Radbourn, who later earned his nickname, "Old Hoss," from his ability to pitch so often. For forty of the Grays' last forty-three games, Radbourn trotted to the mound and gnashed through the discomfort. His fifty-nine victories in 1884 established a record that never will be broken, nor will any pitcher come near the 678⅔ innings he threw.

Nobody benefited quite as much as Radbourn from the new change implemented in 1884: the legalization of overhand pitching. In baseball's prior four decades, rules mandated that pitchers throw either sidearm or underhand. The advent of overhand pitching was a seminal moment for baseball, unlocking the body's fullest potential to throw hard while inviting the injuries that accompany it.

Which is not to say the previous deliveries exempted players from harm. This is a great myth, one easily disproved even with the paltry historical record of arm injuries in the nineteenth century. Pitchers of that era did not throw with great velocity, so the sheer load of innings, and the potential for those innings to stretch on, thanks to copious errors committed by gloveless fielders, ended careers with regularity. Of the eighteen players with at least one five hundred–inning season before 1884, two-thirds were finished pitching by age thirty. Tommy Bond was practically done at twenty-four, a year after starting thirty-five consecutive games for the 1879 Boston Red Stockings. George Derby's wonderful rookie season with the Detroit Wolverines in 1881 ended with shoulder pain and a dead career two years later.

Baseball did learn something. The five hundred–inning pitcher was extinct by 1892, the four hundred–inning starter by 1908. Teams changed their strategy of relying on one or two men for almost every inning of every game. The new restraint did little to stop injuries from proliferating. To make matters worse, sports medicine barely existed in the early 1900s. The man nearly every injured player sought wasn't even a doctor. John "Bonesetter" Reese was a Youngstown, Ohio, mill worker whose supposed ability to heal through muscle, tendon, and ligament manipulation brought him great renown and a client roster filled with Hall of Famers. Cy Young, Walter Johnson, Christy Mathewson, Pete Alexander, Addie Joss—the best pitchers around the turn of the century and into the 1920s sought treatment from the Bonesetter, whose formal training consisted of three weeks at medical school before he dropped out because the sight of blood nauseated him.

Reese's work with soft tissue foretold much of what's done by athletic trainers and massage therapists today. Other treatments for sore arms, meanwhile, dove headlong into quackery and continued to prevail for decades. When Chicago Chi-Feds lefthander Ad Brennan lost velocity on his fastball in 1914, a doctor accused his inflamed tonsils of infecting his shoulder muscles via an infection traveling through the bloodstream from the mouth to the shoulder. Karl Spooner was far from the first pitcher whose arm injury was blamed on oral hygiene. Ridiculous though it may sound, doctors demonized the tonsils, teeth, and other parts of the mouth as the arm's greatest hazard. Three abscessed teeth were yanked from the mouth of Red Sox star Lefty Grove at the beginning of the 1934 season to help heal his sore arm. He turned in the worst season of his career. Grove returned in 1935 looking like his Hall of Fame self, validating tooth extraction and prompting a litany of copycats. Four years after Grove, lefthander Lee Grissom tried to cure chronic arm soreness by one-upping him with the removal of four teeth. "The teeth pulling didn't hurt me," Grissom later said. "But it damn sure didn't help my arm none."

Surgery grew commonplace after the successful removal of third baseman Pepper Martin's bone chip in 1934. At least six pitchers had bone chips taken out before the 1939 season, including Hall of Famer Carl Hubbell. Robert Hyland, the orthopedist nicknamed "Baseball's Surgeon General" and an expert at bone-chip removal, hypothesized that arm issues were due to "the development of trick pitching"—sliders, screwballs, forkballs, knuckleballs. Syndicated writer Harry Grayson warned of an "epidemic of arm injuries" and wrote that pitchers suggested "it was caused by the lively ball forcing them to bear down on every pitch." Bonesetter Reese blamed high-velocity fastballs for elbow injuries and breaking balls for shoulder woes.

Evolution is a funny thing. The technology, the advancement, the progress—everything today reinforces the idea that we know more and are better positioned to understand the problem at hand. And maybe we are. Maybe we're closer to figuring out the arm. That doesn't take away from the fact that most baseball men are still saying the exact same shit they did seventy-five years ago.

IN 1959, *SPORTS ILLUSTRATED* RAN a cover story about arm injuries. The main headline: "The Pitching Crisis." Mentioned as one of many cautionary tales was a man named Paul Pettit. His arm had changed baseball.

A decade earlier, the seventeen-year-old Pettit was among the best-known baseball players in Los Angeles, a hard-throwing, six-foot-two, two-hundred-pound left-hander who in one high school game struck out twenty-seven hitters over twelve innings. Like other gifted pitchers of the time, Pettit threw every day. When one of his friends in the housing project where he lived begged off to go home for dinner, Pettit found another to play catch. He pitched for his high school team during the week and on Saturdays, plus an American Legion team Sundays. When he was fifteen, a semipro team in nearby Torrance offered him a spot in its rotation, and he jammed that into his schedule, too. "I knew a couple times I wasn't really in good shape when I threw," Pettit said. "I remember one winter I played for a team over in Hermosa Beach. I didn't throw during the week. I was playing basketball. And I went out and threw on Sunday. That wasn't good."

Nobody knew better at the time, least of all a film producer named Frederick Stephani. He wanted to make a movie about a major league pitcher. One featuring a star player would cost too much, so he concocted another plan: he would lock the finest amateur pitcher into a ten-year contract and harvest the rewards when the player signed with a major league team. On October 19, 1949, Pettit agreed to an $85,000 deal with Stephani, who figured with no amateur draft and teams salivating for young pitching he could fetch more money. Three months later, the Pittsburgh Pirates made Pettit baseball's first six-figure bonus baby, paying $100,000 for his rights. Stephani took the extra $15,000 and the title of baseball's first player agent. He never made the movie.

Pittsburgh assigned Pettit to Double-A New Orleans, where he threw a 154-pitch game in which he walked eleven and struck out nine. He labored through the 1950 season, losing velocity on his fastball and forcing him to reconsider how he pitched. "I was working on a curveball," Pettit said. "I needed one that was a little faster. And I messed up my elbow."

Pettit went to Baltimore to visit George Bennett, the doctor believed to have first identified a UCL tear. He had worked in sports medicine for nearly forty years and had seen every kind of sore arm. Ten years earlier, Hall of Famers Dizzy Dean and Lefty Gomez traveled to Baltimore the same day so Bennett could save their arms. Dean's career lasted two more starts and Gomez scratched out two substandard years. Even the best doctors can't undo damage already done.

Bennett cleared Pettit to keep throwing. "I went back, and there wasn't really any therapy to give me," Pettit said. "No cortisone. I was anxious to get back. I would just throw and throw. And I'd start favoring the elbow. Then my shoulder and elbow both were hurting."

Neither ever improved. Pettit threw 30⅔ innings in the major leagues, won one game, gave up pitching at twenty-one, reinvented himself as a power-hitting outfielder, and bounced around Triple-A for another seven years. Pettit is eighty-four today, too old to harp on his misfortune, except once a month when he goes to the Navy Golf Course in Los Alamitos, California, the place where Tiger Woods cut his teeth, and spends the afternoon with about a dozen other ex-ballplayers who excel at the art of embellishment. However spurious Pettit's stories sound to his friends, they contain enough truth to cause the listener to feel sorry for him. Baseball's ignorance killed his arm, and those who did survive engaged in the ultimate victim-blaming.

"A sore arm is like a headache or toothache," Warren Spahn, the future Hall of Famer, told *Sports Illustrated* for the 1959 story. "It can make you feel bad, but if you just forget about it and do what you have to do, it will go away. If you really like to pitch and want to pitch, that's what you'll do."

For every Warren Spahn, every freak who managed to throw tens of thousands of pitches and live to throw tens of thousands more, there were countless Paul Pettits, boys with golden arms that turned into pyrite—and not on account of mental weakness or extinguished passion, as Spahn suggested, but because of obliviousness. While the surgical innovations of Hyland, Bennett, and others relieved pain and allowed pitchers to continue throwing, never did they address the root issue: What causes arm problems?

"When I played, everything was corrective," Hall of Fame pitcher Jim Palmer said. "It wasn't proactive, it wasn't prevention. That didn't make sense to me." In 1965, Palmer injured his rotator cuff at twenty and thought his career was over; he couldn't throw faster than 80 miles per hour. He went to Robert

Kerlan, who didn't have a solution, other than for him to pitch in Puerto Rico during winter ball and hope his arm responded. As Palmer recalled, a friend working for a pharmaceutical company suggested he take Indocin, an anti-inflammatory drug. He swallowed three a day and started throwing 95 miles per hour again. He doesn't know why or how. Palmer didn't need surgery, pitched another sixteen seasons, and threw more than four thousand innings for Baltimore, eight of them in game two of the 1971 World Series. Like Koufax, he needed 168 pitches to grind through it. His arm only got stronger, and Palmer won three Cy Young Awards over a four-season stretch soon thereafter. He was *H. erectus*, the survivor.

Palmer's teammate in the Florida Instructional League, and the better performer there, too—an Orioles prospect named Steve Caria—never made it past Double-A because of arm troubles. Dave Ford was supposed to be the next Jim Palmer, a big, strapping, hard-throwing right-handed pitcher. He lasted fifty-one games in the major leagues and last threw a big league pitch at twenty-four, his shoulder shot. Palmer remembers dozens more.

Young arms failed everywhere. From 1967 to 1971, the Cincinnati Reds brought an unparalleled cache of hard-throwing kids to the major leagues: Gary Nolan, Don Gullett, Wayne Simpson, and Ross Grimsley. All four were done in by arm injuries before their twenty-ninth birthdays. The death rattle of the complete game sounded with the 1980 Oakland A's, who rode their rotation of five twentysomething pitchers so hard that four of them didn't make it past 1983. The luckiest of the group, Steve McCatty, lasted five more years.

The year Sandy Koufax retired, a nineteen-year-old made his major league debut in September. He would last longer than the Reds' quartet, longer than the A's quintet, all the way into the mid-1990s, when he would retire as the paragon of durability. Whenever pitchers today draw criticism for their coddling, the discussion inevitably goes back to him, and it's always in the form of a question.

"Why can't they be more like Nolan Ryan?"

To this day, NOLAN RYAN'S delivery is studied and dissected like a work of art rich with hidden ciphers. He pitched for twenty-seven seasons, faced more than twenty-two thousand batters, and still threw in the mid-nineties as a forty-six-year-old. Ryan was not the best pitcher ever, far from it, but he pitched forever, and that makes him a deity.

Here is a little-known truth about Ryan: he was a god whose arm hurt. In 1967, when Ryan was twenty, a doctor recommended he undergo surgery to fix the pain. Ryan refused. Eight years later, Ryan had bone chips removed from his right elbow. Come 1986, Dr. Frank Jobe suggested that the thirty-nine-year-old Ryan undergo Tommy John surgery to mend a torn UCL. He refused again and pitched for seven more seasons until his UCL forced him into retirement in 1993.

What allowed Ryan to survive remains a mystery. Surely genetics factored in. While his mechanics were considered clean, Ryan changed his delivery multiple times in his career, and his UCL issues speak to some flaw. If he had an obvious freakish ability, it was to defy medical advice and keep strong with no loss of effectiveness. His usage was unparalleled among modern pitchers. In his career, Ryan threw somewhere in the vicinity of 90,000 pitches. In 1974 alone, it was an estimated 5,700—a start every fourth day and nearly 140 pitches every turn. His pièce de résistance came June 14 of that year, when Ryan went thirteen innings, walked ten, struck out nineteen, and threw 235 pitches. In 2015, only 66 of the 4,858 starts featured pitchers throwing more than half as many pitches as Ryan did that day.

The survival-of-the-fittest mentality that ruled the game during Ryan's heyday has vanished. His ethos: throw, throw some more, and when you're done throwing, throw again. He equated it with running: if you get tired at the five-mile mark, go six and then seven and eight, and the body will adapt to meet the greater workload. This is an inapt comparison. The arm better resembles its hinged counterpart, the knee. As much as extreme running builds up endurance and cardiovascular fitness, it can be death on the knees.

Ryan sees a happy medium. It does not exist by nannying pitchers.

"I think the system has hurt pitching," he said. "They don't know what they're capable of doing. They don't know what their ability is as far as endurance, and the number of pitches they can throw. Who's to say 110 pitches is right or wrong? They prove what they're capable of doing. We've gone from when I was with the California Angels carrying nine pitchers to carrying thirteen now. That's crazy. More than half your team is pitchers. Why should you do that?"

Every argument about pitch counts suffers from survivorship bias, and it's part of why the debate agitates those who did hold up. Nolan Ryan's arm was an engine on its 100,000th mile without an oil change and still purring, hungry for more. Asking why a pitcher can't be more like Nolan Ryan is like asking why some rookie guard can't play more like Michael Jordan or a hockey player just called up from the American Hockey League can't score more like Wayne Gretzky.

As CEO of the Texas Rangers, Ryan instructed his team's pitchers to throw more. Never in his six seasons did the Rangers finish higher than ninth in team ERA. However much Ryan wanted to find a magic bullet, to have pitchers throw, throw, throw their way to success, it was incompatible with how baseball's youth culture raised them. And, in a way, Ryan understood that.

"These kids are being overused, the dominant kids," he told me in 2009. "When I say overused, if you don't have the foundation for it, you're not conditioned for it. If you have a something in your delivery that's putting undue stress on it, and you're also talking about kids that are in growth spurts, you don't have the muscle structure to handle their skeletal structure, so they don't have the timing."

While his understanding of bones and muscles and ligaments is cursory at best, Nolan Ryan—the greatest advocate for major league pitchers needing to throw more—believes kids should throw less. Even he sees the problems in how baseball treats Harley Harrington and every other child thrown into a youth culture that looks nothing like it did even a decade ago.

CHAPTER 5

Young Guns

AT A BASEBALL TOURNAMENT ON his fifteenth birthday, Anthony Molina threw a fastball clocked at 91 miles per hour. About a year later, before the state of Florida offered Molina the ability to drive a car by himself, a gaggle of scouts sat behind a chain-link fence as Milton Ramos, a future $650,000 bonus baby of the New York Mets, dug in against Molina. Radar guns steadied, anticipation palpable, Molina did what few sixteen-year-old arms had ever done. Every reading said 95 except the one on the Mets scout's gun. His said 96.

Scouts are inveterate gossips, and word of the high school sophomore from a Miami suburb circulated through the baseball world quickly. It was May 2014, and I was looking for a high schooler who threw hard and could illustrate the peril in keeping his gift healthy. I asked a scout friend, figuring he would pass along a junior, someone from the class of 2015. Instead, he said, "There's a kid named Anthony Molina. Created a lot of buzz already."

Even better, Molina had received an invitation to the Perfect Game National Showcase, one of the most important events on the amateur baseball calendar. I planned on traveling to Fort Myers, Florida, to see the showcase, a gathering of talent that draws scouts, executives, and coaches from across the baseball world. Another scout friend described it as "a cattle call where the cows pay two hundred dollars to be there." Perfect Game was a running joke, gallows humor, really, because some people believed it was killing baseball.

Showcase events like nationals barely existed before Perfect Game. Neither, for that matter, did the infatuation with kids like Anthony Molina. Lusting after a sophomore in high school used to be a no-no. Too much could happen between then and his draft year. Perfect Game helped legitimize and monetize the hunger for outstanding kids. One of its partners, a company called Skillshow, which makes glossy highlight videos for high school athletes, handed out a flyer at nationals with promotional material that said, "Due to the increased availability of information in the computer age, the recruiting process is beginning much earlier than ever before. College coaches are starting to identify prospective recruits as early as 7th and 8th grade!"

It was during Molina's ninth-grade season that the University of Miami offered him a full scholarship. He accepted, though it was just a backup plan, because arms like Molina are worth seven figures to major league teams. The first fifty-five picks of the 2015 draft were offered signing bonuses of at least $1 million. If Anthony Molina was hitting 95 as a six-foot-five, 175-pound beanpole of a sophomore, his fully grown self might hit triple digits. The last right-handed high school pitcher to throw 100 miles per hour was a Texan named Tyler Kolek. The Miami Marlins drafted him second overall in 2014 and paid him $6 million to sign.

Perfect Game nationals at JetBlue Park, the spring-training home of the Boston Red Sox, was simply another opportunity to whet the appetites of scouts and send them back to their bosses raving. Nationals kicked off showcase season with aplomb. A military-grade radar system tracked every pitch to the tenth of a mile per hour and broadcast it on the scoreboard. The stakes were obvious. Seriousness and silence prevailed. I literally heard crickets chirping during the games that followed the drills measuring throwing velocity and running speed.

Molina's first, a 92-mph fastball, was returned up the middle for a single. The hits kept coming: a single, a double, another double, and suddenly all the 92s and 93s looked middling. Scouts scribbled notes, undeterred; they figured he would hit nationals again next year and fare just fine—maybe with 96s and 97s.

Halfway up the first-base line, two sections away from the field, Nelson and Olivia Molina feared something was wrong. Nelson inspects homes for a living and wore the aftereffects of a spider bite on his face. Olivia has spent nearly three decades as a secretary at Carnival Cruise Lines. They are working class people, he a first-generation American, she a Cuban immigrant who came to America at four. Tony was their baby and his arm their gift, and when he trudged into the stands after his game, his parents were concerned.

"Your arm good?" Nelson asked.

Molina nodded. Olivia wanted more than a nod.

"How's your arm?" she asked. Molina sat down. "It's all right," he said, and she started massaging his back. Any showcase without pain—any injury avoided—constituted a victory. They sat in the sun, watching the next game, when a man named Roger Tomas approached the three Molinas.

"Arm all right?" he asked. Tomas was Molina's advisor, a code word every amateur player uses for "agent," because those who choose to attend college can lose NCAA eligibility for hiring professional representation. Tomas's duty was to deliver a healthy right arm to the draft in June 2016.

Already it felt like Molina had done this forever. At thirteen, he was part of a team that played a tournament at the Baseball Hall of Fame in Cooperstown. Molina was six feet four and could dunk a basketball. Olivia needed to bring his birth certificate everywhere he went to prove his age. Around that point, Molina said, "I hopped on the mound and I just started doing good, just dominating. . . . I just started blowing it by kids, and kid after kid would just start walking back to the dugout with eyes wide open."

He was a kid himself, one who liked to fish, didn't like to do his homework, and worried his parents. "We try to keep him from the bad crowds," Olivia said. "I don't know. You know how moms are. We take him to the movies and let him go with his friends. Tell him to be careful. Because things are so bad now. You have to be careful out there. Because you never know who's out to hurt you. And for no reason."

Baseball saw Anthony Molina between those moments, and he was its evolutionary archetype, the product of a system that lusts after the next big thing, fetishizes it. Perfect Game posts national player rankings of every age group starting with freshmen in high school. "Kids obsess over the rankings," Nelson Molina said. Even after his performance at nationals, Anthony Molina was the number one player in the class of 2016.

"He has no clue how talented he is," said Richie Palmer, Molina's coach with Elite Squad, a travel team that hops around the country to play in high-level tournaments. "He doesn't realize he can be a multimillionaire in a couple years."

I've written about baseball for a dozen years now, and I can say with certainty that nothing unites people in the industry quite like the enmity for Perfect Game. The complaints go something like this: What at first seemed like a useful idea—bring all of the best players together in one place so scouts could see talent vs. talent and teams could skimp on travel-budget money—morphed into an outsized machine that profited off the backs of teenage boys and glory-hungry parents. While Major League Baseball chased steroid users and cable TV contracts, the whole of its youth system was co-opted by a small-college coach from Iowa named Jerry Ford. And it was only getting worse.

There are truths and exaggerations and hypocrisies in this assessment. One certainty is that baseball's developmental system is almost indistinguishable from basketball's oft-criticized Amateur Athletic Union apparatus. Travel baseball has become at least a nine-figure industry, preying on parents' insatiable desire to secure college scholarship money and a high-paying major league future for their children. In 2015, Perfect Game robbed the cradle with more than a dozen events for nine-and-under teams. The US Specialty Sports Association, originally a governing body for slow-pitch softball that weaseled its way into amateur baseball, ranked thirty four-and-under teams in 2015—as in, preschool-aged. The hunger for validation in youth sports never ends, and it's exceeded only by someone else's hunger to commodify it.

In order to ascend those rankings, or get noticed by Perfect Game, children must play. So they do, hitting and pitching for up to twelve months in warm-weather states. Year-round baseball is the bane of the medical community, which rues single-sport specialization and advocates participation in at least one other sport to lessen the chances of injuries. A study at the American Sports Medicine Institute found that kids who had pitched competitively for more than eight months of the year were five times as likely to undergo arm surgery. Another study, published by the American Orthopaedic Society for Sports Medicine, linked warm-weather climates with a higher incidence of Tommy John surgery.

The significant rise in Tommy John cases dovetails with the expansion of Perfect Game in 1998 from an outfit based in Cedar Rapids, Iowa, to the talent hotbeds of Texas and Florida. Within six years, Perfect Game was holding twenty-five national showcases, and Dr. James Andrews's youth and high school–aged patients jumped from 4 percent of his UCL reconstruction cases to 26 percent. Andrews now estimates that one-third of his patients are under eighteen, and that doesn't count the hundreds who make an appointment only to be sent home with a rehabilitation protocol. Andrews doesn't call out Perfect Game by name. Next to nobody does. It is a powerful entity, and even top major league officials decline to talk about it on the record. They're all afraid of pissing off Jerry Ford.

In his telling of Perfect Game's origin, Ford was nothing more than a parent who would've paid anything to get scouts to see his son. Ben Ford eventually pitched for three major league teams, though it wasn't because people were flocking to Cedar Rapids to see him. Iowa baseball started its high school season around Memorial Day, a week or two before the amateur draft, and the paucity of scouts who showed up to watch the Iowa Wesleyan College teams that Jerry Ford coached convinced him to start a new business. Between a spartan facility he outfitted for baseball players to train in over the winter and a league for them in the spring and fall designed to draw scouts' interest, Ford built Perfect Game to conquer Iowa, not the baseball world.

At first, it did neither. The baseball industry subsists on reputation, and Perfect Game meant nothing. Ford bled money. "If we would've had any brains, we could've gone bankrupt at any time and gotten out," Ford told me. "I've often told people, had we been in the hardware business or a pizza shop or any other business, we'd have been gone a long time ago. But the thing that kept us going was what we were doing was benefiting a lot of kids. The idea was actually working. We just couldn't figure out how to make any money."

In the fall of 1999, a Cedar Rapids businessman named Mark Hanrahan—"I'm the Fred Sanford of the airline surplus business," he said—walked into Perfect Game's offices. He was indebted to Jerry Ford, who helped teach Hanrahan's son Sean to hit for more power. Perfect Game needed a bailout. The gas company was threatening to turn off Perfect Game's heat. Hanrahan bought a majority share of Perfect Game and funded it through its first growth cycle.

"I'd sit in my office and I'd write checks for $25,000 and $50,000, and that went on for five years," Hanrahan said. "I had blind allegiance to Jerry. I will not say that I knew he would make it and do it as well as he's done, but in baseball he was like nobody I'd ever met. Jerry Ford is a goddamn genius."

Ford wasn't just the strategic mind behind bringing elite youth baseball to the masses. He helped set the price for how much peanuts would cost at the games in Iowa. He tapped away on his computer, one finger at a time, to sculpt Perfect Game announcements. He believed that with time the business would turn around.

By the time it did, Hanrahan had sold his share of Perfect Game to a New Jersey man named Jose Rodriguez. Ford was still running the company and wanted it back. "Jerry loves the game," Rodriguez said. "Jerry is knowledgeable about the game. He has a lot of great stuff when it comes to the game. Jerry is not a businessman. And we'll leave it at that."

Eventually, Ford wrestled Perfect Game back from Rodriguez for an amount neither would discuss, and what grew from it seems to invalidate Rodriguez's assessment of Ford. Perfect Game took in $15.5 million in revenue during 2014, according to Ford, and netted $1 million—double its profit of three years before. And it came in a time of significant investment aimed at total takeover of a market it already owns. Perfect Game is now to youth baseball what Kleenex is to facial tissue. Ford still projected "extreme growth" in the future. "We want that corporate identity to be the M of McDonald's, to be the swoosh of Nike," said Patrick Ebert, Perfect Game's managing editor, on a video posted to its YouTube channel. "So when people see the PG, we don't even need to say it's Perfect Game, because you'll know it's Perfect Game."

On its website and social media accounts, Perfect Game documents showcases, games, and events in breathless recaps. Years before Major League Baseball used radar technology to grok on-field goings-on, Perfect Game employed the Trackman radar system to capture pitching velocity and batted-ball exit speed. It implicitly encourages young players to throw harder, run faster, hit longer, all so they can scale the leaderboards that Perfect Game posts online. Perfect Game's database contains more than one hundred thousand names of past participants. If Harley Harrington sticks with baseball, he'll go to a Perfect Game event soon enough. Everyone does.

Perfect Game's biggest asset—the one that makes its critics cringe—is that Major League Baseball teams find it indispensable. Scouts show up to all the big events, droves of them, to validate a system rife with moral hazard, in which grown men are often forced to pit their own futures against what's best for the athletically gifted children they're using to advance their coaching careers.

Ford doesn't see his enterprise as the issue. "The problem," he said, "is there's this thing called winning. That's what seems to make people crazy, not Perfect Game."

LAKEPOINT SPORTS BRANCHES OUT OVER 127 acres, a sprawling, billion-dollar, mixed-use complex in Emerson, Georgia, about thirty miles north of Atlanta. It boasts soccer fields, lacrosse fields, volleyball courts, a golf course, and sixteen synthetic-turf-covered, scoreboard-equipped, night-lit, full-sized baseball fields. Major league teams are jealous of the place. Perfect Game calls it home.

Every summer, about three weeks after nationals in Fort Myers, Perfect Game holds the WWBA National Championship at LakePoint, the wood-bat tournament that is the glorious fruit of its toil. Never before had Riley Pint attended a Perfect Game event, so scouts knew of him only by reputation. Pint took the mound July 9, 2013, and popped fastballs of 92, 93, 94, 95, and

96 miles per hour. Then he threw a one-knuckle spike curveball that was every bit as good as his fastball. Scouts flocked to sneak a peek. And just like that, after one game, Pint had displaced Anthony Molina as the most exciting pitcher in the class of 2016.

Because he lived and attended high school in suburban Kansas City and never went to Perfect Game events, Pint had spent the previous two years in relative anonymity, even as his fastball hit 90 after his freshman year. Baseball in Kansas is a seasonal endeavor, and rather than spend his winters at indoor baseball facilities, Pint plays basketball. I first met him at a basketball practice at Saint Thomas Aquinas, a private school in Lenexa, Kansas, where he was running circles around his teammates when he wasn't running wind sprints. Pint stands six feet four and weighs 190 pounds, perfectly proportioned for a body that can take on another thirty pounds. He is the argument against specialization, a kid who doesn't touch a baseball once the weather turns.

"My dad is always talking about it," Pint said. "During the winter, when we're taking three, four months off, he says, 'You know there are kids in California who still haven't put down a ball.' It's hard to put down a ball for that long, but he tells me we have bigger and better things ahead."

Pint's father, Neil, pitched in college at Iowa State. Riley inherited his athleticism from his mom, Missy, as well, even if it wasn't evident early on. He still cringes at pictures of him as a twelve-year-old so pudgy that he needed to rub lotion between his thighs daily to prevent chafing. After his freshman year, he grew six inches without shedding a pound, and it was then that Neil realized how he needed to handle his son. He wouldn't be the parent who allowed the pressures of elite youth baseball to stunt his child's development. Don't pay attention to the rankings. Stay away from all but the largest showcases until his senior season. Whereas Molina was the classic travel-ball case, with eleven Perfect Game events before nationals, Pint was a modern anomaly.

"I've always felt like maybe I've erred on the side of being too cautious," Neil said. "But I'd rather do that than say, 'Hey, you blew your kid out.'"

Neil and Missy don't worry about Pint. His grade-point average is a steady 3.5. The most dangerous beverage he drinks is Coke. "I'm trying to stay away from the soda," Pint conceded. He never got into video games. He enjoys history documentaries. "I just like learning about the past," Pint said. "My two favorite subjects are the Vietnam War and World War II. It really intrigues me just to listen. I'm a big documentary guy. I've watched an eight-hour documentary on Vietnam in HD on Netflix about three times." He asks a different girl to every dance because Neil worries that a girlfriend could interfere with school and baseball, his two priorities. "I feel kind of bad sometimes for him," Neil said. "I'm sure he wants a girlfriend."

And then the commiseration vanishes, stolen away by the clock that ticks in Neil's head. Every day is one closer to June 2016, one more that Pint's elbow didn't roar, one more on the path to a delightful choice: life-changing money from a Major League Baseball team or a full scholarship to Louisiana State University, which made the offer to Pint after the WWBA tournament. Pint's friends at Aquinas joke with him about it, asking what it's going to feel like to be a millionaire. "I walk away or change the subject," he said. "It's kind of awkward to talk about."

As good as Pint's knuckle-curve was at LakePoint, the velocity on his fastball bowled over scouts and inspired a story on the Perfect Game website that all but anointed him. Perfect Game's love affair with velocity is much the same as baseball's in general: total and seemingly unbreakable, even as evidence linking the relationship between velocity and injury mounts. The nearly one-third of major league pitchers who average 93 miles per hour on their fastballs are nearly twice as likely—21.2 percent to 11.2 percent—to end up on the disabled list the next season as a pitcher whose fastball velocity fails to crack 90, according to a study from Jeff Zimmerman of the website *Hardball Times*. For those who throw 96 mph—plus, the chances of a DL trip the next year jump to 27.7 percent, according to Zimmerman's analysis.

Molina and Pint hit the 96-mile-per-hour mark as sixteen-year-olds, and Pint didn't stop there. Early in his junior season, one fastball against DeSoto High School hit 98. His advisor, Greg Schaum, sat in the stands with his boss, agent Jason Wood, a former college player at Saint Louis University. Wood, mystified that a high school kid could throw like Pint, asked a question as legitimate as it was rhetorical: "When's enough enough?"

The answer for now came by way of Perfect Game. Anthony Molina needed to make room for Riley Pint. He was the new number one in the class of 2016.

IN MANHATTAN, KANSAS, A TOWN of just over fifty thousand, word tends to travel fast, and so when Braedyn Woborny's elbow started to hurt, he didn't want to tell anybody, except his girlfriend, who then told her best friend, who told her dad, who tweeted that he hoped the recovery went well, at which point Woborny's friends started texting and asking if he needed Tommy John surgery, and he couldn't lie, so, yeah, he said, he might.

"And then immediately," said Joni Bunker, Woborny's mother, "we get not on the defensive, but like, 'We didn't abuse him, we swear.' You feel like you have to go on the defensive, that you're going to be judged. What did you do to him? What did you let people do to him?"

Woborny is not Riley Pint or Anthony Molina. He is my kid, your kid, any kid, a sixteen-year-old sophomore who wears a Manhattan High School hoodie over a T-shirt with the Manhattan Indians logo, a boy who might be good enough to play college ball because he's the rare switch-hitting catcher but never has been to a Perfect Game event. He's got a bit of an arm, too—his throws reach second base in less than two seconds—and it's why he drove two and a half hours on a dank

November 2014 morning to a doctor's office in Blue Springs, Missouri.

While the face of Tommy John surgery today may be Matt Harvey and Stephen Strasburg, cases like Braedyn Woborny better represent the growing elbow epidemic. Every kid playing competitive baseball fears what Woborny heard from his orthopedist in Manhattan, Dr. James McAtee: he needed Tommy John, and there was an opening later in that week, so he should get ready for the procedure. Instead of acquiescing like other kids who see it as a badge of honor, Woborny wanted a second opinion, which Dr. Kevin Witte soon would deliver.

I met Braedyn Woborny, whom everyone calls Brady, at Witte's office with his father, Scott Woborny, his stepfather, Russ Bunker, and Joni, whose face creased into a forced smile as she stared at the paper in front of her. She read the questionnaire aloud for Woborny to answer.

"Pain on a scale of one to ten?" she asked.

"When I'm throwing, it's probably a seven to eight," he said.

Woborny hadn't thrown much lately following a fall tournament that prompted his first visit to McAtee. Rest and some occasional Aleve took care of everyday pain. The next question tried to pinpoint when the injury happened. Woborny shrugged. Joni didn't know, either. Maybe the tournament. Maybe over the summer. Maybe years ago.

"Every game was a doubleheader as a freshman," Scott said. "They'd make him catch the whole game, and then he'd pitch the second game."

"But he wants the ball," Russ said.

"He's a competitor," Scott said.

"How do you squelch that, really?" Joni asked. "There's so many good, positive things to that. As a parent, because trust me, we've gone over and over, you're supposed to protect them. And so as parents, what did we not do? Who could've done better? What could we have done different? . . . We live in

Kansas. I mean, you know? It's not like we're in Florida or live in Texas."

A little before 11:00 a.m., a nurse whisked the family back to a spacious office where Kevin Witte waited. He is one of a growing number of surgeons who, after training with top orthopedists, brought UCL reconstruction to the masses. Joni wanted a pedigreed surgeon to examine Woborny, and Witte's fellowship under Dr. James Andrews qualified.

Witte asked Woborny a few questions to get a better sense of how much he threw, where it hurt, and when the pain started. He nodded along when Woborny copped to pitching one half of a doubleheader and catching the other.

"Before I examine you here, we'll talk about this," Witte said. "So . . . if you're thinking worst-case scenario, I did look at the MRI. You've got some bony changes in the sublime tubercle, which is the part of the ulna where your ulnar collateral ligament detaches. So it actually looks like something that's been bothering you for a while, because you actually almost pulled off a little bit of bone from where that ligament attaches."

Before bones ossify, or harden, they are in danger of being torn away by the ligament, which is why full UCL tears are exceedingly rare before fifteen: the bone suffers the force of the elastic energy rather than the ligament. The site of Woborny's injury—the sublime tubercle is one of the three corners to which the triangular UCL attaches—was rare. Usually such injuries, called avulsion fractures, affect the medial epicondyle, the pointy knob of the humerus.

Witte asked Woborny to lie supine on the blue exam table. He started stretching Woborny's shoulder into internal and external rotation. Witte hypothesized his elbow hurt because of poor internal rotation and showed him something called the sleeper stretch, in which he would lie on his side, pull his arm forward, and slowly elongate the muscles in the back of the shoulder.

"You're only sixteen," Witte said. "It's really young to start doing surgery."

"I agree," Joni said. "One hundred percent."

"I would make you fail conservative treatment first," Witte said. "I actually just had this conversation with my mentor, Dr. Andrews. He called me the other day, because we had a mutual patient who is a sixteen-year-old kid. [He had] changes on his MRI, and they really wanted to go down there and talk to him. So they went down and talked to him, and [Andrews] called me Monday, he was like, 'I just can't do it. Sixteen.' Similar situation. 'If I operated on every sixteen-year-old that came in here with this elbow pain for the first time,' he goes, 'I'd be operating on everybody.'"

It was settled then. No Tommy John surgery for Woborny, not yet. Witte didn't mention that in a 2002 study published in the *American Journal of Sports Medicine*, six of eight patients with avulsion fractures of the sublime tubercle eventually needed surgery after rehab didn't work. Woborny was still a kid. He didn't need to know that.

"I don't want you throwing for six weeks," Witte said.

"Done," Joni whispered.

"Excuse me?" said Witte.

"Done," she said, louder.

In addition to rest, Witte prescribed a platelet-rich plasma (PRP) treatment, in which he draws blood, spins fifteen milliliters in a centrifuge, extracts about two to three milliliters of pure platelets—growth-factor-heavy cells that help heal damaged tissue—and injects them into the elbow joint. "I can't tell you with any certainty that it actually makes a difference," Witte admitted, "but I know it's something else, an adjunct you can add to the conservative treatment options."

As Witte left the room to let them consider how they wanted to proceed, Joni started to tear up.

"Braedyn," Russ, the stepfather, said, "that was the best news you could possibly—"

"Oh, my God," Joni said.

"This other guy said we needed surgery," Scott, the father, said.

As the adults in the room huzzahed, Woborny didn't say anything. There was no sigh of relief, no invocation of a higher power. He would do the stretches and get the PRP. He just wanted to play ball.

WHEN NEIL PINT INFORMED PERFECT Game that his son had chosen to skip its most important event of the year in favor of attending its competitor's, in came the reinforcements. Jerry Ford goes to ballparks all the time. He's a scout at heart, a magnate second, leaving the daily management to his son Andy and the two others who formed Perfect Game's original four, Tyson Kimm and Jason Gerst. The number one player in the country does not turn down a spot in the Perfect Game All-American Classic, held every August in Petco Park, home of the San Diego Padres. Only that's exactly what Pint had done, and Ford came to Kansas City to convince him otherwise.

The Under Armour All-America game happened to fall on the same weekend, and its organizers had called Neil Pint first. It had poached the top player from Perfect Game once before with Byron Buxton, the number two pick in the 2012 draft, and Neil was an easy sell. His extended family, still in Iowa, could drive to Chicago and watch Riley pitch at Wrigley Field. Almost certainly he would start the game, which the MLB Network would broadcast. Neil said yes almost immediately.

About a week later, Perfect Game called. Neil apologized, but Riley couldn't come. He didn't break promises, and he pledged to go to Chicago. Different Perfect Game representatives called his advisors, Greg Schaum and Jason Wood, and even the coaching staff at Louisiana State University. When that didn't work, Ford paid Pint a personal visit and tried to talk with Neil about San Diego, even though Schaum explicitly said not to bring it up.

Perfect Game's inability to tolerate rejection did not endear the company to the Pint family, least of all Riley.

One of the challenges of burgeoning stardom is learning to say no. "I hate it," Neil said. "I'm not good at it. And they know it." His son suffered no such compunctions. "I don't really like when people try to tell me what to do," Riley said. "I do listen to people, but when I'm already committed somewhere, I don't want somebody else coming and talking to me like it'll benefit me more. I've made my decision, and I'm happy with it."

It wasn't that Pint thought too much of himself. He just hated distractions. If an agent tried to recruit Riley away from Schaum, he said thanks but no thanks. Two lieutenants for Scott Boras, the industry's most powerful agent, went to what seemed like every one of his games, wearing Boras Corp. logos on shirts with the Greg Norman shark emblem. Pint paid them no mind. When USA Baseball wanted Pint to headline the eighteen-and-under national team, perhaps the biggest possible honor for an amateur, he said no, because those conversations with Neil about taking care of his arm resonated, and he didn't want to throw too much. The numbers supported Pint's choice: A ten-year study by ASMI showed that pitchers who threw more than one hundred competitive innings were three and a half times likelier to suffer a serious elbow or shoulder injury.

It's not that Pint was incapable of throwing more. He refused to kowtow to the machine Perfect Game had created. If he wanted to make some spending money over the summer, he would babysit. The way Neil Pint protected his son was one thing. The lengths to which Pint went to protect himself were empowering. He was the antishowcase antidote, proof that the right kids could make the system and not vice versa. Pint knew his stuff and believed in it. He didn't need Perfect Game to tell him so.

"Personally, I don't really look at the site," Pint said. "I don't pay attention to it much. The rankings are cool, I guess, to see where you're at, but I don't look at it that much. I know some people who are just excited when they see their name on Perfect Game."

Anthony Molina's name more or less disappeared from the site over the winter. His ascent was fraught with peril in the first place. He went to West Broward High, near his home in Pembroke Pines, Florida, as a freshman. He transferred to American Heritage, a local powerhouse, but left after he got caught with fifteen bucks worth of weed. Molina said he was just holding it for a friend.

"The kid's got a golden arm," said Mike Macey, an assistant at Heritage. "We were going to do everything we can to get him in and make sure he can pitch for us. His head's not screwed on. Mom and dad tried to get him away from that environment. But the kid kept coming back to it."

After spending his sophomore season at Somerset Charter Academy, he returned to West Broward for his junior year. After school on January 13, 2015, Molina punched a local kid in the face and blackened his eye. The kid called it a cheap shot. Molina said it was self-defense. That evening, police officers came to Molina's house and arrested him. Now seventeen, he spent the night in detention. The next morning, Molina was charged with aggravated battery, a felony. He cried. So did his mother, Olivia.

"It's been a nightmare for us," said his father, Nelson.

Olivia worried about something like this. Molina loved to mock and debate his overprotective mother. "Tony is a good attorney, I'll tell you," she said. "He will not back down." He promised he would go to class and do well and stay out of trouble.

"I see two versions of Tony," said Richie Palmer, his travel-ball coach. "I see the great kid with me. And I see the fuckup. It has nothing to do with the arm and everything to do with character."

Six months earlier, at nationals, all that mattered was the arm. It was his identity, his raison d'être, and Perfect Game was betting on it. Before his game, Molina was handed a sheet of blank mailing labels and sent to a table in the empty concourse. He used red, blue, green, and purple Staedtler Lumocolor pens to sign dozens of labels that would be pressed onto special trading cards made by Leaf for Perfect Game. Each card is emblazoned with a number denoting its rarity. For just $29.99 on eBay, anyone could have a gold-bordered, autographed Anthony Molina card—number 37 of 50—with an out-of-focus picture of him from nationals. In retrospect, it would seem like a great day compared with those ahead.

"I deal with five Anthony Molinas every summer," Palmer said. "I try to tell him, 'You're not special,' even though he can be. I've seen guys like him throw it away. And that's the path he's going on."

It especially chaps Palmer because he knows the sensation of pitching, how it can be a hundred little games in one, an unremitting challenge. He loved it more than anything when he played at Broward College in Fort Lauderdale, and then he tore his UCL. Palmer never made it back.

WHEN HE TRIED TO UNDERSTAND why his elbow gave out, Arizona Diamondbacks pitcher Daniel Hudson harkened back to the last game of his high school career. Down 8–0 after three innings, he kept pitching, into the fourth and fifth, on to the sixth and seventh, through the eighth and ninth, six straight scoreless, enough for Princess Anne High to play catch-up and force Virginia's Group AAA state championship game into extra innings. And Hudson continued in the tenth, too, because Jerry Ford was right. Winning makes dolts of grown men whose job it is to take care of kids who know no better. Virginia state rules limiting a pitcher to ten innings a week saved Hudson from himself and the coaches who found vindication in a twelve-inning victory that brought Princess Anne its first state title. Hudson threw 164 pitches.

"At that point," Hudson said, "I'm not thinking five years down the road, either. . . . It's not like, 'Hey, how's this going to feel when I'm twenty-five years old?' It's: 'Fuck it, I want to go win.' The only reason I didn't go out for more is because there's a limit on how many innings you can go in a week."

The overuse didn't stop in high school. No pitch counts exist in old box scores from Hudson's games at Old Dominion University. He's certain he exceeded 120 in most games and often went well into the 130s. Every Friday, it was the same routine: damn the torpedoes, at least seven strong for Huddy.

"Coaches have to win to keep their jobs," Hudson said. "They're going to ride their best pitchers. It's just the nature of college baseball, you know? Most guys are competitive as hell and want to win. I didn't know any better."

The culture of college coaches subjecting pitchers to punishing workloads is nearing extinction. Exceptions exist, particularly at smaller programs, but the pitch-count shame police do a strong enough job of monitoring habitual offenders that they change or run the risk of other coaches sabotaging their recruiting with the truth. Scrutiny on high school kids isn't nearly as strong. In 2014, Dylan Fosnacht, a senior at Rochester High in Washington state, threw 194 pitches over fifteen innings in a district playoff game. Fosnacht refused to apologize. He wasn't planning on playing baseball beyond high school. "Just trying to get a much-needed win for my team," he tweeted at Detroit Tigers ace David Price, who had called Fosnacht "a beast" before suggesting his coach should be fired.

Kids today still are part of the first generation reared via Perfect Game. It started right around the same time as Hudson—born in 1987, into travel ball around 2000—when the business was in full expansion mode, out of Iowa and into the South, then the coasts, then everywhere. The quality of assessments from the organization weren't exactly top-notch back then. Hudson traveled to a showcase in Fort Myers at sixteen, where Perfect Game made a laughable appraisal of a delivery that scouts and personnel people alike long believed would get him hurt: "Short, compact arm stroke in back and good extension out front. Hudson does fall off to first base some on his finish, about the only serious quibble we'd have with his mechanics."

Perfect Game's evaluation skills have grown alongside its business. Now an industry leviathan, Perfect Game can rewrite the story of what it really wants to be and how it wants to be known. Its reputation does not match the company Ford described to me. "I really don't think we are causing anyone to throw year-round," he said. "We certainly don't promote that."

Not actively. Perfect Game does hold year-round showcases, though, and kids who don't have Riley Pint's or Anthony Molina's natural gifts feel compelled to attend events out of fear that their rankings will drop if they don't. Agents trade derisive stories of Perfect Game imploring a kid to show up at a certain event.

Ford truly believes it when he says he wants to grow baseball. In recent years, Ford said, he stepped in during a tournament and shut down a top prospect whose coach was about to pitch him twice in one day. Ford can't micromanage every game, though. Perfect Game's worst crime was accidental: it hatched an industry with inadequate oversight.

When that happened once before, Major League Baseball donned its big-government cap and intervened. The youth system in Latin America has been a wilderness of corruption for decades, with trainers pumping teenage boys full of steroids and taking 30 percent cuts of their signing bonuses. Slowly, baseball wants to transition the system into a league-controlled entity that can monitor not just the kids' finances but also their arms. The prospect of Major League Baseball going after Perfect Game in a similar fashion is not far-fetched. Two of the sport's highest-ranking power brokers told me that transferring the youth apparatus to Major League Baseball's hands was a priority, although wresting control from an established company with such reach would take years.

Perfect Game could help its cause by prioritizing players' health, even if that stunts the extreme growth Ford expects. Ford could de-emphasize year-round baseball if he so desired. And he could commission an app that allows coaches, families, or kids to enter pitch-count data so a player's entire record is accurate and available. Perfect Game can be a leader.

Instead, it's creating showcases for nine-year-olds.

In early 2015, Perfect Game announced a spin-off called the Series, which consists of three types of events: scouting combines, tournaments to find the best kids from a geographic area, and a national tournament pitting those local teams against one another, ages nine to eighteen. With the Series, Perfect Game reinforces every ugly stereotype about itself, from too young to too soon to too much.

Ford tries to rationalize it. By keeping showcases local, families wouldn't need to travel as much. Measuring kids before they hit double digits also provides Perfect Game a compelling benefit: the ability to build a powerful database of information willingly given by children. "Let's say this data has meaningful components to it," Ford said. "Let's say your son, a seven-year-old kid, shows us traits that Mike Trout had at the same age. What that means to me is we need to keep that kid involved in baseball. We lose so many kids to other games because, quite honestly, the other games are sometimes more exciting or accessible to those kids."

I didn't walk away from my conversation with Jerry Ford thinking Perfect Game is any more evil or greedier than the rest of the world that fattens itself on youth baseball. Just that he was lost in his idealism. Of all people, Ford should be hypersensitive to the issue. His son, Ben, the one for whom he created Perfect Game, needed Tommy John surgery in 2001. Instead, Ford sits by as the Perfect Game generation keeps on breaking, just another person absolving himself of responsibility.

NELSON MOLINA EXPECTED THE PHONE call. The baseball community is too damn gossipy to have kept Anthony Molina's arrest secret. On the line was a coach from the University of Miami. He was pulling Molina's scholarship offer. Because the commitment was verbal, Miami had no obligation to Molina and could dump him whenever it pleased. All this time Nelson spent worrying about Tony's elbow, and it was his fist that ruined things.

"They said he should've walked away," Nelson said of the incident that landed his son in jail. "Everything has been set up to fuck Tony." He took a deep breath. "I'm sorry for my words. It's hard. Tony's the type of kid everyone loves. He's like a magnet. Everyone goes to Tony. But you hang around in the wrong places . . ."

Nelson never stopped sticking up for his son. The weed episode "was a misunderstanding" and the transfers "not a big deal." Molina's travel-ball coach, Richie Palmer, said, "The dad's the biggest problem. He's an enabler. I try to talk to him, let him know you can't be like this with him. Tony's not stupid. He's a sharp kid. He's smart. And unfortunately, he's a big problem. The dad refuses to be a hard-ass with him, which is what the kid needs." A few days after the incident, Palmer said he heard from a friend who said he saw Molina cutting school. "I just dog-cussed him," Palmer said. "I got tired of him lying to me. 'You're probably going to be working at IHOP across the street cooking for me and my daughter instead of being on my TV.'"

Not once did Nelson consider moving away or shipping Molina off to boarding school somewhere. He took a few months away from baseball before Nelson called to tell me: "He's coming back." Molina's grades were up. He was practicing with Elite Squad again, even as his lawyer, Lyon Greenblatt, planned Molina's defense. He hoped to get the felony battery charge reduced to simple battery so Molina could enter a diversion program instead of juvenile detention. In the worst-case scenario, if the case went to trial, Greenblatt was considering using the stand-your-ground defense. He said video existed of the alleged victim wielding a knife on another occasion and that Molina punched him as he reached into the same pocket from which he had previously pulled the blade.

Though scouts nattered away about Molina's bad makeup—the nebulous quality that combines personality, attitude, willing-ness to accept coaching, and general demeanor—the episode did little to diminish his standing among the showcase class. Under Armour had called asking him back to its All-America Game—this time alongside Riley Pint. Molina heard from USA Baseball, too, and of course Perfect Game expected him to show up at na-tionals. He might not throw 96 or 97, as the scouts hoped, but he needed to maintain his ranking. "I don't want to see him get any lower because of this," Nelson said.

He did drop, and maybe that wasn't such a bad thing. Between June 2012 and October 2014, Molina went to twenty Perfect Game events. That was twenty times throwing to the radar gun, twenty times trying to justify being number one, twenty times being peddled by all of the adults—family, scouts, agents, event coordinators—ostensibly there to protect him. However cosseted arms may be, rest for ones with just-closing growth plates never qualifies as a bad idea.

For the first time, Riley Pint would ramp up his summer schedule with events in between babysitting gigs. He planned to hit five Midwest tournaments and the WWBA with his Mac-N-Seitz team, fly in for a day to pitch at Perfect Game nationals and the Area Code Games, and headline the Under Armour game at Wrigley. After that, Pint expected to shut down for three months and start training for his senior season earlier than before, in No-vember or so. He decided not to play basketball his senior year after a couple of twisted ankles, a concussion, a dislocated finger, and a shot to the nose the previous season. No sense in risking it, not with the rising clamor.

Early in the 2015 Major League Baseball season, the Milwaukee Brewers spiraled to a 4–16 start. Fans grew resigned to them picking first overall in the draft. *Brew Crew Ball*, a blog devoted to the team, took the opportunity to stump for its choice: "Riley Pint has a name fit for the Brewers."

"Not to sound cocky or anything," Pint said, "but I do want to get drafted number one overall. That's my goal. And if that doesn't work out, I can go to LSU and play for an amazing program."

Because Pint is a history buff, he knew the number of right-handed high schoolers that went with the first overall pick: none. Eight right-handers were chosen second, some successful (Josh Beckett, J. R. Richard), some spectacular busts (Jay Franklin, Tommy Boggs). The latest two were Jameson Taillon, who underwent Tommy John surgery, and Tyler Kolek, whose 100-mph fastball in high school raised suspicions about his long-term viability. The only three left-handed high schoolers taken number one were David Clyde and Brien Taylor, both of whom were out of baseball before their twenty-seventh birthday because of arm problems, and Brady Aiken, whose career didn't even start before he needed Tommy John.

Train and pray. That's all Pint could do. His coaches praised his mechanics and scouts liked his smooth delivery. Not once had his arm hurt. Nonetheless, Neil Pint paced every time his son started a game, the clock still ticking, June 2016 too far away to count days but close enough to dream about.

In early May 2015, Saint Thomas Aquinas traveled to Blue Valley West, a high school in the nouveau riche south Kansas City suburbs. Nobody with a radar gun showed. Those would come in waves next spring, area scouts and cross-checkers and maybe even some general managers. Their absence wasn't necessarily missed. Pint struggled to command his fastball. A couple of ground balls with legs reached the outfield. He issued a four-pitch walk. His first-baseman missed an easy out with a brain fart. And suddenly he trailed 5–0, a victim of death by paper cut. He left after fifty-one pitches, and Aquinas soon thereafter got mercy-ruled. "Worst I've ever seen him," Neil said.

Which, he suggested, wasn't a bad thing. The night before the game, Pint spent a few hours with his friends playing basketball. Neil wondered about the wisdom in that, especially with a game early the next day. He didn't belabor the point. He wants Pint to make more of his own decisions and recognize their consequences. You know, a normal adolescence.

Normalcy long ago vanished for kids like Riley Pint. Nothing illustrated this better than the line of questioning after the game, when Pint circled around the dugout and caught the eye of his father.

"Your arm OK?" Neil asked. Pint nodded.

"You good?" asked Schaum, his advisor. Pint nodded again.

His mom was sick the night before, so he walked into the stands to see how she was doing.

"How's your arm?" asked Missy. The words sounded familiar to Pint and boys everywhere inside the baseball machine. It's the exact thing Olivia Molina said to her son almost a year earlier at nationals, the first question, always the first question. They don't want to be like Braedyn Woborny's mom, wondering if they didn't do enough, stuck in the maze of second-guessing, their million-dollar lottery ticket gone like flash paper.

Eventually, the questioning shifted elsewhere. Neil wondered when Pint was going to get a haircut—the edges of his sideburns were starting to curl around his hat—and if he needed any food or Gatorade or something else. Pint politely answered, the frustration of the rare bad game evident. Neil knew better than to keep pushing.

"As long as you're healthy is all," he told his son. "Right?"

CHAPTER 6

Overuse, Underuse, and No Use

NOBODY IN BASEBALL KNOWS HOW to create a firestorm quite like Scott Boras, agent to the stars and seasoned arsonist. What unfolded in September 2015 was no surprise, then, because little stokes Boras's ire like a perceived misuse of the pitching arm, and Matt Harvey's was about to become the biggest story in the game.

In Boras's thirty-five years representing players, only a handful of arms were as glorious as Harvey's. He pitched for the New York Mets, and as they were barreling toward the National League East division title, Harvey's innings count continued to creep up. He was no ordinary twenty-six-year-old right-hander; Harvey was one of the game's best pitchers, and that he was in his first season back from Tommy John surgery made his performance that much more impressive.

Following a seventeen-month layoff, Harvey threw 166⅓

innings through early September. That's when Boras sounded the alarm bells. He said doctors advised Harvey not to exceed his previous high for innings in a season of around 180. The Mets fired back, saying they wanted Harvey to keep pitching, and the New York tabloids weighed in ad nauseam about his dedication, and Harvey published a story online saying the innings limit was malleable, and at the end of ninety-six hours of nonstop Harvey discussions, the arm once again stood front and center, capable of dividing a franchise and its star.

Boras didn't know if staying beneath the 180-inning mark would keep Harvey healthy, and no doctor would dare say so definitively. Trying to protect an arm worth tens of millions of dollars, maybe hundreds of millions, is folly. You guess. You hope. And, if lucky, your guesses and hopes get you through the year, as Harvey's did. He threw 189⅓ regular-season innings with the Mets, enough to pass the threshold, far fewer than he might've without New York skipping his turn in the rotation twice.

"Any player in this game wants to play this game for a long time and be healthy," Harvey said. "It brought up a concern. As a human being, besides being an athlete, your career and your health is always a natural thing to worry about."

Harvey is what Riley Pint and Anthony Molina and every other kid on the showcase circuit strives to be, and it's one reason his arm is so scrutinized. Harvey was one of baseball's most popular players, and his arm bore the brunt. Baseball, as usual, was wading into the unknown with his arm, and whether Harvey sustained his long-term health or not, he was another data point, another chance for baseball to make a legitimate breakthrough.

"Much like space travel, we're just putting a lot of this in orbit for the first time," Boras said. "Before we get to Apollo, we're going through Project Mercury. Right now, giving pitchers extended rest and saying it's not just innings accumulation but the amount of rest you get. Maybe there's another way to say we can utilize this talent and protect it by using this model."

The model cared as much about 2016 and '17 and '18 and beyond as it did 2015. Though Harvey's innings limit applied to the current season, his future—the great unknown—didn't just loom over the decision. It reminded baseball how little the sport really knows.

THE FIRST SIGNS OF A shift toward more oversight with young pitchers started in the late 1980s and early 1990s, even as managers wore Bobby Witt and Al Leiter and Ramón Martínez and Cal Eldred and Alex Fernandez with 150-pitch starts. The last three hundred–inning season was now a decade in the rearview mirror, and rising salaries forced teams and players to focus more intently on preserving healthy arms. Better training, weight lifting, and arm-care programs became routine, if still rudimentary. Baseball finally began to realize that turning nineteen-year-old wunderkinder like Gary Nolan and Don Gullett into twenty-five-year-old also-rans was malpractice.

If doing more of something is bad, the thinking now went, doing less must be better. The widespread adoption of the five-man rotation gave starting pitchers an extra day of rest but didn't demonstrably help keep pitchers healthier. When Russell Carleton of *Baseball Prospectus* studied every start from 1950 to 2012 to learn whether an extra day of rest helped a pitcher perform better, the answer surprised him. "There was no indication that pitchers did better or worse based on how many days of rest they got," he wrote. "What *was* significant was the number of pitches that the pitcher had thrown in his previous start."

After a game in the range of 140 pitches, a pitcher's next outing suffered mildly. Today, keeping a starter in that long warrants Congressional intervention, thanks to a dermatologist in Chicago whose research ushered in baseball's pitch-austerity plan.

In the mid-1990s, well before he got his medical degree, Rany Jazayerli was a Johns Hopkins undergraduate and an unapologetic Kansas City Royals fan. At a used bookstore's dollar bin, he stumbled across a copy of *The Diamond Appraised*, written by Craig Wright and Tom House and published in 1989. Wright was one of the first statistical analysts to infiltrate a baseball front office—he wrote most of the book's essays—and House was a former big leaguer turned pitching coach. Jazayerli bought the book because Bill James, the godfather of sabermetrics—the analysis of baseball statistics that today suffuses the sport—wrote its foreword. The authors took aim at everything in the game, all of the fallacies and thoughtless tripe that passed for critical thinking. More than a quarter century after its publication, the wisdom of *The Diamond Appraised* still shines brightly.

Wright didn't just rail against problems; he tried to offer solutions. In lamenting the fortunes of Nolan and Gullett and others, he proposed a change to the system. "In trying to protect the modern pitcher," Wright wrote, "we can no longer rely on innings pitched as our sole measure of a pitcher's workload. We also have to consider how often he's pushed past his endurance level within his starts."

He suggested focusing on the number of batters faced, which wasn't entirely novel. In the late 1950s, Paul Richards, the manager and GM of the Baltimore Orioles, had eased rookie pitchers into the major leagues with reduced workloads before pushing them above the two hundred–inning mark. The rest of baseball didn't catch on until after Richards died and Wright's book, gathering dust in the dollar bin, happened to inspire the right person.

During his first year of medical school a few years later, Jazayerli joined four others from the pre–web 2.0 baseball Internet community of geeks, diehards, and know-it-alls to publish a book in 1996 they called *Baseball Prospectus*. However off-brand and amateur its appearance, it was a revolutionary declaration of independence from the wrong thinking of the past. *Baseball Prospectus* was the twisted, snarky progeny of Wright and James.

Two years later, as Jazayerli watched the Florida Marlins tax Liván Hernández with 150-plus-pitch starts and keep rookie Jesús Sánchez in for 147 pitches, he thought back to Wright's idea that batters faced mattered more than innings pitched. One could approximate pitch count from the number of batters—plate appearances tended to average about 3½ pitches—which allowed Jazayerli to make it even more granular. He wanted to quantify the harm done to an arm by the exact number of pitches thrown.

"The creation of any new baseball statistic is an act of arrogance," Jazayerli later wrote, and yet there it was, on the *Baseball Prospectus* website June 19, 1998: "Pitcher Abuse Points: A New Way to Measure Pitcher Abuse." Jazayerli did not see all pitches as equal. There was no way throwing 95 pitches in consecutive starts equaled a 150-pitch start followed by a 40-pitch outing. There had to be a point at which one pitch was more harmful than another. Jazayerli's original theory assigned pitcher abuse points, or PAP, for pitches over 100. One point for every pitch from 101 to 110. Two points for each from 111 to 120. Three for 121 to 130. And so on, all the way up to Nolan Ryan's 235, and the 211 thrown by Brooklyn Dodgers left-hander Joe Hatten on September 11, 1948.

His PAP article ran the summer that twenty-year-old Kerry Wood lit up baseball with 100-mph fastballs for the Chicago Cubs. Wood underwent Tommy John surgery the next spring. Between the Wood surgery and Jazayerli's demonization of high pitch counts, the issue of how much a pitcher throws wove itself into the fabric of every game. TV broadcasts today track pitch counts on a graphic next to the score. Box scores include pitches thrown by starters and relievers. Even if Jazayerli's PAP article wasn't the impetus behind the evolution, it captured the zeitgeist with impeccable timing.

By focusing on pitches, baseball, in the throes of its number-centric revolution, could revisit its history. Pitch counts for the Brooklyn Dodgers existed from 1947 to 1964 because of a man named Allan Roth. His first day of work at Ebbets Field, April 15, 1947, was overshadowed by another debut: Jackie Robinson. Dodgers general manager Branch Rickey had hired Roth as the game's first full-time statistician. On bespoke seventeen-by-fourteen-inch sheets of paper, Roth tracked every pitch thrown, hopeful that the data would reveal some tiny advantage to exploit. From platoon splits to home-and-road results, it did, and the Dodgers won three World Series and played in five more during Roth's time with the team. He failed to link overuse with arm injuries, even though the Dodgers had plenty of both.

The most egregious pitch counts belonged to Koufax. In a 1961 game against the Cubs, he threw 205 pitches in a thirteen-inning complete game. Another thirteen-inning outing a year earlier required 199 pitches. The Dodgers rode Koufax as they pleased. Over the ten-year period Roth tracked his starts, Koufax exceeded 150 pitches 6.9 percent of the time, 140 pitches 13.8 percent, and 120 almost 40 percent of his appearances.

Roth's data provided insight into not just how the Dodgers operated but all of baseball. In recent years, noted sabermetrician Tom Tango developed a formula to estimate past pitch counts that stands up remarkably well to Roth's actual Dodgers numbers. It uses batters faced, strikeouts, and walks, and it illustrates the ebb and flow of usage by the decade far better than innings pitched. The upper boundary on a modern pitcher is around four thousand pitches in a season. Four-thousand-plus-pitch seasons were prevalent in the 1920s and '30s, dipped in the '40s and '50s, made a comeback in the '60s, and peaked in the '70s. An estimated twenty-two pitchers exceeded four thousand pitches in 1970. It's almost as many as the entirety of the 1990s. There are legends in that group: Bob Gibson and Tom Seaver, Steve Carlton and Fergie Jenkins, Gaylord Perry and Jim Palmer. And there are those whose arms betrayed them: Gary Nolan and Larry Dierker, Chuck Dobson and Mel Stottlemyre, Dave McNally, and, after his only four thousand–pitch season, Tommy John.

Since 2000, only Randy Johnson (twice) and Liván Hernández (once) have thrown four thousand pitches in a season. Nobody in baseball cracked the 3,500-pitch mark in 2015. Baseball took a well-intentioned idea—limit young pitchers' workloads to prevent them from getting hurt because of overuse—and applied the doing-less-must-be-better philosophy to every pitcher, as though handed down on Mount Sinai by the baseball gods. "It's gone so far beyond what I was hoping would happen, I'm kind of flabbergasted," Jazayerli said. "I'm just astounded. It's a credit to the game that it considered it. But maybe it overshot things."

When a starter reaches one hundred pitches today, the bullpen almost inevitably stirs. I've wondered, as have many in the intervening years, why one hundred happened to stick as that line of demarcation and figured it was our infatuation with round numbers. Jazayerli fell for that spell, too, and gave *Baseball Prospectus*'s implicit blessing by assigning PAP after the one-hundredth pitch.

"The one thing I feel guilty about was that one hundred is this magic number," Jazayerli said. "One hundred was just a starting point. When I made it a baseline for PAP, I was just thinking that pitches one through ninety-nine aren't going to hurt you. So let's start at one hundred and go from there."

The arbitrariness dissatisfied Bill James and other prominent sabermetricians who criticized PAP. Jazayerli and Keith Woolner, an influential colleague, collaborated on a newer, sounder version in 2001 that doubled down on the concept. Instead of adding one point every ten pitches, they suggested PAP grew cubically with every single pitch over 100. A 110-pitch outing, then, equaled 1,000 pitcher abuse points, while a 120-pitch start meant 10,000. Using this methodology, they found players with above-average PAP were three times likelier to be injured than those who had thrown the same number of pitches but had fewer PAP.

The winnowing of pitch counts already was well under way. By 2002, the number of 120-plus-pitch outings was nearly halved from four years earlier. In 2015, pitchers exceeded 120 pitches just thirty times, a more than 90 percent reduction from the year in which Jazayerli first wrote about PAP. Only four pitchers have thrown 140 pitches in a game in the last decade: two of them came in no-hitters, and the other two were from the rubber-armed Liván Hernández.

Pitch counts have dropped to the point that Jazayerli wrote that

PAP "became obsolete." And yet here we are, two decades after he read *The Diamond Appraised*, pitchers throwing less and blowing out more. The arm confounds even the smartest people and inspires radical ideas, such as the best pitching prospect in a generation sitting out the playoffs in 2012 because maybe it would keep his arm healthy.

THE FRONT DOOR OF THE Boras Corporation offices in Newport Beach, California, is like something straight out of *The Wizard of Oz*, impossibly tall and swinging open to reveal a hidden world. There is the conference room with more TVs than Best Buy, the outdoor lounge area with a pool table, and the ultimate showpiece: Scott Boras's office, the hub of the sprawling building because what's done inside this one room pays for everything else.

On the conference table rested a blue binder, the reason I came here in the first place. The title page said: "Strasburg UCL Reconstruction (Tommy John) Timeline." Boras's infamous binders usually teem with data meant to convince teams to drop nine figures on his top-end free agents. This one was different. It contained dozens of sheets of paper that defended the most controversial, debated decision in recent baseball history: the shutdown of Stephen Strasburg.

Before he talked about that, Boras wanted to show off the two glass cases against his office's back wall. Inside one was a signed baseball from every member of the three thousand–hit club, all the way back to Cap Anson in the 1800s. The other contained balls autographed by every three hundred–win pitcher. There's Nolan Ryan and Tom Seaver, Steve Carlton and Warren Spahn, Lefty Grove and Old Hoss Radbourn. The collection is a tribute to longevity in a sport that specializes in aborted careers.

"We're in a perishable business," Boras said. "That's why the rarity of winning is so difficult. Because you have to not only diagnose his talent, you have to diagnose his durability and you have to have good fortune to get all of that."

Boras is the most successful sports agent ever, the driving force behind mushrooming player salaries that now average more than $4 million a year. He's brilliant and blustery, principled and self-righteous, beloved by those he helps and loathed by everyone in baseball who holds the purse strings. Nobody is better at bending people to his will, no matter how grandiose his demands may be. Every person in baseball knows Boras revels in his own hyperbole, and most of them still lap it up anyway. He walks the walk, and upward of $3 billion in contracts negotiated does the talking.

When Boras cloisters himself in his office with his three phones, in front of framed pictures of him with clients, across from a whiteboard with black and red markers, in an ergonomic chair that rolls up to a Mac with a small TV monitor, he considers the future of the game dear to him. The game is different than it was when he started advising players in the early 1980s, when the successful Tommy John surgeries numbered one.

In the seven years after the original procedure, Dr. Frank Jobe performed seven UCL reconstructions. Not one of those players made it to the major leagues after the surgery. He had waited until 1978 to try it a second time. "I wasn't sure it would hold up," Jobe said. "When he kept winning games, I said, 'We've got an operation here.'" Enter Brent Strom, a middling left-handed pitcher who, after going third overall in the 1970 draft, bounced from the Mets to the Indians to the Padres. He calls himself the Buzz Aldrin of Tommy John surgery. "They were very, uh, how shall I say," Strom said. "They were very excited to do the surgery."

Because Strom didn't have a palmaris longus in either wrist, Jobe used a tendon from his leg. The surgery itself went as well as John's, and Strom returned to the minor leagues with Houston in 1979. He pitched three more years, stagnated at Triple-A, and retired at thirty-two. It wasn't until a prospect named Tom Candiotti made it to the big leagues in 1983 that Jobe had his second success. More followed quickly. Reliever Don Aase, operated on by Jobe's colleague Lewis Yocum in 1984, returned to the major leagues. Paul Molitor, a future

Hall of Famer, was the first position player to make it back—and the first to do so in less than a year. Dr. James Andrews, the Alabama surgeon who would take Jobe's place as the most famous orthopedist in America, operated in 1985 on a twenty-two-year-old Double-A pitcher in the Toronto organization. David Wells would go on to play twenty years in the major leagues and retire with the eighth-most innings pitched among starters over the last three decades.

In 1986, twelve years after he pioneered Tommy John surgery, Jobe shared his findings in a landmark paper in the *Journal of Bone and Joint Surgery*. Orthopedists around the world marveled at the procedure's ingenuity and effectiveness. And yet over the next quarter century no obvious common thread among the postsurgery successes revealed itself, leaving Boras to wonder how he could keep Strasburg healthy the second time around.

He was a right-handed pitcher whose fastball hit triple digits in college, prompting the Washington Nationals to give him a record $15 million guarantee after taking him with the first pick in the 2009 draft. Just twelve starts into his major league career, Strasburg tore his UCL. Immediately, the organization, Dr. Lewis Yocum, and Boras began discussing how to map out the next two years. Boras's involvement wasn't surprising. He sees himself more as an attorney and advocate than an agent, and the last thing he wanted were decisions about a $100 million arm made by those without a stake in the full scope of Strasburg's future.

Boras was an early adopter of the pitch count. In Jeff Weaver's rookie season with Detroit in 1999, Boras urged the Detroit Tigers to keep him under a strict maximum of 110 per game. The Tigers obliged. During Rick Ankiel's first full season a year later, Boras asked the same of the St. Louis Cardinals. After Ankiel approached 120 pitches in three May starts, Boras called the Cardinals out in a chat on ESPN.com. Even though general manager Walt Jocketty protested to the *St. Louis Post-Dispatch*—"We don't allow agents to run our organization"—Ankiel didn't exceed 111 pitches over his remaining twenty-one starts.

Almost immediately after Strasburg blew out on August 21, 2010, Boras commissioned the binder. It wasn't just a schedule of rehabilitation milestones. It explained the rationale behind what would happen two years later: the Nationals shutting down Strasburg on the cusp of the first postseason baseball in Washington since 1933. No one questioned the importance of Strasburg's long-term health. At the same time, franchises don't often put a key player's future ahead of their own long-awaited return to prominence.

Boras's binder provided the argument in favor. It looked at pitchers from 1980 to 2003, the first quarter century or so of the five-man-rotation era, and focused on those who logged heavy innings early in their careers. Forty-seven pitchers exceeded four hundred innings prior to turning twenty-four years old, and ten of those threw more than six hundred innings. Of the four hundred–inning group, only six went on to throw more than one thousand innings past their thirtieth birthdays. And just one of the six hundred–inning group survived to pass the thousand-inning mark: Greg Maddux, heralded for his clean delivery and ultraefficient innings.

Never mind that even if Strasburg did throw a full season of innings in 2012, he still would've finished the year about a hundred innings shy of four hundred. And that instead of giving Strasburg occasional rest to spread during the season that might have allowed him to pitch into October, Washington wanted to follow the plan it used when starter Jordan Zimmermann blew out his elbow a year earlier: throw every fifth day and end the season at the 160-inning mark, no matter when that came on the calendar.

Never mind that Zimmermann was a different arm, a different body type, a different delivery—that what works for Pitcher A is the furthest thing from guaranteed to work for Pitcher B. With their injury timelines almost identical, Strasburg copycatted nearly everything Zimmermann did, from the end-of-season rehab stint in the minor leagues the year after the surgery to the amount of work in the full year back to the shutdown date.

Strasburg watched the Nationals lose their first-round play-off series in 2012 after finishing with the best record in base-ball. Their starting pitchers threw twenty-four innings over five games. Give two of those starts to Strasburg and maybe the out-come is different. Maybe not.

It's all a fanciful guess, the same as Strasburg's health going forward. Since 2012, he hasn't suffered another major arm injury. Perhaps the Nationals did the right thing, even if they haven't won a playoff series since. Had Strasburg abided by a different schedule—throwing a curveball July 2, 2011, instead of July 1, as the binder dictated—he might've gotten injured again. Had he pitched in October and the Nationals won the World Series, he might be healthy still. Everything is hypothetical, stuff for a counterfactual dimension, though if enough Zimmermanns and Strasburgs succeed adhering to the Nationals-Boras plan, others will adopt it soon enough.

Washington's confidence in Tommy John cases is evident. The Nationals chose high schooler Lucas Giolito—at one time the favorite for the number one pick in the amateur draft—sixteenth overall in 2012 after he needed UCL reconstruction. He entered 2016 as the best pitching prospect in baseball. In 2014, Erick Fedde of the University of Nevada, Las Vegas, dropped to the Nationals after undergoing Tommy John, and they didn't hesitate to pluck him. Each received a signing bonus of more than $2.5 million.

"It may be a rite of passage for all we know," Boras said. If he can convince an owner to spend $210 million on a pitcher, as he did in January 2015 when the Nationals signed Max Scherzer, surely he can convince himself that catastrophic elbow damage is baseball puberty.

HALF A CENTURY REMOVED FROM his last pitch, Sandy Koufax paused to consider the one question I felt he could answer as well as anybody. He is a generational fulcrum for baseball, someone who ties together two vital pieces of the game, not unlike the ulnar collateral ligament itself. The question: How did we get here? And by here, I meant to this place—to this evolutionary landing spot—where almost the entirety of the baseball establishment is frightened by its lack of knowledge about the one asset that costs more than anything.

"The big change is medically and the number of players," Koufax said. "And the fact that longevity is possibly more important than winning. In those days, you didn't make any money unless you won. The whole team. If you won, everybody got a raise. Not much, but everybody got a raise. Today, if somebody is paying you that much money, don't get hurt. Don't do anything stupid."

The money. Of course it's the money. Over his twelve seasons with the Dodgers, Sandy Koufax earned around $450,000. That's about $3.5 million in today's money—one-sixtieth of what Max Scherzer got for five fewer seasons. More than half Koufax's money came in his final two years, and to get the raise to $125,000 he earned in 1966, Koufax needed to hold out during spring training with Don Drysdale and play salary chicken.

If it took teaming up and threats to pay one of the greatest pitchers ever a salary of $900,000 in today's money after a year in which his arm was so bruised it looked like a camouflage fatigue, it's easy to imagine how affordable the rest of the pitchers were. Cheap salaries meant interchangeable players, giant margins of error, no fear of depreciation. The one salary suppressant left today is loss aversion; in what amounted to a loss-less market, teams could treat pitchers however they wanted, and the lack of a players' union left pitchers vulnerable to the whims of their managers, coaches, and owners.

When salaries started to spike in the '80s, so, too, did caution, whether it was five-man rotations or pitch counts. Money did what it can do: frighten the investor, especially when it's going toward such a volatile commodity. "People are scared," said John Mozeliak, the GM of the St. Louis Cardinals. "They're making this huge investment in a young arm and they're not quite sure what the secret-sauce recipe looks like, so they're going tentative."

Alex Anthopoulos and the Blue Jays weren't the only ones turning young horses into geldings. At the same time, the Baltimore Orioles were weaning nineteen-year-old Dylan Bundy on professional baseball. Baltimore chose Bundy with the number four pick in the 2011 draft and gave him a major league contract that guaranteed $6.25 million. At six feet one and two hundred pounds, Bundy did not possess the classic, long-and-lithe pitching body. He was a thick, muscled, mature, defies-his-age type—a kid who could rocket to the major leagues as a teenager.

Bundy was an Oklahoma high school legend. As a junior in 2010, he pitched twice in the same day and threw 181 pitches. His father, Denver, said: "We trained to do that." It started when Bundy was six years old and jumping rope. He progressed to digging ditches and chopping trees before he turned ten and peaked as a teenager with weight-room pyrotechnics and three-hundred-foot-plus long-toss sessions. Denver Bundy wanted to build a machine capable of handling extreme pitch counts, no matter how foolhardy it may have been to burden a seventeen-year-old with it.

Once Bundy reached the minor leagues, Baltimore shackled him with a pitch count he hadn't seen since grade school. While throwing 181 pitches seemed ridiculous, limiting a physically mature, advanced talent to three innings a start, as Baltimore did in his first three starts, made just as little sense. He barely sniffed forty pitches in those outings, and I asked Orioles GM Dan Duquette to make sense of it.

"What we're trying to do is condition him for the long haul to increase his volume and innings and also help him improve his command and the consistency of his pitches," Duquette said. "We will monitor both the timing and workload and the amount and the rest, because we'd like him to build up to be a thirty-five-start-a-year pitcher who can be a workhorse."

Bundy took five, six, seven, eight, sometimes nine days between starts. His heaviest workload over the season's first four
months was eighty-four pitches. No evidence existed to suggest
this was the proper way to treat a pitcher like Bundy. Baseball was
testing pure hypotheses on its six-million-dollar man.

When he debuted in the major leagues that September as
a teenager, Bundy looked every bit the superstar-in-waiting,
throwing two scoreless innings of relief. Going into the spring of
2013, Bundy was a few minor league starts away from cracking
the Orioles' rotation. Then he felt a pain in his arm. Rest didn't
help. Rehab didn't work. In June, a little more than two years
after Baltimore drafted him, Dylan Bundy underwent Tommy
John surgery.

The elbow scares teams because no matter what they try, it
breaks. Throw a lot of pitches and it breaks. Limit the pitches
and it breaks. Implement a piggyback rotation like the Houston
Astros, in which two "starting pitchers" throw back-to-back in
the same game, and it breaks. The more teams learn, the more
they try, the more frustration mounts because nothing is working. Perhaps solutions exist down the granular path Rany Jazayerli paved. It's not just about pitch count but pitches per inning.
And it's not just about pitches per inning but the velocity of those
pitches. And it's not just about velocity but the spin rate. And it's
not just about the spin but how tired the arm was when spinning
the ball. And not just how tired the arm was but how the rest of
the body compensated for it, from head to toe and every little link
of the kinetic chain in between.

We could build three hundred–inning pitchers again. I firmly
believe this. With the advances in training, the improvements
in nutrition, the knowledge passed along from Bennett and the
Bonesetter to Jobe and Kerlan to Yocum and Andrews to ElAttrache and this generation of doctors, we could condition baseball
players at every level to throw, throw, throw. Here's the catch:
The upshot does not match the price. It would force baseball to

acknowledge that many arms will break so a handful of survivors can reach what amounts to little more than an arbitrary round number. Baseball won't traffic in collateral damage, won't sacrifice the many for the one. It made that choice long ago, and it was the right one. Three hundred innings is not a sorely missed benchmark. It's a false idol.

Its pursuit left us with the desiccated arms of Mark Fidrych and Ernie Broglio and Steve Busby, and the sense is that the arm is less than it used to be. It leaves teams spitballing, glomming onto concepts like the one offered by *Sports Illustrated* writer Tom Verducci, who for years has suggested year-over-year inning increases of more than thirty are dangerous for young pitchers. Sabermetricians claim to refute his hypothesis annually, the legacy of Craig Wright alive and well, though the conclusions ought to contain a caveat: pitching by its nature is dangerous on the arm.

The confusion filters down to Koufax, and he's not sure what to believe. He wants pitchers to throw more, but he sees the year-round throwing in which pitchers today partake, and he isn't certain his generation threw more over the course of twelve months than modern pitchers.

"People train all winter, this and that," Koufax said. "Is that good? I don't know."

The edges of Koufax's lips curled outward, his face puzzled, and he raised his left arm in a shrug. His moneymaker moves without pain, like Dr. Kerlan told him it would, and he never regretted the choice, not even during his two favorite times of year, spring training and the World Series. The wisdom he gained in a life away from baseball taught him that the arm is something neither he nor Dr. Kerlan nor any professed expert could fully comprehend, not until better diagnostic methods exist. There are things about it that we know, truisms proven over years.

It's the things we don't that make it so frightening.

The ultimate endgame is a meeting. It is Scott Boras and some lawyers in suits, and reams of paper with numbers on them. It is Matt Harvey, one of baseball's best pitchers, the Dark Knight of Gotham, reduced to nothing more than a risk valuation.

"I sat with an insurance company for three and a half weeks to figure out an insurance policy for Matt Harvey," Boras said. "What is the reason? His psychology. I'm not doing this because I think something's wrong with the player. I need psychology. I need a pillow so he sleeps well. I'm going to pay for it. And pay dearly."

Even Boras, somebody who speaks in absolutes, won't do so about the arm. Ultimately, he believed the Mets handled Harvey in a proper fashion, and he still bought a policy in September 2015 that would pay out millions of dollars in case of an arm injury that affected Harvey's expected free agent contract or ended his career. Though it was macabre, like a baseball morbidity table, it was nothing new.

Over the last thirty-five years, Dan Burns saw baseball pitchers through the same prism: risky. He works at Pro Financial Services, a Chicago-based insurance company that specializes in coverage on pro athletes. (It did not handle Harvey's insurance contract.) Burns estimates he has written policies for thousands of pitchers. His job is to understand what he's insuring against, and nobody can tell him why pitchers are getting hurt. After the rash of Tommy John surgeries early in the 2010s, he hoped for change that never came. "It was not a blip on the radar," Burns said. "I don't know how long this trend is going to continue. Nothing I've seen points to it stopping."

So Burns writes up policies, and teams take them out on their highest-paid pitchers, and, in rare cases, someone like Matt Harvey pays a literal premium for the privilege of pitching past his innings limit. "[Insurance] does help your mind a little bit in the future," Harvey said.

The financial future, whether through the policy or on the mound, is guaranteed. When the Detroit Tigers offered pitcher Max Scherzer a six-year, $144 million contract in 2014, he turned it down. Unknown at the time, Boras had spent the previous seven months negotiating a tax-free $40 million insurance payout for Scherzer in case of injury. The policy cost $750,000. The Washington Nationals gave Scherzer a seven-year, $210 million deal. His $750,000 bet paid $66 million.

Sandy Koufax was right. Baseball is about the money. Even if the sport can't figure out how to use pitchers correctly, it damn sure knows how to pay them.

CHAPTER 7

Pay the Man

At around four o'clock in the morning on December 8, 2014, Theo Epstein was mildly buzzed, severely sleep deprived, and looking to shell out $155 million. During the previous month, he made a video, sent gifts, wrote letters, and basically used every last morsel of his famous charm to convince Jon Lester to take his money. Now, sitting in a high-floor suite at the Manchester Grand Hyatt in San Diego, his jeans stained with Jägermeister, his patience eroded to the rawest nerve, Epstein alternated between euphoria and delirium. If he couldn't spend his money before the sun rose, he was going to get into a fight.

Epstein is the prince of baseball. A decade ago, he was the boy-wonder general manager who piloted the Boston Red Sox to their first World Series championship in eighty-six years. Now he was the president of baseball operations for the only franchise more woebegone than Boston: the Chicago Cubs, who hadn't won a World Series since Teddy Roosevelt was in the White

House. Almost everybody in baseball likes Epstein and his disarming sense of humor, his eternal pragmatism, and his appeal to both the intuitive and the analytical sides of the game. He's the guy who could sit at lunch one day with the jocks, the next day with the nerds, and not only look comfortable in both places but own the table.

Among the few men in the business of baseball capable of wresting that power from Epstein, two were in the suite. Seth and Sam Levinson, a couple of Brooklyn-born and -bred brothers who ran the ACES agency, lived for nights like this. They played to every sibling stereotype. Seth was the older one, brandishing his law degree, always crunching numbers, in full command of a room whenever he walked through the door. Sam was his perfect complement, the ultimate schmoozer, as good with equipment vendors as he was with executives. He was the one who kept pouring the drinks.

Over the previous quarter century, the Levinsons had negotiated more than $1 billion in contracts for a coterie of All-Stars and MVPs they represented. Lester—thirty years old, left-handed, a paragon of durability, two hundred–inning seasons a given, his arm scar-free—had the biggest price tag of them all. He had clinched the 2007 World Series a year after a cancer diagnosis and was among baseball's five best pitchers in 2014. The Levinsons had spent the previous month leveraging teams and offers with an eye on baseball's annual Winter Meetings, where they would sequester themselves in their hotel room and let a historic deal come to them.

"They get you into their world, into their suite," Epstein said. "It's two in the morning, three in the morning, and they just keep going. They wear you down, and it's almost like you start hallucinating and they become vampire-like guys who convince you that they're right."

Epstein and his consigliere, Jed Hoyer, the Cubs' general manager, didn't usually spend the Winter Meetings boozing deep into the night. On this night, they shared laughter over drinks slugged and spilled, the latter courtesy of an ACES agent named Peter Pedalino, who told a joke, delivered the punch line, and, in the midst of slapping Epstein on the back, proceeded to knock a red Solo cup of Jäger on his jeans. If grogginess and a dry-cleaning bill were the tax on the $155 million the Cubs were ready to drop, so be it.

Already Epstein and Hoyer surged past the $150 million ceiling they set at the start of the pursuit, certain it would get the Levinsons to say yes. It didn't. And that started to piss Epstein off. He wanted Jon Lester, wanted him despite algorithms that warned against such desires given the high rates of failure among the small sample of thirty-and-older players with long-term contracts and the truth about Lester's arm that neither the Cubs nor any other team knew.

Early in the free-agent process, Lester flew into Cincinnati to visit Timothy Kremchek, the doctor who had performed Todd Coffey's first Tommy John surgery. If any serious problems in Lester's arm existed, better to find out first and prevent a nightmare scenario in which he agreed to terms with a team, only for him to fail the physical and neuter his market. An MRI revealed slight fraying on Lester's rotator cuff, typical weathering on an arm used as much as his. The ultrasound on Lester's elbow confirmed the presence of something he long suspected lurked inside: a bone chip. The UCL itself looked fine, thankfully, and the range of motion Kremchek measured through manual testing was better than expected, but a little grenade floated near his ligament, and at some point it would warrant surgery.

For a week or so every spring, the chip bothered Lester, only for the pain to disappear as his arm worked into game shape. He didn't consider it an issue, and he figured teams wouldn't, either. Maybe that was naive. Maybe it was realistic. He wasn't going to reveal it until it was absolutely necessary, and with a deluge of teams interested in giving him nine figures, Lester played coy, even as the Cubs tried to close a deal. Epstein thought the Levinsons were stalling, so he started to push, pester. Epstein's usually unflappable demeanor gradually became a sleep-deprived, emotional buzz saw. Sam Levinson stood up, engaged Epstein, and a screaming match erupted, about nothing and everything, about Lester and even Julio Lugo—really, Julio Lugo—a former Red Sox shortstop and ACES client Epstein had signed to a regrettable four-year, $36 million deal in 2006. They were two alphas at the top of their professions, adversaries only because the rules pitted them against each other. They said what needed to be said, and then Theo Epstein said, "Let's just fucking end this fucking thing," and then Sam Levinson agreed, and the next day, after he shook off the cobwebs of the previous night, Levinson called Jon Lester and asked if he wanted to be a Chicago Cub for the next six years. Twenty-four hours later, a Major League Baseball team bet almost a sixth of a billion dollars on one arm.

No matter how much I learned during three years trying to understand the arm, it still stupefied me every time a team gave $100 million to a pitcher. Baseball is rich. Players must get a certain cut of revenues. Thus, pitchers get paid. It is a simple equation, simultaneously true and wildly unsatisfactory because of the arm's guiding principle: it probably will break. I needed to see how teams got to this juncture, how a player handled everything that came with it, both sides of the most inefficient market in professional sports: baseball free agency.

So on November 13, 2014, I called Jon Lester. He'd agreed to let me follow his free agency from the inside, to watch the process and understand what compels a team to lavish nine figures on a pitcher with nearly twenty thousand pitches on his odometer. I wondered about his arm, too, because even though he passed the age-thirty threshold with no problems, he would slide into an MRI tube before he put pen to paper on his contract, and it would reveal just how much wear and tear a team is willing to tolerate. Between Lester and right-hander Max Scherzer, a pair of presumed $100 million-plus pitchers were hitting the market after the two most catastrophic years of arm injuries on record, an ugly streak after which then–commissioner Bud Selig and Major League Baseball vowed to figure out the arm. Teams aren't nearly as motivated to solve the mysteries of the arm once and for all as they are to go all-in on free agent hurlers and cross their fingers.

For his foray into free agency Lester had to thank Carmine, the computer program that helps shape the Boston Red Sox's decision making. Before the 2014 season, the Red Sox and Lester agreed to negotiate on a long-term contract extension. He wanted to re-sign, even if he had to give the team a hometown discount. Boston had drafted him, developed him, stuck with him as he beat non-Hodgkin's lymphoma, watched him get married and have kids. Even if he was most comfortable in a deer blind, camo'd like a soldier, bow or rifle in hand, Lester felt at home in Boston. Wanderlust wasn't his thing.

Then came the Red Sox's and Carmine's first offer: four years, $70 million. Opposing executives were mystified. Lester's teammates were horrified. The Red Sox vowed they would never give a pitcher in his thirties a six- or seven-year deal, and such prudence brought them rancor external and internal. It wasn't viewed as a lowball offer; it was a joke, the mighty Red Sox too stubborn to budge on a homegrown kid who embodied so many of the organization's values. Far inferior pitchers received far bigger contracts, and here were the Red Sox, taking Carmine's actual suggestion—$68 million over four years—and bumping it a whole 3 percent.

As much as Lester tried to rationalize the offer—every negotiation has a starting point—he couldn't explain it. He didn't want to hear that long-term deals for pitchers in their thirties are among the very worst investments a team can make. Lester rejected the offer, even if it felt like the absolute height of ingratitude to say no to tens of millions of dollars. He grew up in Puyallup, Washington, a city of about forty thousand southeast of Tacoma. Lester's dad, John, was a cop and his mom, Kathie, drove asphalt trucks and snowplows. "You're talking about seventy million dollars," Lester said. "Seventy million is a lot of money. And no matter how you talk about it, you sound like a typical athlete. It's not a slap in the face. It wasn't.

"It's not about the money," he said. Lester stopped and snickered at his own cliché. Except he swore it would be true, even if the Major League Baseball Players Association depended on players like Lester to set new salary thresholds. "I'll know where I'm going," he said, "when it feels right."

He wanted what was best for his family, especially following an ugly incident in Oakland, where he landed in a July 2014 trade after Boston's bungled first offer and failed attempts at further negotiations. The wife of an A's player was assaulted at a home game, and it scared Lester and his wife, Farrah, who knew only the relative safety of Fenway Park for them and their two sons, Hudson and Walker. Lester wanted a team that would prioritize his charitable work, too, especially his NVRQT campaign that raised money to combat childhood cancer. And he wanted to win, his two gold World Series rings anxious to be joined by a third.

"There's a happy medium," Lester said. "What people need to understand, too, is if you're talking 120 and 140, in the greater scheme of my life then, what is $20 million going to do? Nothing. My life does not change. I live the same life regardless. I get what the union's saying. You don't want to go backward. Guys like Scherzer can push the market."

Teams lined up to take their crack. On the first day of free agency, Epstein and the Cubs overnighted a DVD to Lester. The Kansas City Royals, one of the lowest-revenue teams in baseball, wanted in. Same with the Toronto Blue Jays and Detroit Tigers. The Atlanta Braves were Lester's secret dark horse, the team he hoped would express more interest than it had in the early going. He and Farrah just bought their dream home in Atlanta's northern suburbs, near where the Braves were building their new stadium. Lester also could see himself wearing a New York Yankees jersey, the history of the franchise so rich.

He didn't know what to think about the Red Sox. They said they wanted him back. Carmine was wrong. So was Boston's ownership. Even though Lester understood why the Red Sox traded him to Oakland, it hurt him. And here they were, the unabashed and apologetic aggressors. They wanted the first official meeting, a request Lester granted. He would open the front doors of his home, and in would come the Red Sox trying to do what they'd screwed up once already.

"I'm sure there will be some awkward moments," Lester said. "It's kind of like when you get divorced, you meet your ex-wife for the first time, and want to talk about everything and figure out where it went wrong."

HERE'S WHERE IT WENT WRONG: the Red Sox looked at the arm rationally in a marketplace without oxygen for rational thought. Logic dictated that no team should hand out five- or six- or seven-year deals to pitchers entering their decline phase. Logic's enemy happens to be scarcity, and so few pitchers like Jon Lester existed that even the Boston Red Sox, one of baseball's proudest franchises, resorted to groveling in hopes he would come back.

"I want to apologize that we're even here." Those were the first words of the meeting on November 14, 2014, from Tom Werner, the Red Sox chairman, who was joined by principal owner John Henry, president Larry Lucchino, COO Sam Kennedy, and GM Ben Cherington—the five highest-ranking people in the Red Sox hierarchy.

Werner was a dealmaker, at home in a setting like this, a spacious living room with a group surrounding a table. He lived for this. By the time he was thirty, the Harvard-educated Werner was running a TV production company that would launch *The Cosby Show* and make him hundreds of millions of dollars. He later bought the San Diego Padres, sold them after an embarrassing dismantling, slinked his way into Boston's new ownership triumvirate, and basked in three World Series titles since 2004. The success bolstered an ego already inflated; three months earlier, Werner had made an unsuccessful power grab, trying to wrest baseball's open commissioner job from the favorite and ultimate appointee, Rob Manfred. Now, Werner found himself in front of a far easier audience than thirty billionaires: Lester, Farrah, Seth Levinson, and two other ACES agents, Keith Miller and Josh Yates.

The Red Sox tried to leaven the conversation. "Listen, Jon," Kennedy said, "if you sign back, I was talking to the CEO of Dunkin' Donuts. We'll get you free coffee for the rest of your life." To which Miller replied: "Can the agent get free donuts for life then as well?"

When Cherington started to talk, Lester sat rapt. He was a worthy replacement for Epstein as GM, intelligent enough to navigate the political complexities of a team with an ownership Cerberus. Running the Red Sox's baseball-operations department was one giant booby trap. Autonomy was only as good as the whims of the owners. Cherington had bitten his tongue raw in 2012 as the ownership's handpicked manager, Bobby Valentine, self-immolated and torched the Red Sox's season. The initial offer to Lester had been another classic tone-deaf move.

"Listen, we believe relationships can get better and stronger with bumps in the road," Cherington said. "No marriage is perfect. That's why we're here, and we want to put everything behind us."

The awkwardness soon abated. Lester was reminded why he loved Boston. Then it was Larry Lucchino's turn to speak. Lucchino is one of baseball's most polarizing figures, known as much for his loutishness as his business acumen. He liked to bloviate, often to his team's detriment; he was the first to call the Yankees the "evil empire." But he sparked baseball's retro-park revolution when, as president of the Baltimore Orioles in the early 1990s, he facilitated the construction of Oriole Park at Camden Yards. Under his stewardship, Fenway Park went from dump to jewel.

Following the 2008 season, the Red Sox longed for first baseman Mark Teixeira. Lucchino, Henry, and Epstein flew to Dallas for dinner with Teixeira and his agent, Scott Boras, convinced they could hammer out the particulars that night. Before the appetizers arrived, Lucchino, sitting across from Teixeira, told him no team would beat the Red Sox's $162 million offer, so there was no sense in shopping for another team. Shortly after dinner ended, Boras was on the phone with the Yankees. Teixeira signed with them a week later for $180 million.

At Lester's house, Lucchino tried to play humorist. "We know that you love Boston," he said. "We know your kids love Boston. And, heck, Jon, you're a Southern cracker despite being from the West Coast." Everybody laughed. Some of the chuckles were more uncomfortable than others. Lucchino talked about the support system the Red Sox would have in place—how they were bringing back Bob Tewksbury, the team's former sports-psychology coach who was working at the Major League Baseball Players Association. Cherington shot a dirty look Lucchino's way. That wasn't public yet. The Red Sox were sworn to secrecy.

The one voice nobody had heard pierced the quiet. John Henry is the Red Sox's majority owner, the analytical complement to Lucchino the lawyer and Werner the politician. Henry had made billions trading commodities, and since buying the Red Sox in 2002 had expanded ownership's empire to include an English soccer team, Liverpool, and a three-car team in NASCAR. Even though he once said Lucchino runs the Red Sox, Henry ran Lucchino. His words in an April 2014 *Bloomberg Businessweek* story had stuck with Lester. Henry, riffing on a paper presented at the annual MIT Sloan Sports Analytics Conference that reaffirmed the value of young players and slagged those paid for past performance, was quoted as saying: "To me, the most important thing this study shows is that virtually all of the underpaid players are under thirty and virtually all the overpaid players are over thirty. Yet teams continue to extravagantly overpay for players above the age of thirty."

Henry now claimed he had been misunderstood. "We have no biases for players signing in their thirties," he told Lester. The Red Sox have spent the second most money in baseball behind only the Yankees since Henry bought the team, he noted, and the resources existed to continue that. No more transition years, like 2014, when the Red Sox's reliance on young talent contributed to their last-place finish.

Cherington went for the close: Even though the Red Sox did prefer shorter contracts for older players, they wanted to dispense with protocol for Lester. Cherington pulled out a folder with a white envelope.

"This is for you, Jon," he said.

Lester took the envelope and thanked Cherington. Everyone else stood up and exchanged pleasantries. The meeting was over. After the Red Sox brass left, Lester tore at the envelope and pulled out a piece of paper. His eyes flitted across the page, looking for the offer: six years, $120 million. Two more years and $50 million more, all because of two bets. The first was that Lester had bet on himself. The second was that baseball believed in his arm. Because of Lester's time in Boston, the Red Sox were the only team in baseball that knew something might be amiss inside his elbow. And they still offered him one of the ten biggest contracts ever for a starting pitcher.

THREE DAYS BEFORE LESTER'S MEETING with Boston, the Levinsons had been in Mesa, Arizona, at the Cubs' opulent spring-training complex. They locked down specifics for their meeting—Epstein and Hoyer wanted to host Lester in Chicago—before heading to catch a few innings of the Arizona Fall League game being played inside the stadium.

Epstein stood in between the Levinsons in the concourse, directly behind the home-plate seats where scouts and other personnel sat. He looked down and recognized Ben Cherington, who sat alongside lieutenants Brian O'Halloran, Zack Scott, and Jared Porter, the team's director of pro scouting. Cherington could be serious, so Epstein pulled out his phone and tapped a text message to Porter.

"Do the Levinsons have any good clients?"

"Lester," Porter replied.

"Oh," Epstein wrote, "I heard he's good."

"Morse, Badenhop, Janssen, McGowan," Porter continued, ticking off four other ACES free agents.

"Look back and to the left," Epstein wrote.

Porter turned around and saw a smiling Epstein, his left arm around one Levinson, his right arm around the other.

Over the previous dozen years, Epstein had carved himself a unique place among baseball executives. He was not the Houston Astros' Jeff Luhnow, a wheel-reinventing swashbuckler intent on upending the system. Nor was he the Arizona Diamondbacks' new GM, Dave Stewart, a scouting hardliner who believed numbers were best left inside calculators. And he certainly was not a cross-cultural icon like Billy Beane, with Brad Pitt clamoring to portray him in a movie. Epstein took a sliver of each to form the archetypal modern GM: he was just as comfortable arguing the value of analytics all day as he was breaking down an on-the-ground scouting report or joining Eddie Vedder for his fiftieth birthday party in San Francisco.

The cult of Theo was powerful. Hoyer had left the GM job with San Diego—a position with more decision-making power—to join Epstein in Chicago. He was the conscience on Epstein's shoulder, the confidant who challenged him most, as close to an equal partner as Epstein would allow himself. When they arrived in Chicago for what would be a massive rebuild—a top-to-bottom reimagining of how the organization runs, with a sell-off of every valuable asset they couldn't sign to a team-friendly long-term deal and a focus on larding the team with hitting prospects to counteract the offensive drought they saw beginning to plague the game—they first needed to implement a new worldview. The Cubs scrapped the idea of a hierarchical office and set it up more like a boiler room, open and democratic, willing to accept every idea so long as it could be challenged and dissected by the brains with which they stuffed the room.

Never did Epstein and Hoyer figure one of those ideas would be Jon Lester. There weren't many sure things in baseball, but Lester re-signing with Boston was one. Then came the offer in the spring of 2014, and the moment it leaked, the Cubs recognized just how game-changing it was. "We'd look at the free agent list and be like, 'Eh, Lester is never going to be a free agent,'" Hoyer said, "and so it really wasn't until the whole thing in spring training that we said this actually could happen. Even then, I don't think we really thought it would."

Still, it warranted due diligence, and when Epstein and Hoyer asked their scouts, analysts, and other bright minds in the organization, they agreed almost unanimously: Lester was the target, more than Scherzer or the other front-end free agent starter, James Shields. Lester checked almost every box on their wish list. Left-handed pitchers age better. Strong mix of pitches without an excessive reliance on velocity. "Perfect mechanics," Epstein said. Off-the-charts makeup. Playoff dominance. From the start, Epstein and Hoyer figured Lester would fetch at least a six-year deal, so in the annual survey sent to all Cubs personnel, they asked: "Under any circumstances would you ever go six years, $100 million-plus on a free agent pitcher?"

Answers ran the gamut. Coaches, minor league managers, and scouts were more of the hell-yes variety while in-house sorts weren't quite as keen. Depending on the day, Epstein and Hoyer found themselves on both sides. "Unless you think you've got it all figured out, which no one does in baseball, you have a lot of back-and-forth in your own head about it," Epstein said. "You try to balance different factors. You wake up one day like, 'We've got to sign Lester,' you wake up another day, 'We're never signing a pitcher in his thirties,' and it's an internal struggle. Jed and I had the back-and-forth with each other. We changed each other's minds. It's a process of getting to the least bad answer."

For all of the front office's success so far—the emergence of the greatest collection of prospects in the game was enough to make a lot of people forget the Cubs' 286 losses over their first three seasons in Chicago—Epstein and Hoyer were far from infallible. They operate by a mantra: "We don't know shit." The biggest contract they'd ever given to a pitcher was to Daisuke Matsuzaka, a six-year, $103 million deal with the Red Sox, for which they got 668 middling innings before his UCL gave out. The history of the $100 million pitcher, from Mike Hampton to Barry Zito to Johan Santana, was littered with disappointment.

On a conference call with Cubs chairman Tom Ricketts and his siblings Laura, Todd, and Pete, Epstein and Hoyer laid out the strategy. All their young, cheap players gave them room to splurge on the frontline starter their farm system lacked. So here's how Lester fit. Here's the market. Here's the personal connection. Here's the downside. Here's why he's the right guy at the right time. Here's how high they'll go. Here's the first offer.

Settling on that number took time. Unlike Carmine, the Cubs' computer system, named Ivy, looked at Lester in far friendlier fashion. It said $120 million over six years was more than tolerable. The Cubs could adjust the model to rationalize $150 million, the ceiling Epstein and Hoyer suggested. Their ability to hunt for bargains convinced the ownership that Epstein and Hoyer could root out the extra $30 million elsewhere. The Rickettses told them to go get Lester.

Step one: the perfect pitch for their perfect pitcher. For more than a year, the idea of a Cubs infomercial bounced around the office. They had considered making one to lure Robinson Cano, the jewel of the 2013–14 free agent class, until they came to a grim realization. "We had nothing to put in the video," Epstein said. The rise of homegrown talent like Kris Bryant, Addison Russell, Jorge Soler, and Kyle Schwarber, along with the emergence of ace Jake Arrieta, the hiring of the first-rate Joe Maddon as manager, and the unveiling of the renovation that would bring Wrigley Field into the twenty-first century, changed all that. "We've got a pretty good story to tell," said Epstein, who supervised multiple cuts of the video and fired off emails with changes and fixes throughout October.

On November 4, the first day of free agency, Lester received a DVD copy of the video along with a letter from Epstein and Hoyer that said: "We are not going to hide the ball: you are exactly the type of pitcher AND person we want wearing a Cubs uniform." The fifteen-minute video might as well have been titled *Propaganda Explicitly for Jon Lester*. "Everything we did," Epstein said, "was just meant to appeal to a deep layer of Jon and Farrah's psyche that maybe they weren't aware of."

In the video's first two minutes, Epstein talks about how the team staffs a twenty-four-hour on-call doctor and nurse for families in case of emergency when the team is out of town. First baseman Anthony Rizzo touted Tom Ricketts as an Everyman who drinks beers with the fans. Epstein extolled the spring-training complex in Mesa. Ricketts itemized the Wrigley Field renovations and improvements. Quotes from writers Buster Olney, Rany Jazayerli, and Dave Cameron exalted the team's young core. Ryan Dempster, a longtime Cub and teammate of Lester's in 2013, waxed on about how the Cubs' large number of day games allowed more time with family. Helicopter shots of the busy city and the quiet country an hour away were aimed at Lester's rural tastes. And around the eleventh minute, Rick Sutcliffe, a Cubs star in the '80s and now an ESPN broadcaster, popped up to say: "I don't think I can even put into words what Chicago is going to be like when they win the World Series." The video ends with clips from a commercial for the video game *MLB 12: The Show* that imagines the hysteria of a Cubs championship, with parties in the streets and a jubilant vendor kissing a fan.

The day of the meeting started with a whimper. Lester's flight from South Carolina into Chicago was delayed for three hours. He and Farrah hopped in a car at O'Hare, which the Cubs stocked with a case of beer and a handwritten note apologizing for their travel issues. After leaving their bags at the hotel, they were dropped off at the Cubs' makeshift offices across the street from the under-renovation Wrigley Field and spirited into the one presentable space, a conference room with modular clocks, soft carpeting, recessed lighting, and a thermostat set at 72 degrees. At Hoyer's suggestion, Lester's career batting statistics—.000, hitless in 36 at bats—had been posted on a faux scoreboard. It got a hearty laugh from Lester and Farrah, the perfect icebreaker. Twenty minutes into the meeting, she was sipping a glass of wine, Lester, Epstein, and Hoyer were drinking beers, and it felt like old times to everyone. Ricketts was supposed to present first, but he had skipped the meeting because he refused to miss his daughter's school play. The Lesters appreciated that.

Cubs charity czar Connie Falcone explained how the team could support NVRQT, traveling secretary Vijay Tekchandani boasted that the Cubs would travel the fewest miles of all teams in 2015, and media relations director Peter Chase promoted the virtues of the Chicago press corps compared with that of Boston, where Chase once worked as well. Epstein and Hoyer then broke down the Cubs player by player, trying to explain their vision and allay Lester's anxiety over joining a team with a losing tradition.

"We were exceptionally honest about where we are in the life cycle," Hoyer said later. "We told him that we're going to be very young. We didn't try to sugarcoat it or say we weren't. . . .

You're going to have to live through some growing pains with some young hitters, but that what we're growing has a chance to be pretty special."

The day ended at chic RPM Steak, where Ricketts met the group in a private room and immediately bonded with Lester over their mutual love of hunting. Throughout the day, Epstein and Hoyer had noticed a different Lester than the one they knew in Boston, one more mature and comfortable with himself. He opened up, knocked off one-liners. Their dream pitcher was even better than they remembered.

Following dinner, Epstein, Hoyer, and the Levinsons hung around to talk business. Epstein's plan: get the Levinsons drunk and figure out what they really wanted. Tequila shots and beer flowed. Though the Levinsons never cracked, Epstein and Hoyer got the sense that $150 million would win them Lester. And so they felt confident about the initial offer they planned to present: six years, $135 million—nearly twice as much as the Boston offer that made this day possible.

ONE WEEK AFTER THE MEETING, Epstein and Hoyer sent another package to Lester. Inside was a camouflage hat featuring the Cubs' logo and a letter that showed just how unconventional they were willing to play in order to convince Lester to come to Chicago: even though the Levinsons hadn't yet responded to their initial offer, the Cubs told Lester they planned to increase it anyway.

"This is a bit of an unusual negotiating strategy, but we don't believe in playing games or stringing things along when we know what we want," the letter said. "You are our absolute top priority and we don't want to leave anything back."

The Cubs didn't know their first offer was still the highest. Detroit committed to five years and $100 million on the nose. While Toronto offered the highest annual salary at $25 million a year, it refused to go beyond five seasons. Atlanta, with whom

Lester met, indicated it would max out at six years, $120 million. Each was a respectable offer. Just not enough for where the market was going.

"We knew 135 wasn't going to get it done," Epstein said. "I thought 150 was our walk-away. So we did go back and forth a lot on, 'We want to make a move, we don't want it to be too big because we need to leave some room, but we don't want it to be too small and piss him off.'"

The goal: dazzle Lester enough that he would sign before the Winter Meetings, preventing another team from making a Godfather offer higher than the comfort zone the Cubs had already stretched. The day before Thanksgiving, the Levinsons set up a phone call with Lester, Epstein, and Hoyer during which the Cubs asked how interested he would be in signing now. The ploy failed. Lester asked for space instead.

Within twenty-four hours, the Cubs' fears were substantiated. Los Angeles Dodgers president Andrew Friedman called the Levinsons on Thanksgiving Day and said his team loved Lester but needed time to figure out how serious it could get. The San Francisco Giants, World Series champions three times in the previous five seasons, suffered from no such equivocation. They wanted in. Lester picked the brain of friend and 2013 Red Sox teammate Jake Peavy, now a Giant, about San Francisco's merits. Madison Bumgarner, the World Series hero in 2014, raved about the organization, the fans, everything. When star catcher Buster Posey showed up at Lester's house along with GM Brian Sabean and manager Bruce Bochy on December 1, the Cubs–Red Sox duel looked like it would have company.

"We have a new team to consider," Lester told me, and excitement tinged his voice even as the process wore on him. At the ugly-Christmas-sweater party he and Farrah hosted—Lester wore a cardigan wired with blinking lights—friends tiptoed around the question of where he'd end up because they understood the stress. It wasn't just the text messages from reporters chasing completely incorrect rumors thrown out on Twitter by a teenage kid. It was the idea that within a week, he would choose where he spent the next six years of his life, a hard enough decision for anyone, regardless of the money. And the knowledge that when he did sign the contract, he no longer would be Jon Lester. He would be $150 Million Man Jon Lester, his contract permanently attached to his name.

The Giants' interest spooked the Red Sox and Cubs into their own maneuvering. On December 5, John Henry and his wife, Linda, flew a private jet to Atlanta to meet with the Lesters. They brought two bags filled with presents for the boys and a case of Opus One wine, about which Henry raved. The get-together lasted an hour, of which fifteen minutes was devoted to talking business. Henry intimated three times that the Red Sox probably wouldn't be the highest bidder.

The Cubs, already the highest, finally made that second offer the same day: six years, $150 million, with another $250,000 a year to cover personal jet service to ferry Farrah and the boys to and from Atlanta. The family travel bonus was symbolic; they knew Lester wanted to be wanted. Epstein wrote one final letter to Lester the next day. With the Red Sox sending in Henry to close their deal, the Giants priming their own huge offer, and the Dodgers seemingly lurking, Epstein couldn't stop typing on his iPad. This would be his last message to Lester before the Winter Meetings started, and he wanted it to be memorable.

Going to Chicago has "been a wonderful rebirth for all of us, one of the best decisions we've ever made," Epstein wrote. Chicago offered Lester the same opportunity: to become part of something novel, this idea that he, his old bosses, and a bunch of kids could slay a century of disappointment. Of all the appeals to his psyche, this one resonated the most with Lester, who said every time we spoke: "It would be pretty cool to win there." This challenge was Epstein's best bait, stronger than Boston's familiarity and San Francisco's rings.

"If you do decide to join us in Chicago," the last sentence of Epstein's message read, "we look forward to taking care of your family, to great fun to be had together, and to the biggest celebration in the history of sports!"

WHEN JON LESTER NEEDS PEACE, he takes Interstate 85 south into Meriwether County and goes hunting. On December 8, he drove to his farm with a Mathews bow, a stand that locks onto a tree, and the promise of silence. He needed all of it to help him with the biggest choice of his life.

"As soon as you make the decision and you're up there in the press conference, you're always gonna kind of second-guess it," Lester said. "You're human. You're going to ask if you made the right decision. And you'll never know until you play the whole thing out."

He returned from his hunting trip without an answer, so he and Farrah compiled a two-sided list, a technique his father taught him. On one side were the pros, on the other the cons. He compared and contrasted to figure out what was truly important, to avoid emotional intervention, to force a choice. And if he could rationalize living with the cons of that decision, he would stick with it, knowing that nothing is perfect.

Boston was home, a place with his best friends in baseball, the team with which he won two World Series—familiar, comfortable, easy. It was also unwilling to pay what the market thought he was worth, and no matter how many times the Red Sox apologized, the pain of his departure never flagged. San Francisco was the minidynasty, its ballpark built for him to throw two hundred strong innings, the city a jewel, and it threw a late trump card: if Lester committed to the Giants, the team indicated a willingness to give him a seventh year and a deal in the neighborhood of $168 million. San Francisco was also a five-and-a-half-hour flight from Atlanta, twice as long as the other two cities, and the prospect of hauling Hudson and Walker across the country bothered him. If it were about the money, he'd have gone to San Francisco.

It didn't feel right. Chicago was exciting, a new beginning, with intimations of immortality, with big money and two men he trusted who were promising him the world. On the other side of the ledger was the potential for a bust with a group of kids he'd never met.

"When it came down to it, it's still Red Sox and Cubs," Lester told me. "It's like your first love. No matter what happens, you always kind of go back to that person. You fall back on that. Regardless of what the money and years were, it always came back to Boston for the comfort, knowing where spring training is, knowing the guys in the clubhouse, the training staff. All that stuff. And then you have to sit there and ask whether you're really going to choose the unknown—this new city, this new place, that's never won."

First he needed to hear from Boston. Out of respect, he gave the Red Sox last right of refusal because, unlike the Cubs, Boston hadn't budged from what it handed Lester in the envelope nearly a month earlier. Chicago bumped its offer a third time, to the $155 million that caused the fight between Epstein and Sam Levinson, plus a seventh-year option—another $15 million that would vest if Lester pitched two hundred innings in 2020 or four hundred between 2019 and 2020. The Red Sox's final offer matched the Cubs' initial one: six years, $135 million. Boston knew it was $20 million short. It did not matter. This was the Red Sox's number. It would not move.

Lester had made history in Boston, winning the final game of the 2007 World Series. Now he planned on making more in Chicago. It was over. Just like that. The conflict, the agita, the indecision, all gone in a clink of champagne glasses with Farrah.

"The biggest thing that made me believe in the Cubs was Jed and Theo," Lester said. "They made me believe in what they believe in."

He and Farrah gathered the boys and headed to dinner at Chops, a steakhouse near their home, where the manager, a Yankees fan who a few months earlier bet Lester a dollar he would sign with New York, asked, "Are we here to celebrate or are we here for dinner?" Lester's answer was to order a $400 bottle of wine.

The calls to his agents and the Cubs prompted a raucous scene in the Levinsons' suite, where Epstein, Hoyer, and Maddon, all there for the Winter Meetings, gathered to celebrate—minus the Jäger. Telling other people wasn't nearly as easy. Lester's first call went to Dustin Pedroia, the Red Sox's second baseman.

"As soon as he answered, he knew," Lester said. "I lost it. I apologized to him. It's supposed to be one of the happiest times of my life, and I'm sitting there apologizing to one of my buddies."

He rang David Ortiz and Mike Napoli and Shane Victorino, linchpins of the Red Sox's 2013 World Series win, along with Ben Cherington and Boston manager John Farrell. As much as they hated his choice, each understood. The Carmine offer created this mess, and the retooled Red Sox would enter the 2015 season with Pablo Sandoval and Hanley Ramírez, Rusney Castillo, and Yoan Moncada— nearly $320 million worth of bats—but no ace. They would finish in last place in the American League East division for the second straight year.

Toward the end of the night, the calls made and drunk on the thought of a new adventure, Lester wanted to celebrate with one last bottle of wine. He uncorked it and took a sip. John Henry was right. The Opus One tasted like heaven.

ALL OF THIS—THE LETTERS, THE gifts, the VIP treatment, and, ultimately, $155 million, every penny of it assured—for an arm that went through the showcase circuit and four years in the minor leagues, nine more in the major leagues, and a dozen spring trainings. I shouldn't have been surprised. Free agency supercharges the right brain in left-brained people.

Watching it unfold with teams blind to the inside of Lester's arm made it even more intriguing until the Cubs essentially shrugged their shoulders at the problem. Elbow injuries are so pervasive that a team run by two of the smartest men in the game, primed to make a strong run at the World Series over the next five seasons, was willing to guarantee nearly $26 million a year, at the time the second-highest number ever for a pitcher, to somebody it knew needed surgery.

"The chip doesn't bother me at all," Epstein said. "It's not going to be debilitating. It can only fuck you for part of the season with bad timing." To him, a bone chip was like a hamstring strain or an oblique tear, an injury with a finite recovery time and minimal long-term implications. And he was right: on the spectrum of elbow injuries, bone chips are what teams hope for when a pitcher complains of soreness. Recovery from bone-chip removal takes two to three months and doesn't involve the mental and physical drain of Tommy John rehabilitation. It's surgery, though, and it would add Lester to the brotherhood of scarred elbows, the long list of those at greater risk for a future injury.

"If the Cubs want me to get it removed, I'll get it removed," Lester said. "If it's not bothering me and we don't want it to, I won't. It's one of those deals where I don't want to get cut on unless I have to. I don't want to get cut on to remove something that isn't a big deal. You never want to do surgery, regardless of how routine it is."

It's not like the Cubs usually played fast and loose with the arm. When they went to Los Angeles to see free agent Masahiro Tanaka after the 2013 season, they declined to rely solely on Dr. Neal ElAttrache's report. They were the only ones to bring their team doctor so he could perform an examination. Both ElAttrache and the Cubs' doctor, Stephen Gryzlo, said Tanaka's elbow looked healthy. His UCL showed a partial tear less than six months later.

One of the lessons Epstein has learned in his thirteen years running a baseball team: "You can't go into an MRI expecting it to be pristine." Even when Gryzlo said his comfort level with Lester dictated only a three- or four-year contract—few team doctors ever will recommend a pitching contract longer—Epstein chalked it up to caution. Doctors exist to be skeptics. Executives exist to win baseball games.

"I think we talk ourselves into it to a certain extent, but if you're brutally honest with yourself, you recognize that you don't know," Epstein said. "There's so much more that we don't know than we do know. That's the reality. And whether you do know it or not, you're one phone call away."

One phone call away. When P. J. Mainville's name pops up on caller ID, Epstein doesn't want to pick up. Hundreds of times a year he'll get calls from Mainville, the Cubs' head trainer, and Epstein hopes every time it's not the worst-case scenario.

"My heart stops every time," Epstein said. "You're just praying it's not a 'Jake felt something in his shoulder today.' 'Jon felt something in his elbow today.' 'It's probably nothing but we're going to shut him down and get MRIs tomorrow.' That's the worst part. Your organization, your franchise, changes with one phone call. That's the worst part. You can weigh all the mitigating factors and it doesn't matter. You're still one phone call away."

One phone call away, just like the arm is one pitch away. No matter how fragile and expensive, the arm is a Faustian bargain with which all thirty teams begrudgingly live.

"We're one phone call away on a $150 million investment, and that's the reality," Epstein said. "So, no, we're not going to sleep well. But we're really happy we have Jon Lester."

CHAPTER 8

The Second Time Around

At the lowest moments of his rehabilitation, Daniel Hudson would log into his email account and search for a message hidden in the depths of his in box. When it popped up, Hudson knew he shouldn't click on it. He did anyway. He scrolled down and saw the memo from Billy Ryan, the assistant general manager of Hudson's team, the Arizona Diamondbacks. It was a contract offer.

The Diamondbacks had presented it to Hudson in March 2012, following his first full season with the team. The twenty-four-year-old had thrown 222 innings, won sixteen games, and posted a 3.49 ERA. Hudson didn't outright dismiss the offer of $15 million for five years. He didn't spend much time considering it, either, not out of greed but because it was startlingly under-market. Starting pitchers like Hudson could make $15 million a season if they stayed healthy. Jon Lester's first full season, at age twenty-four, looked eerily similar to Hudson's: He threw 210⅓ innings, won sixteen games, and posted a 3.21 ERA.

Hudson thought he would be like Lester. All good pitchers do. Invincibility is a shared trait among elite athletes, and it colors their every decision. Turning down the money was the right choice, and Hudson knew that, and yet when he pulled up the email he would read it over again and again, stare at it, think about the paychecks that could've been.

"I should probably delete it," Hudson said.

He still hasn't.

FIFTEEN MONTHS AFTER HE RECEIVED the offer, eleven months after his elbow blew out, Daniel Hudson flew to Jacksonville, Florida. It was June 4, 2013, and the first test for his new arm came against the Double-A Jacksonville Suns at Bragan Field. As much as their swings would give a sense of how Hudson looked, the better indication would come from a man named Yogi.

Behind home plate sat Bill "Yogi" Young, his radar gun trained on Hudson. The old scout trusts his gun. He treats it right. Never dropped it, not once. Sends it out for recalibration every year. Keeps it out of the rain. "I take very good care of my baby," Yogi said. For twenty-six years, he aimed all different models of radar guns at baseball players around the country, and nothing has worked as well as his Stalker Pro II, which he paid $1,300 to have rush-delivered to Texas for a Double-A game in 2008 after his older model crapped out. His Stalker is the one thing in life that never lied to him.

That's why the number that flashed across its LED screen confused Yogi: 95. The first pitch Daniel Hudson had thrown to hitters in nearly a year was a fastball, gripped across the horseshoe-shaped seams, flung from a three-quarters arm slot, spinning at about 2,300 revolutions per minute, sizzling past Jake Marisnick, who took it for strike one.

I saw Yogi glance to his left, eyebrows aloft. Another scout named Mike Brown returned the look. Neither knew quite what to say.

"Wow," Yogi said.

"Ninety-five," Brownie said.

"I guess everyone should have Tommy John surgery," Yogi said.

Less than a year earlier, around the time Todd Coffey was going under the knife for his second Tommy John surgery, Hudson had needed his first. During a game he started for the Diamondbacks, Hudson felt a pop in his right elbow after throwing a fastball. He wanted to pitch through it. His arm refused. The UCL had ruptured. Hudson suffered through endless days of rehabilitation, all leading to his return with the Double-A Mobile BayBears for the first of four minor league tune-up starts before he could rejoin Arizona. His audience consisted of three thousand fans, a fraction of that watching on the Internet, and two incredulous scouts. Hudson couldn't believe the 95, either; his fastball sat in the low 90s during the live batting practice sessions before his rehab assignment.

Everything that day had gone right. Hudson spent most of the morning certain the pouring rain outside would scuttle his start, but the clouds cleared by midafternoon, the sun bathed the field, and Hudson readied himself for the first of four or five minor league starts before he returned to the Diamondbacks' rotation. He slung a number 13 jersey over his shoulders and lounged in a locker room's metal folding chair, headphones clamped to his ears, the wails of an electric guitar stoking his competitive fire. The ripe locker room smelled like the minor leagues, the opposite of an antiseptic major league clubhouse, where Hudson had spent parts of the previous three seasons as a burgeoning star.

His lone concern was trivial. One of a rehabbing major leaguer's responsibilities is to embellish the locker room spread beyond the perpetual snacks of fruit, cereal, and peanut-butter-and-jelly sandwiches. Hudson didn't know what to buy. He paced the room, looking for a clubhouse attendant to make the food run, worried more about BBQ vs. Italian than himself vs. the Jacksonville Suns. "Danny Hudson," Yogi said, "is one of the best kids in the world." Yogi called him Danny, even though Hudson's wife called him Dan, his baseball card called him Daniel, and everyone else who knew him called him Huddy. Danny just felt more personal.

Yogi knew all kinds. The baseball rats and the pompous shit heels, the ones too smart to play ball for a living and the ones too dumb to do anything else, the drunks and the teetotalers, the churchgoers and the commandment slayers, the good kids who didn't have enough talent and the bad kids endowed with too much. Hudson fit no baseball stereotype. His biggest vice was golf. He didn't cheat on his wife. He was a regular guy with a gifted right arm. Hudson first met Yogi in Great Falls, Montana, in 2008, where the Chicago White Sox, who drafted him in the fifth round, had sent him to play for their rookie-league affiliate. Yogi, a Sox scout since 2000, had gone to Great Falls to gather reports on the team and sit behind home plate with Hudson, who charted the pitches of his fellow starters on his days off. He followed Hudson after the White Sox traded him to Arizona, cringed when Hudson blew out, and wanted to be there to see his return.

Now, after the first 95-mph pitch, Hudson settled in with two more fastballs. He fed Marisnick his best pitch, a changeup, then followed with another fastball and a slider that cracked Marisnick's bat. "Breaking ball looks better," Yogi said. Hudson cruised through the next two hitters and finished the first inning with eighteen pitches and nary a blemish.

"He's back," Yogi said to Mike Brown. "All the way."

Hudson started the second inning with a 92-mph fastball and got an easy out. The next hitter saw a 92-mph fastball and doubled. And the next slapped a 91-mph fastball for an infield hit. And the next stared at 90-mph fastballs, one of which flew high and outside when the catcher set up low and inside, and drew a walk. Hudson stepped off the mound, adjusted his cap. The bases were loaded.

"He's not right," Yogi said.

"He's not letting it go," Brownie said.

They saw subtle differences. Hudson squinted for signs from the catcher. It wasn't his vision; his left eye is 20/20, and he wore a contact lens to correct his right. Something was stealing his focus, and squinting forced him to concentrate. Nobody in the stands noticed, but good scouts decode every clue. The body language. The mannerisms. They cross-reference their hunches with their technology. "The gun verifies what you think," Brownie said. "That's the ultimate truth detector."

Hudson was back up to 92 on his first pitch with the bases loaded. The next couple dropped to 90. A slider limped to the plate and the resulting force play allowed a run. Two down. Up next was pitcher Nate Eovaldi, a prospect and Tommy John survivor himself whose fastball in the second inning topped out at 99. Yogi's gun clocked Hudson's first two fastballs to Eovaldi at 89. The third was 88. Eovaldi swung through it to end the inning, and Hudson lurched off the mound and into the dugout.

Yogi glanced at Brownie again. Both knew something had happened. Neither dared speculate what. It could be small—an oblique strain, maybe, or a twisted ankle. They scrawled down a couple of final notes and pocketed their pens. That last pitch—that 88—hung in the air like the smell of burnt toast.

A moment later, my phone beeped to break the silence. It was a text message from Hudson.

I had to come out. Feels like shit. Just feels dead and tight all over.

FOR SOMEONE COMING OFF UCL reconstruction like Hudson, any setback sets off a panic. The injury in Jacksonville could have been inflammation or scar tissue or a tweaked muscle. No one really knew what the hell had just happened.

In Phoenix, Arizona, Kevin Towers, the Diamondbacks' general manager, watched MiLB.com's live stream of the game in Jacksonville on his computer. Towers embraces his reputation as a loose cannon among GMs; his email address includes his nickname: "Gunslinger." Nobody in the organization liked Hudson more than Towers. He tried trading for him when he was GM of the San Diego Padres and succeeded when he took the Diamond-backs job. He saw so much of himself in Hudson. They were both six feet four, both right-handed pitchers, both unrelenting competitors on the mound, on-field Hydes to their everyday Jekylls. Both wear scars on their right elbow, too.

Towers got his in 1985. It's a gnarly one, thick with bumps and ugly with wear and tear, a foot-long reminder of the distance Tommy John surgery has come. Fewer than fifty players had undergone the surgery in '85; perhaps ten thousand baseball players of all ages across the world have done so since. Towers needed arthroscopic surgery three times on the elbow after his Tommy John and finally gave up and retired at twenty-seven. He didn't want to think about what had just happened to Hudson. Towers turned off his computer. "You knew it couldn't be good," he would say later, "just because he's such a warrior."

Andrew Lowenthal, Hudson's agent, watched on the computer from his home in Livingston, New Jersey. Lowenthal had cold-called Hudson in 2007 when he was a sophomore at Old Dominion University in Norfolk, Virginia. Agents comb lists ranking high school and college players, and spend years recruiting in hopes that a personal connection develops. Hudson took a liking to Lowenthal, even though Hudson spent the next few days after they met for dinner hunched over a toilet bowl on account of some bad shrimp alfredo.

Over the next five years, Lowenthal negotiated Hudson's $180,000 signing bonus, played occasional psychologist, and kept him on a clear career path—the one that could lead to the tens of millions of dollars that teams paid quality starting pitchers. He advised Hudson to turn down the contract; three months later, Hudson blew out. Jacksonville was the first step back toward what could be generations of well-heeled Hudsons. Now this. Lowenthal didn't know what to say. He figured Hudson didn't want to talk and sent a text message: "Saw you came out. Everything OK?"

Kris Hudson watched her son on her computer in Virginia

Beach, Virginia. During Hudson's childhood, Kris stayed at home with him and his younger brother, Dylan, while Hudson's father, Sam, worked for the military in information technology. From the time Hudson turned ten, he spent most of his weekends at baseball tournaments, with Kris typically his chaperone. Mother and son were too much like each other, obstinate and feisty. They fought about him staying up to watch TV, about him finishing his dinner, him taking the car. Once, Kris let him have the keys—by chucking them at him. Hudson grew up, recognized the similarities, learned to appreciate them, and told his parents almost everything. Now Kris and Sam sat in their bedroom and worried about their son's surgically repaired elbow. "He's twenty-six years old," Kris said to her husband. "What else is he gonna do? He hasn't gone back and finished his degree. He's talked about nothing else in his life but playing baseball."

Sara, Dan's college sweetheart and now his wife, watched on her computer in Chandler, Arizona. They had married less than a year earlier. She had quit her job as a labor-and-delivery nurse to play full-time baseball wife, though she fit none of the stereotypes. Devilishly funny, even caustic, Sara was the marriage's alpha dog, which took some doing because Hudson is no wallflower himself. She usually got what she wanted, whether renovations on their house or what to eat for dinner or how soon they were going to get pregnant, which was very. She liked things under control, so when Hudson didn't jog out to the mound for the third inning, her fears ignited. Not again, she thought—not the frustration and depression and anxiety, the toll rehabilitation takes on a man, on a marriage, on a family's finances, especially when both know what could have been had he just signed the contract. "I just want to know if he thought it happened again," Sara later said. "If it was like the first time."

Nobody knew, not yet, not even Yogi Young and Mike Brown, who sat in the stands, trying to stay focused. They anticipated the worst, because baseball had conditioned them to do so, reminded them over and over that the sport's splendor is exceeded only by its cruelty. Brownie texted his boss, Matt Arnold, the Tampa Bay Rays' director of pro scouting, and asked whether he should write a report on Hudson. The answer was no. Not if he's hurt again.

"It's like being on the threshold of a rainbow," Brownie said. "You're right there, and then it's gone."

AFTER THE GAME, THE KID with the video camera wanted to interview Daniel Hudson for the Jacksonville Suns' YouTube channel, and even though his elbow hurt like hell and he was worried his career was over and he wasn't thinking right, he said OK, because that's how he is. Hudson stood in front of a brick wall outside the BayBears' clubhouse. The kid, at least a half foot shorter, tilted the camera up.

"Daniel," the kid started, "you made your first rehab start with the Mobile BayBears tonight. Just, first of all, easy question: How'd you feel out there?"

Awful, he could've said, because he did. His arm hurt the entire second inning. It was sore on the back side and tight everywhere. It wasn't one pitch. It was all of them. No life on his fastball, no bite on his slider, no action on his changeup. Nothing. Hudson didn't hear anything pop and conditioned himself to deal with pain, so he kept throwing. Inside the dugout, the BayBears' trainer, Kevin Burroughs, saw the look on Hudson's face, nervousness replacing the typical glower. At the first opportunity, he had hustled Hudson into the clubhouse and back to the trainer's room. Burroughs ran a valgus stress test, a three-part examination of Hudson's elbow that hunts for signs of ligament damage. All three came out negative. Usually there's pain, apprehension, wincing, a jumpy arm. Hudson sat silent as a monk while Burroughs dug into his elbow, even though it was throbbing. He had grown used to his arm hurting.

Instead, he told the kid: "Felt OK. Uh. You know. It could've gone a little better than it did. But for the most part, it was pretty good."

"What was the plan for you tonight?" the kid continued. "Was the plan for you to only go a couple of innings and see how you felt?"

No, he could've said, that was not the plan. The plan was for ninety pitches, not forty-eight. The plan was for six innings, not two. The plan was for this to be a quick layover on his return to the big leagues, where he belonged. The plan was most certainly not for his arm to go dead in his second inning back, to leave him here, on a trainer's table that felt more like a desert island, with the trainer reminding himself not to say what he really thought because Hudson didn't need to hear it.

Instead, Hudson told the kid: "Yeah. Just see how it felt. Play it by ear and go from there."

"Was the decision to take you out a feel thing on your part," the kid went on, "or was it your manager coming to you saying, 'Hey, that's enough'?"

It was me, he could've said, because it felt terrible, on the field and in the trainer's room and by his locker, where he spoke with Sara, explaining what happened, saying he didn't know much. A local newspaper reporter came in and asked the same kinds of questions, and Hudson evaded those as well, which made him feel terrible. He didn't like lying; he just didn't want to explain that his elbow might've blown out again. He wasn't supposed to think that. He couldn't help himself. While the physical scar on his elbow had long ago healed, the emotional one inside him felt fresh as ever.

Instead, Hudson told the kid: "It was probably both."

"Do you know what the next step for you is in the rehab process?" the kid inquired.

Get drunk, he could've said, because that was the plan. Back in Phoenix, the Diamondbacks were booking Hudson a flight home for the next day. He'd probably get back too late to see Michael Lee, the team physician, so he'd have to wait another day for that. And even if Lee's tests found no more than Burroughs's did, Hudson would probably still hop into an MRI tube to rule out ligament damage. The wait scared him, and if that meant passing the time with some 7 and 7s, he'd drink.

Instead, Hudson told the kid: "At this point, it's more day by day and how I feel."

For another minute Hudson prattled on with clichés and non-answers and misdirection. Only his face told the truth, something the scouts could've seen. It was pained and wounded, beaten and defeated. He would know his fate in less than seventy-two hours. Until then, he would wait.

"Daniel," the kid said, "thanks for your time."

"Yeah," Hudson said, "no problem."

IN MARCH 2013, THE BASEBALL card company Topps released its retro-printed Heritage set. Daniel Hudson was card number 149. He recognized the picture. Hat cocked back on his head, left hand unbuttoning his jersey, mouth agape. He sent out a tweet commemorating the occasion.

At least he could laugh at himself. Blowing out an elbow treats baseball players to all sorts of indignities, beginning with the moment it happens. Standing on the mound, the focal point of the forty thousand people in the stadium, and then pacing around because something is wrong. Handing the ball to the manager, knowing you won't pick up another for at least four months. It's pain on top of pain, especially for the pitcher who can suss out the problem. Right after the photographer snapped that picture of Hudson, the Diamondbacks' manager, Kirk Gibson, and the team's training staff arrived at the mound.

"My elbow is fucking done," Hudson said.

He was right. His UCL was completely torn. Dr. Lewis Yocum, protégé of the originator of Tommy John surgery, fixed it as he had hundreds of others and sent Hudson home with explicit instructions not to do anything with his right arm. He wore a cast and then a restrictive brace and tried to follow every step of the rehab protocol and pledged to never let his impatience get the best of him, no matter how antsy he got.

Boredom, on the other hand, beat down Hudson. He created a shortstop named "Daniel Hudson" in the video game *MLB 12: The Show*, even though he was in the game already, because it didn't feel right to play as himself when he wasn't actually playing. If Sara happened to be home when Hudson was killing time on his PlayStation, she would wait for it to utter his name in a speedy animatronic lilt—*"DAN-yul HUD-sin"*—before yelling, *"DAN-yul HUD-sin*, take the trash out!"* He killed time golfing, the challenge of man against course replacing man against man, the competitive rush of staring down a hitter, knowing nothing in the world would stand between him and an out. It's why he didn't like going to the ballpark; not only did Hudson feel useless, he was jealous of his friends getting to do what he so desperately wanted.

Hudson earned his way to the major leagues. He wasn't much of a prospect until his senior year at Princess Anne, when he grew four inches and his fastball ticked up from 87 to 94. No team drafted him, so he took a partial scholarship to Old Dominion, a half hour crosstown. He was an out-of-shape baseball player who, at his first workout, took about twice as long as his teammates to complete a running drill. "Guys, I can run," he said. "I'm not a bad runner. I just literally can't move my legs." They laughed, ran him into shape, and watched him win freshman All-American honors. He entered his junior year as a potential first-round pick until he struggled. Between that and his unique arm action, Hudson's stock fell.

When the White Sox drafted him, Yogi's first report to the team noted "some mechanical flaws and varied arm slots that are very correctable." Almost every scout pinned a red flag to his report on Hudson because of the arm action. "I have awkward mechanics to begin with," Hudson said. "Low arm slot. I don't have the greatest-looking delivery. Post-throw it's ugly." All of which might be worth correcting if he gave much of a damn what others thought.

He didn't, and history vindicated his indifference. Scouts assign prospects grades on a 20-to-80 scale, with an average of 50. In Great Falls, Yogi had put down a 50 for Hudson, with a future upside of 60—best-case scenario, an occasional All-Star. By 2012, when Hudson was shredding the National League with sixteen victories and a 3.49 ERA, Yogi called his fastball a 70, an elite offering. A pitch that had hovered between 88 and 92 miles per hour upon his signing jumped to the high 90s. Against San Francisco in 2011, Hudson popped a 98 on the stadium gun. When a collector showed up for a random drug test that night, Hudson half-jokingly worried that someone had spiked the new acne cream his dermatologist gave him to take care of some pesky zits.

Losing Hudson tormented Towers. It wasn't just his arm. "He's just a freaking warrior," Towers said. He knows no higher compliment. Towers built the Diamondbacks after his own image: grit over talent, attitude over aptitude, character over all. In the middle of the Diamondbacks' playoff push in 2011, Hudson threw an absolute stink bomb against Houston, which lit him up for eleven hits in three innings. Gibson walked to the mound, and Hudson started yelling at him: "Why the fuck are you taking me out of the game?" The Diamondbacks were in the midst of a twenty-five-games-in-twenty-six-days stretch. "Just let me wear it," Hudson said. "I'll wear it for two more innings." Gibson laughed. As a player, he'd turned managers' hair gray with his own recalcitrance. Good thing Gibson was cue-ball bald, because this was payback.

"If you were to model your staff after a guy for his demeanor, his determination, Daniel would be one of those guys," Gibson said. "It was a huge blow for us when we lost him. It was huge. He's a unique individual." During the team's internal meetings when executives projected their roster three years into the future, Towers excitedly penciled in Hudson as part of the 2015 rotation. Hudson couldn't return soon enough; Towers hated his pitching staff. "I'm tired of it," Towers said. "I hate guys that make excuses. I don't need pussies."

In late April 2013, Towers and his consigliere Mike Fetters

watched a game inside the Diamondbacks' clubhouse. Over a two-week span, their bullpen would blow the lead in eight games. This was one of them. Hudson, who often spent time during the games doing rehab work, sat with Towers and Fetters to watch the end of the game. He didn't last that long. When the Diamondbacks lost the lead, Hudson yelled, cursed, and showed himself to the exit. He refused to watch any more failure.

"Oh, fuck, Fet," Towers said. "We've got to get this guy back."

THE CURRENTS LOUNGE INSIDE THE Hyatt Regency Jacksonville is a paint-by-numbers hotel bar, with a few flat-screen TVs, a menu of mediocre food, and a broad liquor selection to help people forget they're drinking at a hotel bar in Jacksonville. Hudson ordered a drink to wash down his loaded nachos with extra sour cream. He picked it up with his left hand.

"I'm sorry you came down to see only two innings," he said to me.

What do you say to that? That it's OK? That everything's going to be all right? Bars may be home to more honest words than anywhere, but some truths can wait. Hudson spent the last eleven months thinking about nothing but his arm and how it betrayed him once. Pitchers coming back from Tommy John spend every bit of mental energy convincing themselves to stop worrying it's going to happen again. And here he sat, three hours after an 88-mph fastball, his right arm limp on the bar top, scared it actually might have. He didn't need to talk about that.

Anything else sufficed: the ballgame on one of the TVs, guns made using 3-D printers, music, how his granny back in Virginia gave not a single, solitary damn about what anyone else thought. How much he wanted kids. How he worried he couldn't have them. Every fifteen or twenty minutes the bartender checked in to see if he was good. Hudson said he was. His demeanor said otherwise.

He lived the parts of Tommy John so few understand. The optimism and fear, the strength and weakness, the triumph and failure—all the pieces that constitute its greater reality. Elite athletes traffic in hyperachievement, and Tommy John surgery forces them to quit the pursuit of it cold turkey. It feels Sisyphean until the moment they're back on the mound, the place they're more comfortable than any in the world. Nothing beats a major league mound, a ten-inch-high Kilimanjaro that few get to climb. Nobody in team sports commands a game like the pitcher. He dictates the pace and controls the tempo. A goalie in hockey or soccer can win a game with superior reaction. A pitcher *prevents* action. There is great power in that.

Earlier that day over lunch, Hudson had talked about reclaiming his domain. This was so much more than a minor league game. It validated those days when his arm hurt so badly he was afraid it would fail him again. He never told Sara about the pain. "I didn't want her worrying," Hudson said. He didn't say anything to his parents or the Diamondbacks' training staff, either. He told only his little brother, Dylan, because he could keep a secret.

It started when he threw breaking balls from the mound for the first time in April 2013. Soreness shot through his forearm and elbow. He knew he should have said something to Ken Crenshaw, the Diamondbacks' athletic trainer, or Brad Arnsberg, the pitching coach the organization had hired especially to nurse him back. Except there was supposed to be soreness, and it would go away, and it did, and when it returned, it was somewhere else, down along the flexor muscles in the forearm, which made him think that was normal as well, even though it hurt not just when he was throwing but when he was simply drying his hair with a towel. And perhaps, even then, the soreness was appropriate. The impossible mystery of the pitching arm was that no one knew for sure what Hudson did to make his arm hurt. At this bar, on his third drink, the night young enough for a few more, he damn sure didn't know himself.

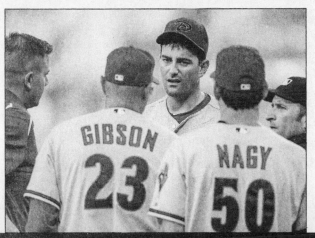

Daniel Hudson with manager Kirk Gibson and pitching coach Charles Nagy after he first tore his ulnar collateral ligament. Hudson long feared an arm injury because of his unorthodox delivery but never imagined what he would need to endure to return to the major leagues. (*Daniel Shirey/USA TODAY*)

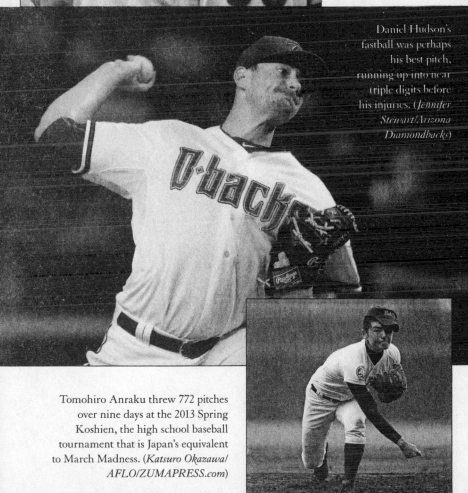

Daniel Hudson's fastball was perhaps his best pitch, running up into near triple digits before his injuries. (*Jennifer Stewart/Arizona Diamondbacks*)

Tomohiro Anraku threw 772 pitches over nine days at the 2013 Spring Koshien, the high school baseball tournament that is Japan's equivalent to March Madness. (*Katsuro Okazawa/ AFLO/ZUMAPRESS.com*)

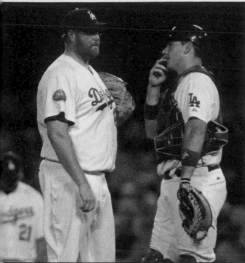

Todd Coffey with Dodgers catcher A. J. Ellis during the outing in which he blew out his right elbow for the second time. Coffey kept his shoes from that night and vowed to wear them the next time he walked onto a major league mound. (*Kirby Lee/Image of Sport–USA TODAY Sports*)

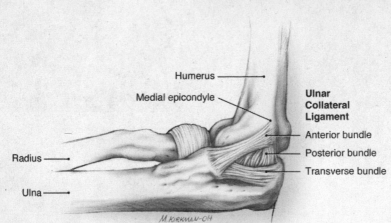

Cleveland Indians minor leaguer Casey Weathers prepares to throw a weighted ball against padded plywood with his coach, Kyle Boddy, who oversaw his return to organized baseball. Long controversial, training with overweight and underweight balls has become more common in recent years. (*Driveline Baseball*)

Diagram of the elbow, including the three bundles of the UCL. Doctors believe the anterior bundle endures the vast majority of stress on the ligament during the overhand throwing motion. (*Myriam Kirkman-Oh*)

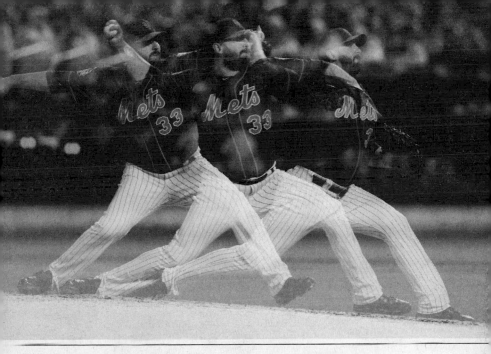

The return of Matt Harvey from Tommy John surgery, in which he rehabilitated for five months longer than typical, was among the most successful to date. (*Brad Penner/USA TODAY Sports*)

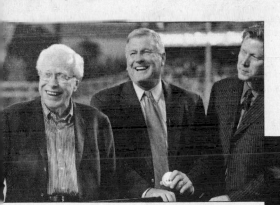

The Los Angeles Dodgers honor Dr. Frank Jobe, the pioneer of Tommy John surgery and regarded as the best sports orthopedist ever, as John (*center*) and Orel Hershiser (*right*) look on. (*Kirby Lee/Image of Sport–USA TODAY Sports*)

After throwing 164 pitches, Daniel Hudson celebrates a Virginia high school state championship with Princess Anne High coach Jimmy Hunt. (*Kris Hudson*)

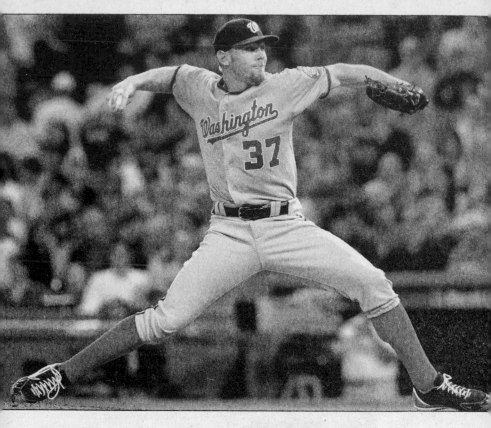

The position of Washington pitcher Stephen Strasburg's elbows—in the so-called Inverted W—is believed by some to have caused his torn UCL. No evidence definitively links the Inverted W to arm injuries. (*Bob DeChiara/USA TODAY Sports*)

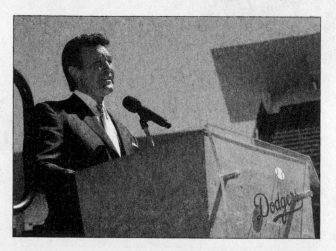

Dr. Neal ElAttrache, the surgeon for Todd Coffey, speaks at a memorial service at Dodger Stadium for Dr. Frank Jobe, his mentor. (*Los Angeles Dodgers*)

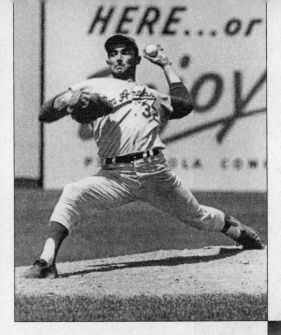

Sandy Koufax, one of the greatest pitchers in history, was forced to retire at age thirty because of arm injuries. (*Malcolm Emmons/USA TODAY Sports*)

Super-agent Scott Boras, who represents Matt Harvey and Stephen Strasburg among many other top pitchers, has called Tommy John surgery "almost a rite of passage." (*Kirby Lee/USA TODAY Sports*)

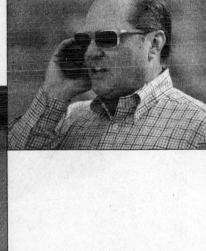

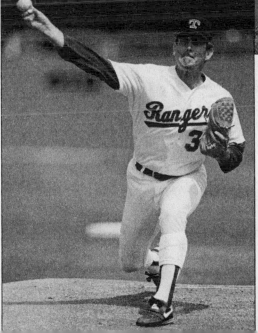

Nolan Ryan's near-unparalleled durability was hardly as easy as it seemed. He suffered from arm pain throughout his 27-year career but never underwent Tommy John surgery despite doctors' recommendations to do so. (*USA TODAY Sports*)

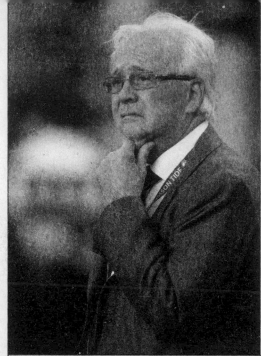

Dr. James Andrews remains the biggest name in orthopedic surgery, and his think tank, the American Sports Medicine Institute (ASMI), the center for some of the most cutting-edge research on arm injuries. (*John David Mercer/USA TODAY Sports*)

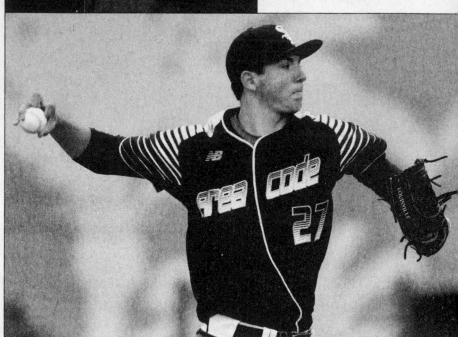

Scouts believe that if Riley Pint can stay healthy, he will be a first-round draft pick and a multimillionaire at eighteen years old. (*Scott Kurtz*)

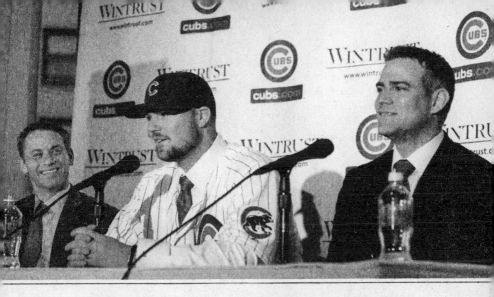

Jon Lester with Chicago Cubs general manager Jed Hoyer (*left*) and president Theo Epstein (*right*) at his introductory press conference on December 15, 2014. The Cubs paid $155 million for Lester despite the risk of long-term deals for pitchers. (*Steve Green/Chicago Cubs*)

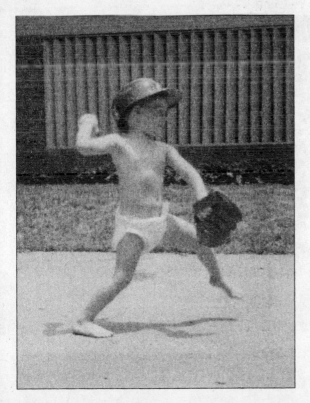

Todd Coffey brings to life the cliché that he was throwing a baseball while still in diapers. He never stopped, even as people doubted him all the way to the major leagues. (*Todd Coffey*)

Even pushing 300 pounds, Todd Coffey still managed to confuse hitters with a heavy sinker and a biting slider. He's even better known for his sprint to the mound than for his work on it. (*Todd Coffey*)

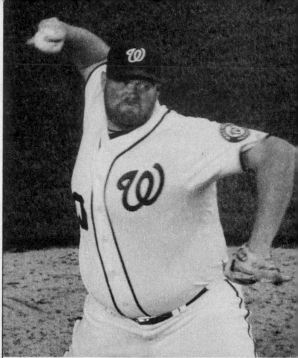

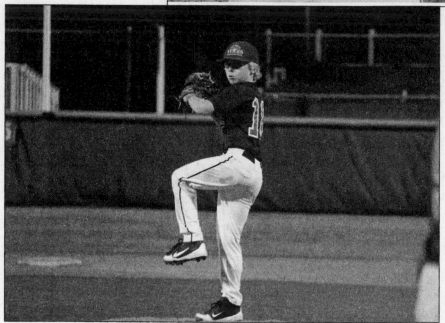

Parents of children like Harley Harrington struggle to balance winning with arm health. Baseball's broken youth system incentivizes winning, even if it means putting young arms at higher risk for injury. (*Martin Harrington*)

Maybe it was just inflammation or scar tissue or something else. Maybe it would go away with some soft-tissue work using a fascial abrasion tool, a cast-iron implement that hurts like mad when a trainer scrapes it across your skin to loosen muscles and feels like heaven when the muscles comply. Anything but the other maybe.

Seven months earlier, just as he was starting to throw, Hudson had marveled at his good fortune. Not an iota of soreness. Not a single setback. He knew better than to trust that. Beware the pitcher who's free of fear. "That's what I keep telling myself: It's going too well right now," Hudson said. "Something bad is going to happen, but it hasn't happened yet."

WHEN HE WOKE UP THE next morning, Daniel Hudson's right arm wouldn't move. It was bent at the elbow, 95 or 100 degrees, swollen and hard. He tried to straighten his arm. No luck. He started gathering his belongings from around the room, left arm functional, right cocked like he wanted to salute a commanding officer. Packing took a little longer than usual. Eventually, Hudson's arm loosened up. He tried to keep it moving, though the closer he extended it to zero degrees, the more the previous night's discomfort returned.

"This waiting game sucks," he texted me. He was at the airport, and even if his elbow felt different than the first time, Hudson remembered the emptiness in his stomach from the year before. He blew his arm out for the first time in Atlanta, and the flight home to Phoenix, where an MRI machine and a diagnosis awaited, was the longest five hours of his life. This flight was even longer, this injury more mysterious, this discomfort greater. Hudson dug into a John Sandford novel on his iPad and shuffled his musical selection, hopeful that an assault on his senses would put the flight on fast-forward.

He landed in the late afternoon, too late to visit Dr. Lee but early enough to grab dinner and a couple of drinks with Sara. She asked how his arm felt and he didn't say much. She didn't pry. He appreciated it. When Hudson woke up the next morning, his arm actually moved. It felt better except when fully extended. Sara felt relieved. Just a minor complication, maybe a few weeks or a month. She wasn't normally this optimistic; she just knew that optimism was necessary.

The appointment with Lee next day was encouraging. He loaded Hudson's elbow into different positions, put it through the standard stress tests, felt around for the telltale signs of a blown UCL. Lee found nothing alarming. "Doctor doesn't think it's anything more than inflammation," Hudson texted. "Gonna get an MRI to be sure though."

Hudson's MRI was over by 7:30 p.m., almost exactly forty-eight hours after he left the game in Jacksonville. Lee told him not to bother bringing the scans back to his office. He figured they'd talk about it at the stadium the next day and go over an updated rehab plan and timetable. At home that night, Hudson pulled pictures printed from the MRI out of a folder and stared at it. "I don't know why I'm doing this," he said to Sara. He had no idea what he was looking at, let alone what he'd be looking for.

The next morning, at 8:30, Hudson's phone buzzed. He looked at the number. He recognized it from a text message the day before as Dr. Lee's. In between the first and second buzzes, Hudson's mind raced, questions flooding his psyche, chief among them: Why would he call now when he said he'd look at the results at the ballpark?

Hudson flipped the screen of his phone toward Sara. He told her who it was. Before he tapped the green answer button, he knew. So did she.

"I'm fucked," he said.

HIS VOICE TREMBLED. IT WAS 10:53, a couple of hours after he'd heard. He'd had a good cry already, a heaving, sobbing, why-me of a lament in Sara's arms. He wasn't the shit heel or the dummy. He didn't disrespect the game or treat the privilege of playing baseball with anything less than his finest effort. Not that he believed any of those things mattered. Baseball wasn't casting judgment on him. The arm is just merciless.

"I guess the graft just wasn't strong enough," Hudson told me. He didn't know many details. When Lee said the UCL was torn again, Hudson went into a fog. Lee sounded like Charlie Brown's teacher. Hudson responded the same to everything: "Uh-huh." Hudson dropped his phone to the floor when the conversation ended. Everything was for nothing. He was Sisyphus.

Sara later called Lee for details. Like every orthopedist, Lee could explain only what happened. If he knew why—if anyone knew why—baseball's greatest scourge might disappear, or at least be manageable and not some booby trap set to go off at an indeterminate time. The graft, a tendon taken out of Hudson's wrist like in the original Tommy John surgery, had snapped just like the one with which he was born. It had retracted about a centimeter, which caused fluid to rush to the back of his elbow and cause the stiffness. Neither Lee nor Burroughs, the trainer in Jacksonville, could diagnose the tear because Hudson's body went into full-on protection mode; the muscles in the area surrounding the UCL instinctively tightened around the trauma, stabilizing the elbow, and Hudson's unusual ability to weather the discomfort hid from everyone else what he suspected. "They told me I have a high pain tolerance," Hudson said.

Physical, at least. The mental toll grew with every conversation. Ken Crenshaw, the Diamondbacks' trainer who had drawn up Hudson's original rehab program, called to apologize. Diamondbacks owner Ken Kendrick and team president Derrick Hall texted their regrets. Josh Rawitch, the head PR man, told Hudson he was going to send out a news release, at which point a deluge of calls came in. He let them kick to voicemail.

Hudson didn't hear from Kevin Towers, his GM. "I was just

sick to my stomach," Towers said. He didn't know what to say. Neither did Andrew Lowenthal, his agent. He talked about getting a second opinion, about how things were going to be all right. "You've got to tread lightly when someone is in that emotional state and be positive as possible," Lowenthal said. "I remember hanging up, thinking that's one of the worst phone calls I've ever gotten. I'll never forget my mother calling me at four in the morning to tell me my cousin had committed suicide. I remember that feeling. This phone call, not to compare it to death, but it was probably the second-worst phone call I've ever gotten."

The worst for Hudson was the first he made that day. Sam and Kris Hudson were sitting in their bedroom. They put the speakerphone on. Hudson couldn't compose himself. He tried to stop crying. Everything hit him during that conversation. The years his parents invested in his career. His rapid ascent to the major leagues, tearing through Low-A and High-A and Double-A and Triple-A, all the way to the major leagues the year after the White Sox drafted him. How he promised to provide for Sara. The contract he turned down. The reality of another year plagued by monotony, chasing this illusion, this mirage, this idea that next time would be different.

"I don't think I can do it again," Hudson told his father, Sam, who suggested he first talk with Sara before making a rash decision. Hudson had done that, and he said the same thing to her, too, that he couldn't do it. "Take your time," Sam said.

So he did. He calmed down. The tears dried. He chatted with Sara again. When he was in Jacksonville, Sara said, she felt nervous. She gets that sometimes, this sixth sense that manifests itself in extreme anxiety. This one was about his arm. She didn't want to bother him, so she didn't say anything.

He tried to rationalize it and came to the same conclusion Yogi Young did a long time ago: "They're all gonna break sooner or later." Hudson's UCL happened to break twice, and he could not let the mystery of why consume him. His mom was right: He was a baseball player. He wouldn't know what else to do. "Finally I stopped being a pussy and figured it out," Hudson said. "My dad didn't want me to make a decision now and three months down the road hate myself for it. Because baseball moves on. With or without you."

Over the next few days, Hudson gathered his life together and readied for another year just like the last. It had been the toughest of his life. This would be tougher. Only three players in major league history had done what he was attempting: return to the major leagues after back-to-back Tommy John surgeries. The first was a relief pitcher named Doug Brocail. He pitched for three years after an angioplasty fixed a 99 percent blockage in a left coronary artery branch. For Brocail, elbow reconstructions were like butterfly stitches. Mike Lincoln, a talented right-handed reliever whose arm bore scars from top to bottom, took almost four years to return to the major leagues from his Tommy John surgeries. The other was a journeyman named Denny Stark. He missed five years and came back for nine forgettable games.

Hudson was younger than they were, better than those guys, except that didn't matter. Plenty of other arms were younger and better, and they couldn't stay healthy, so nobody beyond the kids they faced in high school or those they blew away in the low minor leagues ever bore witness to what could have been. Pitchers who get hurt tend to stay hurt. It's a truth Hudson knew and one he needed to ignore.

He couldn't avoid every fact and figure. Thirteen days after Jacksonville, Hudson flew back across the country, to Pensacola, Florida. There he met Dr. James Andrews, the face of orthopedic surgery whose name to elite athletes conjured up images of the reaper. A visit to Dr. Andrews usually ended with a scar. And nobody in the world sewed up more Tommy John elbows than Jim Andrews.

Almost every patient Andrews cuts gets a pep talk the day before to explain the procedure and ask any questions. While

Andrews usually did most of the talking, Hudson needed some context for what exactly happened to him. He knew the failure-of-return rate of one in six cases. Failure like this, though? Catastrophic, instantaneous failure?

Twenty-seven years earlier, Andrews had created the American Sports Medicine Institute to study things like this. ASMI tried to research everything, though elbows, the body part that made Andrews rich, were a particular point of concern, because he kept seeing kids younger and younger come into his clinic wanting Tommy John surgery. In ASMI's longitudinal study of 1,200 Tommy John patients, just four blew out their new ligament before they returned to pitch in a game.

Hudson wasn't the one in six. He was the one in three hundred, the 0.33 percent, exponentially cursed. He didn't tell people this, because he didn't want anyone to accuse him of using an excuse. The baseball world was rooting for him. Not just the Diamondbacks but the few inside the game who understood the epidemic the sport faced. Hudson would be the test case to show that even after two elbow reconstructions, a pitcher could carve out a long and prosperous career.

The toughest person to convince? Daniel Hudson. He wanted to do this, yes, to prove it to himself and to the world. Only he couldn't escape a question that superglued itself to his psyche. Rarely does Hudson occupy his time trying to answer things he knows he can't. This wasn't some sort of rumination on predestination or an argument against free will. It was how the brain of a broken man responded to the idea that he wouldn't be able to do what he loves for more than two years. It was a dangerous question to ask. It was a vital question to ask. And he asked it more than once.

"What if I'm not supposed to throw a pitch again?"

CHAPTER 9

Rehab Hell

DESPERATION CONSUMED DANIEL HUDSON BECAUSE he remembered every moment of the previous 343 days, all the way back to the beginning of the arduous trip he would need to take once again. Ten days after his first Tommy John surgery, Hudson sat in the passenger's seat of a GMC Sierra that cruised up Interstate 10, his right arm immobilized in a gray contraption that looked more torture device than technological marvel. The truck parked at a medical mall on the outskirts of Phoenix. He was becoming a regular. Earlier in the week, nurses had removed the cast that held his arm in place. Now came the next step: replacing the stitches that held together the skin covering his elbow with Steri-Strips and trading in the iron maiden on his arm—a brace to stabilize it—for something a little less cumbersome.

To the world, Tommy John surgery consists of only two days that matter: the date of the procedure and date of the return. In reality, the days in between matter far more than either. Healing a broken elbow takes at least a year, time that limps along with loneliness and quiet desperation, monotony and boredom. The physical aspect takes care of itself via a fairly standard protocol. The mental grind is the truer test. It changes a man, even when he's certain it won't.

"I know this has been traumatic," Dr. Michael Lee said. He was the Diamondbacks' team doctor, a stratum below the name-brand surgeons like Frank Jobe or his protégé, Dr. Lewis Yocum, who had done Hudson's first surgery. Lee's job wasn't to oversee Hudson's rehabilitation so much as to guide him through the early stages and ensure he hit the mundane benchmarks along the way.

"He actually bathed himself today," Sara Hudson would later marvel. Wherever she went, levity followed. Hudson loosened up around her because her presence demanded it. Sara didn't guide conversations so much as grab them by the arm and wrench them into complicity. Couple that with the fact that she was a registered nurse, and the setting at Lee's office put her at ease, even if it freaked out Hudson.

He hated hospitals. "They just creep me out," he said. Hudson's mom was a nurse, too, and if ever he needed to pick her up at work, he refused to go inside. They are, of course, the very last place an athlete wants to find himself. Until his first Tommy John surgery, Hudson never even had stitches. Just before the anesthesia knocked him out, Hudson told Yocum that if he wasn't throwing 100 miles per hour upon his return, he wanted his money back. It's easy to think a year down the road before the realities of that year strike. Few things can humble a man who wants his fastball to hit triple digits like sitting on a table and squeezing something called the Eggsercizer.

The first day of rehab started a week after the surgery. No longer was Hudson popping codeine-laced Tylenol; it made him itch. The day-to-day toil would be supervised by Ken Crenshaw, the Diamondbacks' trainer, whom everyone called Crank, and that first session gave Hudson a sense of how wearisome his days soon would be. Because his elbow was locked into place, almost all of the work focused on the wrists and fingers. Three sets of two minutes clutching the Eggsercizer, a squeezable, egg-shaped, molded polymer that provides resistance. Same with the Digi-Flex, a hand gripper with spring-loaded buttons for each finger to depress. Hudson then spread his hand into a rubberized web with finger-sized holes and stretched it for three seconds at a time, forty reps in all. Thirty more minutes hooked up to an H-Wave stimulation machine—Hudson called it the thumper, because of the force with which it activated his muscles—preceded another twenty with a HIVAMAT, which helps reduce swelling with low-intensity electrostatic pulses.

Visiting Lee was a nice respite from the Eggsercizer, if a bit painful. Hudson removed the elbow brace, and Lee started to slink the stitches out of his arm. "This one's gonna tug," Lee said. He pulled out a six-inch-long piece. Hudson grimaced. Sara gave him credit for confronting his squeamishness; Hudson didn't once turn away. To distract him, she said: "We need to get you a manicure." His response: "Never happen."

She and Hudson grew up near each other in the Hampton Roads area of Virginia and lived on the same floor freshman year at Old Dominion. She could've gone to Virginia Tech, where her father, Jimmy Milley, was an All-American tennis player. She preferred ODU, a school in Norfolk populated by commuters.

Sara instinctually went into nurse mode during Hudson's examinations, tilting her head to get a better perspective. The inside of Hudson's elbow was bruised and school-bus yellow.

"Look how good it looks," said Jessica Luevano, Lee's medical assistant and point person for Diamondbacks players.

"It doesn't hurt," Hudson said.

"It's amazing," Luevano said.

She laid the Steri-Strips across the wound that later would thicken into a hearty scar. Hudson gently slid on a compression sleeve covered with hair from Buckley, his English bulldog whose tongue hangs out of his mouth like a stray piece of corned beef in an overstuffed sandwich. The old, bulky elbow brace was replaced by a sleek Össur Innovator X, straight from Reykjavik, Iceland.

"This one's awesome," Hudson said.

"Pretty, too," Sara said.

This was a proper implement for a million-dollar arm, set to 40 degrees extension and 100 degrees flexion. Over the next five weeks, Crank progressively turned the dial on the elbow a few more degrees, eventually down to a zero-degree straightened arm and the fully flexed 145 degrees. Hudson would ditch the Eggsercizer and other hand tools and focus more on breathing through his abdomen, improving his posture, and building the rotator-cuff muscles around his shoulder blade. He flexed and extended, pronated and supinated, used rubberized resistance tubing and the muscle thumper, received therapy through old-school massage and newfangled Class IV lasers.

This was just the beginning, harrowing for any Tommy John patient and still invigorating. There's optimism in the early stages, enough to keep Hudson looking for little signs. Like the view from the window in Lee's office building. It stared straight into downtown Phoenix, where Chase Field peeked over the skyline, close enough that he could feel it.

SQUEEZE. RELEASE. SQUEEZE. RELEASE. TODD Coffey buried his hand into a five-gallon bucket filled with uncooked white rice and let the kernels envelop it. It was thirty-eight days after his second surgery. He knelt on the floor of the Los Angeles Dodgers' spring-training facility, the epicenter of players rehabbing from a variety of injuries, and did what the protocol told him to. Squeeze. Release. Squeeze. Release.

If buckets of rice for hand and forearm strengthening were good enough for Nolan Ryan and Roger Clemens and Steve Carlton, Coffey wouldn't argue. As retrograde as the exercise seemed, it beat squeezing and releasing a neon-tinted Eggsercizer. He used buckets of rice after his first surgery, and his new ligament had lasted more than twelve years. "I should do everything the same," he said. Well, except the part where he exited the hospital with five scars. That was not fun.

"I had to take a shit with my legs straight out," Coffey said. "You ever tried to take a shit with both legs straight? Try it. And then try being able to wipe left-handed without being able to bend both knees. It was not fun. Shit everywhere. Literally."

Coffey guffawed not just at the memory but at the ridiculousness of actually sharing the story. Nothing is off-limits with him, nothing too embarrassing. Honesty is his defense mechanism, born of the bullying for being too naive or too fat or too whatever the assholes who razzed him chose to harp on. When Coffey signed and went to rookie ball in Billings, Montana, as a seventeen-year-old country kid who knew no better, a teammate named Eric Cooper said: "If you ever make the big leagues, I'll jump off the Golden Gate Bridge." Cooper flamed out in Low-A "I'd love to find him again," Coffey said, "and tell him to jump."

All of Coffey's former teammates brim with stories. About his wardrobe filled with paisley Robert Graham button-down shirts. Or the time he forgot to latch the top on his cherry-colored Corvette in Milwaukee and watched it fly off the back of the car, only to recover it the next day, get his Brewers teammates to sign it, and trade it in to a dealership for a new roof and some cash on top of it. Even the one that sounds too ridiculous—Coffey's first wife found a video of him on his cell phone having sex with another woman and soon thereafter became his ex-wife—is indeed true.

Coffey's foibles occasionally revealed themselves publicly. Jennifer went into labor about three weeks early and gave birth to a son, Declan, on October 7. Six days later, a mildly sleep-deprived Coffey jumped on Twitter and blasted out to his followers a political critique that lacked in grammatical dexterity what it made up for in passionate conservatism.

@ToddCoffey60: If Obama had his way I wouldn't be able to talk bad about him I like this country the way it is freedom of speech
@ToddCoffey60: Romney all the way
@ToddCoffey60: I think Romney Ryan should get there turn In the last four years Obama hasn't done anything
@ToddCoffey60: And he's trying to turn us in to a socialism
@ToddCoffey60: World ending anyway December 21, 2012 lol

The Internet being the Internet, Coffey got pilloried within minutes. Rather than cop to it, he went to the tried-and-true excuse of every celebrity whose use of social media has turned regrettable: I was hacked.

@ToddCoffey60: Sorry everyone I let my 14 year old Friends kid use my phone to play a game While I was watching the game and just saw what he tweeted
@ToddCoffey60: My friends, 14 yo kid

On election night, at 11:17 p.m., one minute after Fox declared President Obama the winner, Coffey tweeted: "Where fucked." He deleted it immediately, softening his blaze of glory.

@ToddCoffey60: Wow big mistake
@ToddCoffey60: 4 more years of this guy, great
@ToddCoffey60: I'm out I'll be back on twitter in 4 years if we can make it 4 more years.

And @ToddCoffey60 was no more. He nuked the account that day, aware that even in the ultraconservative world of baseball, political ramblings of any variety can peeve a team, and he wanted interest from all thirty once his arm healed.

It's why he did the buckets of rice every day, why he did the same flexion-and-extension exercises as Hudson with a far different goal in mind: to remember how to straighten his arm. More than 400 innings in the major leagues after Tommy John surgery had left a permanent bend in Coffey's right arm. Hard as he tried to straighten it, the furthest it would go was 23 degrees before his surgery. Coffey believed getting even a degree or two more in range of motion would provide extra giddy-up on his fastball and better depth on his slider, and maybe even the ability to throw a changeup.

"Hoffy's gonna teach me his," Coffey said. For two years in Milwaukee, Trevor Hoffman, who retired as baseball's all-time saves leader, had tried to show Coffey the grip for his changeup, considered one of the best in baseball history. It wasn't the typical circle change, held with the hand made into an OK sign, or a split-change, with the index and middle fingers shaped into a V with the ball jammed slightly between them. Hoffman stuffed the ball deep into his palm, with his thumb and ring finger holding it and his index and middle fingers in the air. It imparted a spin similar to his fastball, and with the arm speed on the two pitches the same, the changeup tricked hitters into more than one thousand strikeouts.

This was Coffey: Try something for two years, never get it, and convince himself it's a fait accompli anyway. His optimism was a gift, something he never took for granted. Had he let Eric Cooper's words win—"If you ever make the big leagues, I'll jump off the Golden Gate Bridge"—he wouldn't have logged 461 major league appearances. He might not have any.

It's why when Dr. Neal ElAttrache told him it would be eighteen months until he returned, Coffey scoffed. He respected ElAttrache's opinion, really, but just figured he was going to be wrong like so many others were. "I can't wait to run out of that bullpen next year," Coffey said. "I want to be back right after the All-Star break. That's my goal. It fluctuates depending on how things go."

Like Hudson, he had benchmarks to hit and dates to abide by. He wanted to pitch off the mound April 1, throw in a simulated game May 1, hold a showcase for all thirty teams to see how well he was throwing, and then sign in June. A few weeks in the minor leagues to face live batters, and back he'd be, better than ever.

"I wanted to take these few months slow," said ElAttrache, though he knew better. Coffey sprinted from the bullpen and did parking-lot donuts in his Corvette. Slow was a cuss. He would squeeze and release, squeeze and release, the time between each muscle contraction and his return to the mound a few seconds less.

"Every time the phone rings, when I see his name on it," ElAttrache said, "I hold my breath."

IN 2013, *BASEBALL PROSPECTUS*'S RUSSELL Carleton looked at more than a dozen variables in trying to answer a simple question: what is the best predictor of arm injuries? It wasn't strikeout rates or walk rates or ERA. Not ground-ball rate or fly-ball rate or line-drive rate. Innings pitched? Nope. Pitches thrown? Not that, either. Age? Two-strike counts? Contact made? No, no, no.

"It's clear," Carleton wrote, "that the biggest risk factor for injury is previous injury."

If you've been hurt before, you're far likelier to get hurt again. The general sense among pitchers is that those who reach thirty years old without an arm injury aren't completely insured but far less likely to suffer something catastrophic. Which doesn't preclude first-time injuries from happening, of course; it simply speaks to the double jeopardy pitchers face after they hit the disabled list with an arm injury once. Todd Coffey and Daniel Hudson were living proof of Carleton's conclusion, and others like them lent credence to the idea that injury-proneness is more than the narrative stylings of frustrated fans.

While a sleeve of tattoos covers Chris Carpenter's left arm, on his right are more natural markings, a map of scars that tell his story. Five of them dot his shoulder thanks to a labrum injury, degenerative bone, and scar tissue. His elbow later gave out, and bone-spur surgery begat Tommy John. Carpenter became an arm-woes Yoda, dispensing wisdom to a dozen St. Louis Cardinals teammates who needed Tommy John during his nine years with the team.

"You try everything, which is kind of crazy," he said. "When I was coming back from surgeries, I would do stuff to the point of where sitting there in the winter, reaching across to grab my beer mug watching football on Sunday, I'd feel a little something and think, 'Oh, that was a good exercise.' And so I'd keep doing it."

Everything revolves around the arm. It becomes the focal point of a player's life, like a child who needs constant attention and proper care and special treatment. It wears him out—"Holding your phone gets tiring," Carpenter said—and dominates his thoughts and brings out sides good and bad. It is always there, unavoidable, a constant reminder. Worst, it is already guilty of betrayal, and now he must forgive it and trust that it won't do the same again.

"Is my scar going to rip open? Is my arm going to fall out?" said veteran starter Brett Anderson, who tore his UCL at twenty-three. "You haven't thrown in four or five months. You don't know what's going to happen." Medication dulls physical pain, but nothing eases the mind. The calendar taunts the injured, every minute like an hour, every hour a day, every day a month, every month a year. This is the bond of Tommy John, the lesson passed from player to player, like fables down through the generations.

No current player has reached out to Tommy John himself for insight, because the game overflows with so many surgery veterans willing to dispense it. Things are different now, anyway. Nobody would dare ape John's rehab routine of throwing for forty-five minutes a day. They do their Jobes and tug on rubber resistance bands. The Bodyblade and its longer cousin, the Shoul-

der Tube—two javelin-shaped implements held in the middle—
are popular because their oscillating movements strengthen
muscle. More and more pitchers are throwing weighted baseballs,
as light as two ounces and as heavy as two pounds. Gone are the
days when athletic trainers would fax injury reports once a road
trip. Every minute medical detail gets attention, which highlights
the frustration in the lack of progress at stopping elbow injuries
in particular.

"After you have surgery, your body lies to you for the rest of
your life," said Los Angeles Angels starter C. J. Wilson, one of the
more fortunate cases; his new ligament is on its thirteenth season.
"It's never honest. You'll have days where you go out there and
feel like you're throwing 105 miles per hour, and you look up and
you're throwing the exact same speed. And you have other days
where you feel terrible, and you're throwing one mile an hour
faster."

Daniel Hudson felt the confusion. He knew his arm was telling him something. He just didn't know what to believe.

WHEN BRAD ARNSBERG STARTS TALKING, the words do not come
out in sentences so much as they do verbal tidal waves, anecdotes
piling upon anecdotes, some fairly pithy and others non sequi-
turs, each trying to reach an ultimate truth where everything ties
together, at which point he'll punctuate his thought with a well-
timed expletive, because that's how real baseball men talk, and
Brad Arnsberg, a man who is a lot of things, is unquestionably a
real fucking baseball man.

The Diamondbacks hired Arnsberg, whom everyone calls
Arnie, in the spring of 2013 to serve as their rehabilitation coordinator. "I've never been a coordinator, and I still don't know if I
am," Arnie said. "I don't know if I can coordinate my own life."
His job entailed looking after some of the young Latin American
kids who spent the year working out at Salt River Fields, the Di-

amondbacks' spring-training complex, but in the short term the job description went something like this: fix Daniel Hudson after his first Tommy John surgery.

Arnie spent eight years as a pitching coach for the Montreal Expos, the Florida Marlins, the Toronto Blue Jays, and the Houston Astros. Pitching coaches generally excel in one of two areas: mechanics or psychology. Arnie skewed far toward the mental end of the spectrum. "My main priority is rehabbing some of these kids, and just sitting and BS-ing with them," he said. "That's the best thing I do. I got nothing [else], but I can sure bullshit."

The first day he met Hudson, Arnsberg introduced himself and asked to play catch. He wanted to get a sense of how Hudson's arm was working. He was seven months post-op—past the range-of-motion activities, the tennis-ball throws he started at three and a half months, the 45-foot throws a week after that, and the gradual buildup to 135 feet. The distances are entirely arbitrary, part of a program that exists more because that's how it's always been done and not because 45 feet or 135 feet or any distance in between makes particular sense. Because doctors and trainers still don't know the ideal, every team's program varies slightly.

Two days into spring training, Hudson's shoulder started to hurt. Nearly every Tommy John recovery hits a speed bump, and this was Hudson's. He peeled back for a few weeks, refocusing his time on strengthening the shoulder and refining his mechanics. Most of the work entailed lessons Arnie learned from Tom House, the former major leaguer who is seen as the king of independent pitching coaches. Nolan Ryan used House, and so did Arnie following his own Tommy John surgery.

The New York Yankees drafted Arnie in 1983, and after a cup of coffee in September 1986, he arrived for good in August 1987. In his fourth game, he relieved a struggling starter: the forty-four-year-old Tommy John. By the end of the game, Arnie's elbow hurt. His visit to Frank Jobe confirmed a torn UCL. He returned in 1989 with the Texas Rangers, where House was the pitching coach.

Arnie passed along House's drills to all his charges, Hudson being the latest. He wanted Hudson to hold his glove higher to keep his front side from leaking open, so he put a weight inside it to force him to elevate it. He gave Hudson a plain white hand towel and asked him to pantomime throwing a ball. Critics had long bemoaned the towel drill, not understanding its purpose. Arnie's was simple: he wanted to change Hudson's delivery and force him to get more on top of the ball rather than throw it like a sidewinding slingshot.

Nobody liked Hudson's delivery but Hudson. "The first time I ever saw him throw, I still remember," said Ken Crenshaw, the Diamondbacks' trainer. "We were playing the Mets, and he was struggling in the first inning. Kind of throwing the ball all over. I actually talked to our pitching coach, and it's a little bit scary. You finally get a new guy, and you hear a lot about him, and I'm like, 'Is he going to hold up?' It's always been my concern with him."

Success was Hudson's narcotic. The thought of adding another thing to his rehab—something as crucial as mechanics, which was the one thing on which Hudson figured he could rely—felt like piling impractical on top of impossible.

"That's the way I've thrown for twenty years," he said. "It's going to be difficult to teach my body something different, if we do think that's the way to go. I'm not going to change who I am as a pitcher. If they want me to keep my front side closed or in line, OK, but I'm not changing my arm slot. That's what makes me who I am. It got me to where I am. But honestly, what does anyone use for twenty years that they don't have to replace at some point?"

Considering how much he threw in high school and college, and the unorthodox fashion in which he flung the ball, it was miraculous that Hudson's arm lasted past his twenty-fifth birthday. But what could he do? A pitching coach at a baseball camp at the

University of Virginia had told him it was virtually impossible for a kid to change his arm slot.

"I liked hearing that," Hudson said. "This is what makes me unique and different from everyone else. . . . I get frustrated because they're talking to me about this stuff from a physiological standpoint. You know, I'm a sport management major. I've never even looked at the human anatomy of a body. Like, I trust you that you're telling me something that's good for me. I don't need to know everything about it. If you tell me it's good for me, I'm going to do it. I don't need to know what it's doing to me on a cellular freakin' level. I don't really give a shit about that. I just want to go and pitch."

Pitching is far from a plug-and-play proposition, so Arnie wanted to tell a story. It started with Roy "Doc" Halladay, the Blue Jays ace who won more than two hundred games and a Cy Young Award. Hudson reminded Arnie so much of Halladay, who, he noted, worked hard on his front side, too. Charlie Nagy, the Diamondbacks' pitching coach, nodded along.

"Man, if it's good enough for Doc, I would think it might be good enough for you," Arnie told Hudson. "Because today was really, really good, and I've noticed in your towel sessions this and that, and I'm glad Charlie was here, because if I could improve anything out of here, it would be just a little bit higher. And then if you think back through the evolution of baseball . . ."

Arnie was just getting started, segueing to the mechanics of Stephen Strasburg, the Washington Nationals' triple-digit-throwing phenom, and how his delivery may well be immaterial, because . . .

"I read an article," Arnie said, "and it was the best article I ever read, on the stress and the percentile of stress that's being put on the medial side of the elbow and the shoulder, being the deltoid and the biceps tendon area, and they said when a guy is throwing up to ninety-two to ninety-five miles an hour, let alone a hundred, the stress level that goes on the ligaments and tendons that grasp this rotator together, that grasp this elbow together, are key cogs in it. They're at a ninety-nine-point-whatever. And they've hooked electrodes up. I would think it's somewhat close.

"In other words, my point being is them motherfuckers were gonna blow anyway."

Hudson stood slack-jawed. It was a lot to process, even if Hudson was plenty smart enough to do so. He liked Arnie and trusted him and tried to do what he said, even when the muscle memory of twenty years of pitching revolted against it. Hudson's body fought his brain, and the body almost always wins, especially in the face of a punishing year of rehabilitation.

The desire to return was enough to push him through the shoulder setback, which improved with a cortisone shot. Still, no matter how many Celebrex he swallowed, Hudson couldn't rid himself of the feeling that something in his elbow was wrong. His body, it turns out, wasn't lying to him. The truth was just too much to bear.

EVERY DAY WAS THE SAME for Todd Coffey. Up at ten a.m., glass of orange juice, bowl of oatmeal, cup of yogurt. Hop in the car, get to the gym, jump on the elliptical, work up a nice lather for twenty or thirty minutes. Over to the rehab center. Stretch, loosen up with rubber tubing, chuck a mini medicine ball against a mini trampoline. Back in the car. Two minutes to the field. Uncover the tarp, rake the mound, jog, stretch some more, long toss. Throw. And then back home to paint Blood Bowl miniatures or try to find a good deal on an old Nintendo cartridge or kill time in any palatable fashion possible during an offseason with no baseball.

"Life is repetitive," Jennifer Coffey said—especially in Rutherfordton, North Carolina, smack-dab between Charlotte and Asheville, population of around four thousand. Todd Coffey grew up here. He and Jennifer live in a house originally owned by Albert Tendall Coffey, his granddad, who played for the Rutherford County Owls back in the 1930s and bequeathed his love of baseball to his grandson. After Albert died, Coffey bought the house, renovated it, and made it his offseason home.

Once the 2012 season ended, Coffey was on his own. With the Dodgers no longer responsible for his rehab, he reached out to his cousin, Brendan Waters, who owns a facility called Therapy Plus in nearby Forest City. Waters and a trainer named Michael Melton mapped out what Coffey's next nine months would look like, all the way up to the June showcase. It was an aggressive plan for a Tommy John revision, and particularly for a revision with a flexor repair. The market for healthy thirtysomething relief pitchers was not exactly robust. Baseball is an out-of-sight, out-of-mind sport, and an injured thirtysomething relief pitcher might as well not exist.

"My biggest fear is letting myself down," Coffey said. "To look in my mirror fifteen years from now and say, 'What if I did this?' I don't want to have any wonders or questions about how things would've been different."

So he pushed himself to places he didn't think possible. Ninety minutes of work every day on his shoulder allowed him to throw a ball at five months instead of at the eight-month mark after his first surgery. The elliptical machine became his friend, some sessions stretching past one hundred minutes. "We've literally had to cut him down from doing so much," Waters said. Coffey affixed his iPad to a tripod and filmed every throw off the mound, trying to ensure his mechanics didn't waver. "At our age, there is no mechanical fix," he said. "Our body is accustomed to a certain way. If your arm snaps, it snaps. If I go out there and try to change my mechanics, guess what? My shoulder, my biceps, my back is not used to that. I've been doing the same thing for twelve years. I can't make dramatic changes."

Coffey saw progress. The range-of-motion exercises worked and reduced his extension from 23 degrees to 14. The mound sessions got better and better, enough that Coffey rejoined Twitter on March 15 because he figured the talking his arm did would supersede anything his fingers might relay. After a decade spent on the road, he even felt like a better dad, able to coach one daughter's softball team and take another to a daddy-daughter dance. Hewing to the plan was working.

Eleven months of patience wore out in mid-May, when Coffey finally deviated from the script. He wasn't supposed to know how hard he was throwing. ElAttrache told him it wasn't important. Coffey needed to know if his body was lying to him, though, and some sort of quantification would give him that peace. He told himself at the beginning of his recovery that if his fastball hovered around 88 to 90 miles per hour, he would retire. "I don't want to be that guy who holds on too long and doesn't see when he's done," Coffey said.

The gun arrived May 17, and immediately Coffey took it outside and aimed it at cars driving by. "Had one going forty-two in a twenty," he said. Like Yogi Young, he knew the radar gun would tell him a truth neither his eyes nor his body could discern. One or two miles per hour makes the difference between a major league pitcher and one stuck in Triple-A.

On the first day, Coffey sprinkled a few 87s in with pitches mostly 88 to 89. His pitches sat at 89 the next time out, and he spiked a 90 the time after that, and up they went into the low 90s, each day stronger, every time better, all waiting for the adrenaline kick of a game, which he trusted would add another mile or two. Trusting his arm was dangerous, especially with its duplicitous track record, but Coffey believed. He started to consider the possibilities. Maybe a major league deal instead of having to scrape back through Triple-A. And if it were a big league deal, a team might want to talk about an option for the 2014 season, since there's little sense in bringing a post–Tommy John guy back for just a couple of months.

"All depends on what team it is," Coffey said. "One-point-two-five million to start. I would actually start at one point five and meet around one point two-five, one point three. They would start at a million. Meet in the middle. That would be simple and easy to do."

Relentless optimism fueled Coffey. He just needed to get to his showcase in June healthy, and perform, and the rest would take care of itself. He would be a big leaguer again because that's where he belonged, and Jennifer and Declan and some special guests would be there to see it.

From the day he found out Donor ID 101079556's semitendinosus was holding together his elbow, Coffey wanted to show gratitude to the man's family. For his first game back in the big leagues, Coffey said he would fly the donor's parents or wife or whoever he was closest to into the city where he was playing. First he needed to establish contact, so on March 12, 2013, Jennifer wrote a letter on Coffey's behalf that RTI sent to the donor's next of kin. It talked about who he was and why he was writing and how thankful he was and what a gift he was given.

In July 2012, I needed Tommy John surgery in order to repair a torn ligament in my right elbow. I play baseball for a living and as a pitcher my job depends on the use of that particular ligament. My options were to not repair my elbow and end my playing career or proceed with surgery and have a chance at returning to baseball.

I have been fortunate to be in a profession I highly enjoy and love, especially when it comes to my kids. I have three kids from a previous marriage (12, 9, and 4) who have had the pleasure of growing up watching their father play and will have fond memories of those years. One of my biggest "thank yous" comes from the fact that my wife and I had our first child in October. I wanted to be able to come back from my injury and play so that our son will be able to share in the same experiences and have those same memories.

I cannot thank you enough for a second chance an opportunity that might not have been if it were not for you and your loved one. My family and I will always remember your act of selflessness and utmost generosity.

Wishing you all the best,

Todd

CHAPTER 10

Fear, Loathing, and Rotten Meat

June 3, 2013

On the day before Daniel Hudson blew out for a second time, Todd Coffey decided to "let it eat." This is a favorite phrase of his, one of those colloquialisms that exist only in baseball's weird, insular ecosystem. Like, when somebody is mad, he's not just mad. He's "got the ass." And if somebody's trying to look like he's hustling but isn't, it's not false hustle. It's "eyewash." "Letting it eat" has nothing to do with food. It's about going full tilt, free of care and consequence, and it applies in all facets of life. For example, Drew Storen, a teammate in Washington, once observed about Coffey: "He's a huge paisley fan, and he was not afraid to let it eat a little bit on the outfits."

The finest manner in which a ballplayer can let it eat is with his fastball, and Coffey, nearly one year removed from his surgery, a few weeks from his showcase, finally arrived at that place where he trusted his elbow enough to do so. He cared not where the ball went. Letting it eat wasn't about pounding strikes. It was about pushing himself to a limit he didn't know he would see again.

Nobody near Rutherfordton would catch Coffey aside from a high schooler named David Mendez. So around one p.m. every day, Mendez left Thomas Jefferson Classical Academy, met up with Coffey, and strapped on gear. Michael Melton, Coffey's trainer, stood nearby with the radar gun. Every pitch registered above 90 miles per hour. When he let it eat on the last five pitches, they hovered between 92 and 94.

"I was watching a game last night," Mendez said. "Man, they were throwing like eighty-eight, eighty-nine."

"I know everyone says guys are throwing harder these days," Coffey said, "but I'm telling you. I don't see it when I turn games on. What I did today, I would take into a game."

June 15, 2013

The showcase date was set: July 1 in Phoenix. About two weeks beforehand, Coffey's fastball sat around 91 to 93, and topped out at 94 during a simulated game in which he threw to local high school hitters. His slider tilted like a pinball machine. He never bothered learning Trevor Hoffman's changeup, because he didn't think he needed it. Following the showcase, as major leaguers wound down until the All-Star break, Coffey would ramp up. By the July 31 trade deadline, he'd be ready to join whichever club would have him.

Everything else was great, except for that bit of soreness he felt after the sim game.

"The only place I was sore in the arm was the forearm and the biceps muscles," Coffey said. "Nothing in the elbow. Nothing in the flexor. They said I had such great extension, my muscles were like, 'You haven't been there before. We're going to piss you off.' Not surgery-related sore. Sore from first time ever cranking on it."

Melton wanted Coffey to cancel the showcase. He didn't like soreness.

June 17, 2013

"I made the decision to move my showcase back," Coffey said. "There's really no difference between July first and July fifteenth. July first was a dream. I don't want to sit there and think about July first being so much that I don't listen to my arm or body. Your mind can tell your body to do things it shouldn't do. I want to be smart about this."

July 18, 2013

He didn't make it back in twelve months. The anniversary of Coffey's surgery came and went, just like his scheduled showcases. He'd canceled the July 15 one, too, because the soreness crept into a troublesome spot.

"We were pushing it," Coffey said. "We were trying to get back. And the flexor-pronator muscles flared up. It would take two or three days before it calmed down until I could throw again. Dr. ElAttrache didn't like that."

Coffey went in for an X-ray, and the results were sent to ElAttrache. He saw nothing unusual beyond the scar tissue, inflammation, and general depletion of two-time Tommy John patients' elbows. No chips floating, no spurs hooking, no UCL shearing.

"I'm gonna let my arm dictate it," Coffey said. "I was bummed out. I was bummed because the day had come, and the day had passed. I'm gonna listen to my arm now. I think this year is still doable."

August 12, 2013

Six weeks after he was supposed to throw in a showcase, Coffey ditched the idea of returning for the 2013 season.

"I think a smarter decision is to wash it," Coffey said. "I'll be ready September first, but straight to the big leagues without any minor league games? That's not gonna happen."

After about ten days off, Coffey started tossing the ball again in late July. He was up to 80 percent effort. With a return in 2013 out of the question, Coffey considered his next move.

"I'm gonna go to winter ball," he said.

Coffey had chatted with an old friend, Alonzo Powell, a hitting coach with the San Diego Padres who spent his offseasons coaching the Bravos de Margarita. The Venezuelan Professional Baseball League consisted mainly of Venezuelan major leaguers and young players trying to supplement measly minor league paychecks. Coffey couldn't stand the thought of throwing to high school kids anymore. He needed real baseball.

September 4, 2013

"I'm gonna have to go under the knife again."

Todd Coffey said it so matter-of-factly—almost serenely. There was a bone chip floating inside his right elbow, dangerously close to his new UCL, exactly where his ulnar nerve would've been had ElAttrache and the hand doctor not tucked it under a blanket of muscle and fat.

At least it explained everything: the pain and the decreased velocity and all the issues hampering Coffey during his throwing sessions. He had played catch, building up to a week earlier, when he threw a bullpen session at 80 percent. It hurt. He tried again two days later. "It feels like I'm going ninety over a speed bump," Coffey said.

Lucky for him, Neal ElAttrache was at Duke University with his daughter Nicole, a standout volleyball player on a recruiting visit. Coffey drove about three hours from Rutherfordton to Durham, met with ElAttrache, and jumped into an MRI tube. The scan showed a chunk of scar tissue chiseled off by the daily throwing. During a thirty- to sixty-minute procedure, ElAttrache would remove the loose body, smooth out the scar tissue, and shave down a bone spur on the back of his elbow.

"Six to eight weeks, and then I'll start throwing again," Coffey said. "Dr. ElAttrache said I should be facing hitters in December. It's not going to affect anything as far as this upcoming season."

Winter ball was out. January was the new showcase target, and the prospect of landing a major league contract after nearly two full seasons away from the big leagues looked grim, meaning that Coffey would need to pitch his way onto a team's roster during spring training via a nonguaranteed minor league deal.

"I ain't worried about that," Coffey said. "If I'm healthy it's a no-brainer."

September 20, 2013

ElAttrache removed the bone chip from Coffey's right elbow. The surgery was a success. Coffey found a tape measure and laid the arrowhead-shaped chip across it. It was more than 1.5 centimeters long, a monster. Coffey took a picture with his cell phone and texted it to friends. He was proud of it.

"Finally," he said, "my arm's as good as new."

ABOUT A WEEK AFTER DANIEL Hudson's second surgery, a nauseating smell started to permeate his house. Hudson figured it was some funky garbage, so he emptied every trash can and bombarded them with Febreze. When that didn't work, he wondered if he ran over a rabbit or some varmint with his car, so he wedged himself between the ground and his Infiniti, a flashlight in his good hand, a cast inhibiting his other. Nothing in the chassis, either. The smell in the garage was unbearable, and as her husband's legs stuck out from under the car like the Wicked Witch's from Dorothy's house, Sara finally realized what was causing it.

"I don't want to tell you," she said. Sara was embarrassed, for one, but she also knew of Hudson's fragility, how he invariably traced bad things back to his arm. A few days earlier, she had picked up a couple of blocks of meat scraps that a local butcher saves for dogs. She'd thrown them in the trunk of the car and forgotten about them. The June air—the hottest June on record in Arizona—had turned the meat rotten. It festered for seventy-two hours before Hudson popped the trunk. He ran out of the garage and started to dry heave in the driveway.

Not even the highest-grade industrial solvent could rid the car of the smell, so Hudson started looking at new cars. He wasn't sure what to get. He refused to spend money frivolously just to uphold some stereotype about athletes driving certain types of vehicles. While he was making $518,000 that season, he couldn't say whether the Diamondbacks would bring him back for another, even if GM Kevin Towers and manager Kirk Gibson loved him.

"I don't know what's going to happen next year," he said. "It's getting toward the end of the year. My contract situation is up. I've been thinking about a lot of stuff that could've been. I did turn down a significant amount of money."

The $15 million he rejected was life-changing money, generational wealth if Hudson handled it properly. In the same month Hudson turned down the Diamondbacks' offer, the San Diego Padres signed a pitcher named Cory Luebke to a deal with a guaranteed $12 million. His left elbow blew out two months later. Before he returned to the mound, it snapped again and required a revision. Even if he never threw another pitch, Luebke was a millionaire many times over.

Sara had leaned toward taking the contract. Lowenthal tried to explain the downside. Another season like 2011 and Hudson could get triple the offer. And even if he did get hurt, so did Jaime

Garcia, a pitcher for the St. Louis Cardinals, and they gave him $27 million despite a Tommy John surgery on his résumé. Sara relented. If Dan believed in himself, so did she.

"At the time, it just wasn't the right number," Hudson said. "This is karma coming back to bite me in the ass."

This was just another defeat in Hudson's mind, another bad decision, another dereliction of duty. For the first twenty-five years of his life, everything went right. He was smart, good-looking, talented, personable. He loved playing baseball and was good at it. He married a beautiful, funny, bright, supportive girl. And ever since he turned down the contract—the son of an IT guy and a nurse, spitting at millions of dollars—he found himself spiraling in a fashion he was ill-equipped to handle. He knew it had been the right choice. That didn't mean he could forgive himself for making it.

"I broke down last week," Hudson said. "I feel worthless."

He was back on the couch in his living room, doing his best to avoid leaving home even if inside felt just as hellish as outside, staring at the same tools as eleven months earlier—the Digi-Flex, the rubber web, the Eggsercizer. "The gamut of stuff," Hudson said, "that makes me want to stab my eyes out with a lead pencil."

Hudson still tried to be good at the part of his life he could control. For his birthday, Sara set up a treasure hunt, and he played along, even though he knew the present, because he had a sixth sense for guessing her gifts. They went to concerts on occasion, and to the sporadic party down the street—anything to fake normalcy. She could sense some withdrawal from him, and she understood it.

"Some days, I'll come home, and the trash is full, the dishwasher is still loaded," Sara said. " 'What have you been doing?' 'Oh, nothing.' I know he's been playing video games for three or four hours. It's easy to burrow yourself in your room and play video games and hate the world when you hurt yourself twice."

Sara said no golf this time around, and he didn't argue. She told him she wanted the whole, unvarnished truth about his health, and he promised it. When Hudson bitched about the first surgery, it was the frustration of someone hooked on success who'd never been injured. This was different. Hudson wanted to separate himself from his injury, to not be the poor bastard who blew out back-to-back. Not just because those guys' careers end, but because it defines them, a weakness nobody knows how to solve.

"I don't like being like this," Hudson said. "I was one way for, like, twenty-five years, and this can just turn you into a different person. And I know I was one in three hundred and all that, but I'm trying. I just need to see something now to make me understand why this is worth it."

Hudson thought about seeing the Diamondbacks' psychologist. He never could bring himself to do it. He unburdened himself on Sara, angry and apologetic. They didn't get as low of a rate as he wanted when they refinanced their house. He drank more than usual. She tried not to judge. All the downtime, and he couldn't even give Sara the one thing she really wanted.

"It's funny," Hudson said. "Eric Chavez, when I went on the DL for the first time, was like, 'Don't have a baby.' He's like, 'I went on the DL three times and I had three children.'"

Everything he tried felt like it failed. C. J. Wilson was wrong. It wasn't just your arm that lied to you. It was your mind. Hudson's injury rendered a secure man vulnerable. Little things, stupid things, bothered him. After a weekend away with Sara, he joined the team at Chase Field for a home stand. He arrived at the stadium before anyone, his rehab work early in the day, and relaxed in the clubhouse as his teammates arrived. "Everyone rolls in: 'How you feelin'?'" Hudson said. "What do you think? How am I supposed to answer this twenty-five times? It's not their fault. I'm just so sick of everybody asking me how my arm is. You know how it is. I don't need anybody to ask me anymore."

The dynamic inside the Diamondbacks' clubhouse was changing. At the trade deadline in July, Arizona traded starting pitcher Ian Kennedy, Hudson's closest friend on the team. Not even three full seasons in Arizona, and Hudson was the third-most-tenured Diamondback. Nobody wanted to hear his issues. And it's not like he could walk into Gibson's office and share his pain. At one point during his rehab, Hudson was summoned by Gibson, who told him he couldn't wait for Hudson to return to a pitching staff that lacked the toughness the manager expected. "Everyone in here is a bunch of cunts," Gibson said.

Hudson stopped going to every home game; the clubhouse, where he always felt most at home, turned claustrophobic. When the Diamondbacks were on the road, he didn't always watch. He didn't want to fall back in love too quickly with the thing that had twice now crushed him. "I don't know what my mental state will be like when it's like, oh, shit, let's play catch," Hudson said. "What if it pops on the first throw?"

TODD COFFEY SAVED THE GOOD shit for days like this. From a toiletry travel bag he pulled a tongue depressor and a small plastic container with a fading label written in all-capital letters with no concern for punctuation:

MAY DILUTE 1:1 WITH COLD CREAM IF COMPLAINT OF "TOO HOT" RECOMMEND WEARING GLOVES WHEN APPLYING KEEP HOT MIX AND HANDS AWAY FROM EYES, NOSE, MOUTH MUCOUS MEMBRANES & PRIVATE PARTS ! ! ! ! ! ! ! ! ! ! ! ! ! !

Inside the container was the scion of Sandy Koufax's Capsolin, a balm so potent it scared the heartiest pitchers today. "I don't touch that," said Detroit Tigers starter Justin Verlander, and that was the kindest thing anyone aside from Coffey had to say about the Special Mix Hot Salve from Grubb's Care Pharmacy in Washington, DC.

Coffey called it Hot Cheese, and he loved the stuff. When he twisted off the cap of the container, a nostril-burning odor assaulted him. The Cheese itself was a bright orange-yellow, like coagulated nacho gloop, and when Coffey really wanted a loose arm, he found someone willing to strap on rubber gloves, plunge the tongue depressor into the container, scoop out a thick dab, and massage it in from his shoulder to his wrist.

January 17, 2014, qualified as a Cheese-worthy day. Coffey sat shirtless in the bathroom at Physiotherapy Associates, a rehabilitation center in Tempe, Arizona. At 2:00 p.m., he was scheduled to ascend a portable mound in back of the facility and throw for scouts. One day shy of the eighteen-month anniversary of his surgery—exactly when Neal ElAttrache said he'd be back—Todd Coffey was finally having his showcase.

He took a couple of months off after ElAttrache removed the bone chip; he cranked back into form after Thanksgiving, slogging through Christmas and all the way to January 7 before he declared himself ready. The vital sign for Coffey was the movement of his sinker, and poor David Mendez—who didn't have time to put on a jockstrap and cup when he rushed to catch Coffey during school—needed an ice pack because of it.

"He couldn't catch me," Coffey said. "He wore one right off the nuts. Seriously. Sinker. Off the nuts. He said it was the best one he's ever seen. I beat the shit out of him."

Convinced he was ready to throw for teams, Coffey called Rick Thurman, his agent, and told him to schedule the showcase. "Once we have the showcase, he should be up around ninety-four, ninety-five, ninety-six," Thurman said. "He's got to be there before I put the showcase on. I'd rather push it off for a week or two if you're not a hundred percent." Coffey assured Thurman he was ready.

That morning, he woke up about 9:30, shook off his Ambien fog—Coffey had taken it for years and couldn't sleep without it—and arrived at Physiotherapy Associates about two hours before the showcase was scheduled. Michael Melton, his trainer, Cheesed up his right arm and got a good burn going. For the first thirty minutes, it felt like his arm was self-immolating. It settled into a comfortable warmth, perfect for an arm that needed every bit of help loosening up.

Around 12:30 p.m., scouts started to show up. Coffey didn't expect them that early. Scott Reid, in charge of professional scouting for the Detroit Tigers, introduced himself to Coffey. Others poked their heads inside Physiotherapy to make sure Coffey was there and see if he looked the same as he did a year and a half earlier.

His arm lit up, the rest of his body warm from a quick treadmill run, Coffey asked Melton for the time. It was 1:15. "It's very nerve-racking," Coffey said. "I'm very anxious. I just want to get out there and get it started. Get it over with." He asked Melton to check the time again. It was 1:25.

Coffey decided to go outside and start warming up his arm. "My game plan is just to throw," he said. "Show I'm healthy. Show that I have ninety-one, ninety-two in the tank. To be honest, it's ridiculous to think I'm going to go out there and throw ninety-five." He unlocked a gate, which opened to an alcove with a mound surrounded by netting and a 120-foot diagonal area to warm up. The scouts followed him in to watch his preparation. They chitchatted with one another while sneaking glances at Coffey playing catch with Melton.

He rolled his shoulders in between throws, the heavy sun unlike anything cast during the winter in North Carolina. He started to sweat, at which point he asked Melton to look at his watch.

"It's 1:35," Melton said.

"Only 1:35?" Coffey said.

He couldn't wait much longer. Coffey didn't want to run the risk of his arm tightening up. Thurman had a previous commitment, so he wasn't around to talk with the scouts and map out every step of Coffey's day. The catcher squatted in the practice area to get a sense of the movement on Coffey's throws. He planned on throwing twenty-five pitches if things were good, thirty to thirty-five if they weren't going as planned.

"It's 1:45," Melton said.

Coffey had a secret. He obsessed over the time because the showcase was probably going to be a disaster. A few days after telling Thurman to schedule it, Coffey woke up with soreness in his elbow. He threw again three days before the showcase, and it felt tight. Coffey knew he should have canceled it before flying to Phoenix. He instead trusted his arm and its capacity to recover and respond when it mattered. Five minutes into his warm-ups with Melton, Coffey realized it wouldn't. His range of motion gradually had receded back to more than 20 degrees.

He lifted the netting, walked onto the mound, stood on the right side of the rubber, took a deep breath. As Coffey stood on the mound, ready to throw his first pitch, he couldn't rid himself of one thought: "I'm fucked." His first pitch that mattered in almost a year and a half came at 1:48, twelve minutes ahead of schedule. Every scout trained his radar gun on Coffey, and all but one spit out the same number: 88. The other said 89.

Coffey's sinker settled at 87 to 89. He popped a 90. Only one of his sliders tilted as expected. Coffey lost his footing during one pitch and fell down. Some of the scouts holstered their radar guns and took notes. "Still got bad body," one wrote. The scout didn't know that in 1999, Cincinnati had told Coffey to report to spring training in better shape. He showed up minus fifty pounds. His elbow blew out later that year. Now whenever anyone suggests he lose weight, he says he'd rather not get hurt, thank you, and anyway, Jennifer likes him exactly how he is.

During the final few pitches, Coffey spent more time thinking about how to spin his subpar stuff than the slider he was about to throw. "I was like, 'I've got to do some damage control,'" he said. "When they asked how I felt, I had to tell them I didn't want to peak too soon. You can't show weakness. You show weakness, they're like, 'This guy's a pussy.'"

Jennifer stood behind the scouts, stealing looks at their radar-gun readings, a Louis Vuitton bag slung over her shoulder. On Coffey's twenty-seventh pitch, one scout arrived and wondered what was going on. After two more pitches, Coffey walked toward the catcher and shook his hand. The showcase was over. It was 1:58, two minutes before it was scheduled to begin.

Coffey introduced himself to each of the scouts and thanked them for coming. The scouts stood around, seeming to invite Coffey to converse more with them and give an update on his status. "This is awkward," Jennifer said. She nudged Coffey to gather a few scouts and explain how he was rehabbing from his second Tommy John and expected his velocity to return in full when the adrenaline of facing live batters kicked in. They wondered about his plan, and he said he wanted to sign sometime in the next ten days and head to spring training with the rest of the pitchers and catchers. They nodded and told him they appreciated him traveling to the Phoenix area. And then it was over.

"What was I?" Coffey asked.

Eighty-seven to eighty-nine, with a ninety somewhere in there.

"I think you can throw a lot harder than that," Jennifer said.

"I know I can, too," Coffey said.

Coffey forced a smile. Something wasn't right. He wouldn't admit that now, not in the immediate aftermath of a chance he'd blown in spectacular fashion. This would be just a setback, another good story to tell his donor's family when he made it. Coffey changed out of his workout clothes, fled to his hotel, and showed up a few hours later at Oregano's, an Arizona pizza chain. He wondered what the scouts were telling their bosses, whether the lack of velocity posed a problem.

"I couldn't move," Jennifer said over dinner. "I felt so sick. I thought something was wrong. This was not his level. You can throw so much harder. Is something going wrong with his arm?

I thought you were feeling pain or something. I was surprised his velocity was as low as it was."

Coffey lied and said his arm felt fine. Admitting otherwise—that eighteen months and two surgeries still hadn't fixed him—wasn't easy. He wanted to hear feedback before he assessed the next move. One of the teams, he figured, would sign him on track record alone. He was eager to find out which.

"It's not like, 'This is it, I'm done,'" Coffey said.

"You didn't say that two hours ago," Jennifer said. "You said you were done."

"Noooooo," Coffey said.

"Yes," Jennifer said.

"Done for the day," Coffey said.

THE FIRST PITCHER TO RETURN from back-to-back Tommy John surgeries was named Doug Brocail. To give you a sense of how hard it was, here is the type of thing he says on a regular basis: "Everything went smooth until I had the heart attacks in '06, and that was just a minor setback."

Brocail lounged in a chair in the Houston Astros' bullpen before a June 2013 game, survivor not just of the elbow surgeries but a pair of heart scares that required an angioplasty. He was the pitching coach for the 111-loss Astros, a job he inherited when they fired Brad Arnsberg two years earlier. Daniel Hudson had undergone his second Tommy John surgery three days earlier, and Brocail knew all about it.

"I'd kill to have the kid," Brocail said. "I'm not one of those guys that hears, 'Oh, well, he's had surgery.' So what? I give two shits. I had thirteen of them. Three wrists, seven cleanouts. Eleven, twelve"—he pointed to his elbow—"and a shoulder. That's thirteen. That's just on the arm. I had the two hearts. Friggin' made my comeback, been in the league a month. Bend over to tie my shoe in Tampa Bay and my friggin' appendix explodes."

Brocail is a walking scar, but it did little to stop him from playing fifteen years in the major leagues. The only break he took was from the end of the 2000 season to the beginning of 2004, a three-year sabbatical to mend his UCL. The first time Brocail blew out, he was like Hudson and so many others: stubborn, impatient, problematic.

"I followed the book at the ballpark," Brocail said. "Away from the ballpark, I did a lot of stupid shit I shouldn't have done. Started throwing at three and a half months. And it was my fault. But when you see a guy go through this, I think the biggest recommendation would be: Listen, if you're achy at all, listen to your body. I'm a big advocate of 'nobody knows my body better than me'—until the dumbass sets in. I had a lot of that at the time, and I figured, 'Well, they don't know. I know my body.' Well, I don't know my body as well as I thought I did."

At the sixteen-month mark, on the cusp of his return to the major leagues, Brocail blew out again. He was thirty-five and could have retired with more than $7 million earned. He refused. Players don't let go of the game that easily. You don't quit it; it quits you.

And that's what Brocail faced. Other pitchers had torn their UCLs back-to-back. None had returned from the second. Being a pioneer took patience. He didn't touch a ball for a year. Literally. He loved picking up baseballs, twirling them in the oversized paws that matched his six-foot-five, 250-pound frame, dreaming up new grips and different finger pressures, all the tinkering that makes pitchers pitchers. His willpower won out, and at twelve months, one day, he knew what the leather and seams felt like again.

Hudson wanted to return in half the time of Brocail. He first played catch on December 2, 2013, a little less than six months after his second surgery. He wanted to land in the fourteen- to sixteen-month range that *Hardball Times* writer Jon Roegele found correlated with more successful returns—Hudson penciled in September 3 or 4 as his goal—and five minutes of throwing from forty-five feet that first day marked a familiar baby step. "The first couple throws I was kind of tentative," he said. "After the first couple throws, I remembered how to do this."

Hudson's reward for the milestone: unemployment. The Diamondbacks cut him that day. Hudson knew it was coming. Arizona needed room on its forty-man roster, and Hudson was going on two years' dead weight. He was a free agent, able to escape the clubhouse that felt like a sarcophagus and sign with whoever wanted him. Within the first twenty-four hours of Hudson's free agency, multiple teams reached out to his agent, Andrew Lowenthal, to gauge Hudson's interest.

"I don't want to go anywhere else," Hudson said. "They've been loyal to me. I want to do the same for them. If I make it back, I don't want it to be anywhere else."

Arizona wanted him back as well, and GM Kevin Towers struck a secret deal with Hudson: he would sign a minor league contract, and the Diamondbacks would put him on the major league roster at the end of spring training. The deal would include a team option for the 2015 season, so the Diamondbacks could secure Hudson at a cost-effective price if his rehabilitation went better this time than last. It was almost exactly the deal Todd Coffey dreamt of before his bone chip ended his first comeback attempt.

It took an enormous amount of trust in the Diamondbacks' front office for Hudson to sign what amounted to a handshake deal. He didn't dwell on losing his roster spot. He emphasized the positive parts of staying with the Diamondbacks. Ken Crenshaw, his trainer, knew him and his arm better than anyone anywhere else. Kirk Gibson trusted him. Kevin Towers believed in him. Hudson's name came up often among Diamondbacks personnel, even after the second surgery, and Towers's right-hand man, Bob Gebhard, had a specific role for Hudson in mind. "Gebby thinks he's our next closer," Towers said. "He's got the mentality. He's got the stuff. How hard would he throw if he had one inning?"

Pitchers couldn't dodge executives' desire for velocity, though in this case, Hudson refused to argue with anything asked of him. Time was beating the stubbornness out of him. Hudson progressed from five minutes at forty-five feet the first week to six minutes from sixty the second. "I wanted to stretch it out," Hudson said, "but they didn't want me to, and so I have to listen to them."

On December 13, 2013, Hudson officially re-signed with the Diamondbacks. He would earn $700,000 in 2014 and $800,000 if Arizona exercised his 2015 option. For now, it allayed the fear that paralyzed him over the summer and gave him good reason to stop looking at old emails. He wasn't making millions. And that was OK.

"Sara tells me all the time, 'If you had tried at all, you could have been anything you wanted to be, you know?'" Hudson said. "I didn't want to do anything but be a baseball player. That's all I ever wanted to do."

No one called. The early start and the bad body and especially the velocity at his showcase imprinted Todd Coffey with the very label he wanted to avoid: done, just another guy scraping to hold on to whatever little life remained in his arm. When Rick Thurman didn't hear from a single team, he reached out to all fourteen that sent scouts and heard the same things.

Philadelphia said his arm looked slow. Atlanta had him at 86–90. Miami thought his slider was fringy. Seattle was iffy. Tampa Bay figured he needed more time to get in shape. Scott Reid from Detroit wondered whether he might take a minor league deal. Even if he would've, the Tigers never offered it.

"I shouldn't have had the showcase," Coffey said. It was March 6, six weeks later. He was guilty again of not listening to his arm.

Following the showcase, Coffey had flown to Fort Lauderdale,

Florida, and met ElAttrache to figure out why his arm had locked up. Coffey guessed he had popped through scar tissue, and ElAttrache agreed. There was no structural damage. Following the Tommy John and flexor and bone-chip surgeries, cells rich in collagen—the most common protein in the human body—rushed to surround the inflamed area. The cells weave together to form scar tissue, the body's attempt to buttress injured areas. What scar tissue brings in stability it lacks in malleability, and its loosening—through manual therapy or, in Coffey's case, blunt manual force—is painful and temporarily inhibits range of motion.

Coffey wasn't a pussy or weak or any of the other flaws he feared others saw in him. He was shortsighted, proud, stubborn, the holy trinity for pitchers. At an event held specifically to show teams he was healthy, he had pitched hurt.

"It's happened to all of us," Cy Young winner Max Scherzer said. "It's happened to me before. You're trying to compete out there. You think you can keep going. And you can't. The toughest thing to do is to say, 'I can't pitch. I can't go. I can't give you an extra inning.' That's something I've gotten good at. I know my arm. I know when the situation dictates I'm not going to be at my best. You've got to learn how to do that."

At thirty-three, Coffey still hadn't, and because of it he was back in Rutherfordton, joining Michael Melton for a morning workout, throwing to David Mendez in the afternoon, following spring training from afar for the second straight year. He watched games on MLB Network, wondering what some of the pitchers in camps had that he didn't. His sinker climbed back to 91 miles per hour just that week.

Nothing broke Coffey's outward optimism. Whether he was trying to write his own truth wasn't the point. Coffey didn't have a job, didn't have any prospects, didn't have the stuff he needed—and he continued to believe anyway. That's what the fat seventeen-year-old kid from North Carolina did. The moment Coffey stopped, he let Eric Cooper win.

"How many years does he have left to play?" Jennifer wondered. "He has to be precise and particular and so careful. One more thing goes wrong, and he's done." She never said this to him. And even if she did, he would've swatted it away like a gnat in the summer. Coffey spent his days straddling the not-so-bright line between optimism and self-delusion.

"Every week, we've gained a consistent mile to two," he said. "This week, we've gained a consistent one. If the strength continues to build like it is, next Thursday we'll hit ninety-two, maybe a ninety-three. Do another week, and hopefully it's ninety-three. Hopefully in the next ten to fourteen days do another showcase."

In the next ten to fourteen days, he did not do another showcase. Opening Day passed, another season beginning without him. He was out of sight and out of mind. Coffey kept catching games on TV—Atlanta and Cleveland and Pittsburgh, all teams that had shown interest in the past. As he watched a reliever blow a lead one night, he sighed: "I could get outs with the stuff I have today."

Maybe it would be in the United States, and maybe he'd go halfway across the world. Every player on the sport's fringe at least considers the idea. Hudson and one of his best friends in baseball, Chicago White Sox catcher Tyler Flowers, had discussed the game's capriciousness, how it glorifies players one day and discards them the next. They know their careers in the major leagues could suddenly end anytime. And if that happened, they agreed, they'd consider seeking redemption together in Japan, a culture that reveres baseball even more than that of the United States and pays its stars millions. It was the kind of thing they discussed after a good meal and a few drinks, with their wives nodding along, happy to oblige their husbands' fantasies of Japan and sushi and being a *gaijin*—foreign player—in Nippon Professional Baseball.

In the spring of 2014, as positivity clashed with reality, it was something Coffey considered for a few moments before discarding the thought. He enjoyed his creature comforts: the glow of American TV late at night, the taste of American food. He wanted to play baseball but feared that the culture clash might be too strong.

"Japan," Coffey said, "is a whole different world."

CHAPTER 11

Land of the Rising Arm Injury Rate

Outside the barn, the old man smiled. He could hear the soundtrack of his life around the corner in his makeshift baseball facility. The grunts of teenage boys. The metal pipes thwacking golf balls. The whip-crack of baseball meeting glove. Everything unfolded with militaristic precision on this, the 212th consecutive day of practice, with another 148 in a row left before year's end. The old man didn't bother craning his neck toward the two dozen kids inside. He didn't need to see to know exactly what was happening.

"Baseball in Japan is called *yakyu*," the old man, Masanori Joko, said. "There is a saying that yakyu can explain life. How much you can be patient in the moment and make good use of those moments in life. Even a little pitch can become a big moment. It's important to find those bad moments to save the other experiences. The good moment, even though it's a little good moment, it can connect to a very big moment. You can learn how to connect those little chunks to the better moment. You can say that in life and in baseball."

I came to Japan to learn about yakyu and life and the most fascinating baseball culture in the world, one that holds the arm sacred. Few embodied the spirit of yakyu like Joko. He was sixty-seven years old, with tan skin, sunken eyes, and a full head of graying hair. Even when angry, Joko smiled. He grew up here, the seaside town of Matsuyama, on the smallest of the Japanese islands, Shikoku, and moved back after his wife died of cancer. If he couldn't be with her, he would be with his children.

That's what he called the boys of the Saibi High School baseball team. They made him famous throughout Japan. Every spring and summer, teams around the country travel to Nishinomiya, just outside Kobe, to participate in the national high school baseball tournament at Koshien Stadium, the country's most sacred sporting grounds. For nearly a century, Koshien has hosted twice-annual championships that marry the interest of the NFL, the urgency of the NCAA basketball tournament, and the parochialism of the World Cup. Baseball is Japan's greatest athletic passion, and high school baseball is its purest incarnation.

Saibi reached the finals of Spring Koshien in 2013, thanks to a boy named Tomohiro Anraku. The V-shaped brim of his Saibi cap was the only youthful thing about him. At sixteen, he was noticeably bigger than the other kids, his shoulders so wide that his arms had the stubby appearance of a T. rex's. At Koshien, almost every team chooses its best pitcher and rides him the entire tournament. For Anraku, that meant a nine-day span in which he pitched five games and threw 772 pitches.

This number became famous in Japan and notorious elsewhere. The number 772 symbolized a cultural chasm as wide as the Pacific Ocean. "This is child abuse," said Don Nomura, a longtime agent to top Japanese players.

In Japan, the public crowned Anraku *kaibutsu*—literally, the monster. No finer compliment exists for a baseball player. Only the most fearsome pitchers at Koshien earn the sobriquet. It's not just about dominance or achievement; it's mound presence and intimidation and the core principle of yakyu, fighting spirit, a combination of desire and will. In the United States, Anraku was seen as the latest victim of an anachronistic system that treats arms with reckless disregard. Any coach who dared misuse a teenager's arm to that degree was either stupid, crazy, or both.

"I don't regret it at all," Joko said. He believed in the power of yakyu to make better people. Whatever pain a player felt in practice, it would prepare him for worse pain in life. However dreadful a loss felt, it would train him to better handle the inevitability of true loss.

It's why his children took three hundred swings before workouts and another seven hundred over the course of daily practices that drag on for twelve hours, why their white uniforms were dirtied dark by the end of the day. "Japanese players have less stamina than American," Joko said, so he put them through a drill he named the Saibi Circuit, with lunges and squat thrusts and leg lifts and modified jumping jacks and faux push-ups, all on the sandy, brown-black field.

Joko barked orders. He needed to play aggressor and protector, to be the ultimate *kantoku*—the manager, not just of his team but of traditions and expectations threatened by the vigorous creep of American baseball philosophy. He lived for this. It was the perfect introduction for the next ten days, when I flew around Japan and tried to comprehend what Joko did a year earlier.

In the last game of the 2013 Spring Koshien, Anraku pitched for the third consecutive day and the fourth time in five days. His fastball, which sizzled at 94 miles per hour in his first game, wafted in at 80 miles per hour in the finals. Saibi lost 17–1.

Anraku cried. Then he apologized to Joko.

TWO HUNDRED FIFTY MILES FROM Matsuyama, in a manufacturing town called Koryo best known for its knit socks, a man named Hirokazu Tatsuta peeled away from his small house at two a.m. in an eight-ton truck stocked with three hundred bags of flour to deliver across the country. After he quit smoking, these rides felt a lot longer.

I met Hirokazu in Koryo at the end of his fourteen-hour shift. I wanted to ask about his son Shota. Hirokazu used to take young Shota on some of his shorter trips in the truck. Mostly they talked about baseball. Even in elementary school, Shota towered over the other kids, and Hirokazu tried to nurture the size advantage. They started running together when Shota was in second grade. They played catch daily, after school, when Hirokazu's shift ended. When Shota was nine or ten, he felt pain searing through his elbow, and Hirokazu figured it was the proper time to tell him a story.

Once upon a time, he was a good pitcher. He threw and threw and threw, hundreds of pitches a day. And then after one throw, he felt a pop in his shoulder. It was his last pitch. Without baseball, he didn't know what he wanted to do, so he started driving trucks and never stopped.

Shota didn't understand the moral. It was his dad's job, and that's all he knew, and he was too young to judge, too sweet to fathom his father's regret. And it stayed that way until a team in junior high school rode Shota to a youth tournament title and his elbow barked again.

This time, Hirokazu skipped the parable. "I told my son that you, not the team, have to take care of your arm," Hirokazu said, "and do whatever you need to do."

Thus began Hirokazu's grand experiment, one that would challenge the many institutions of Japanese baseball. Shota Tatsuta would not pitch every game. He would not participate in marathon sessions of *nagekomi*, the daily throwing in order to perfect mechanics that some Japanese players bastardized into marathon sessions of one hundred–, two hundred–, even three hundred–plus pitches. He would not kowtow to a system that left his father hauling product for a living. He would not fall prey to the yakyu ideals that evolved over more than a century after a visiting American professor named Horace Wilson introduced baseball to the country in the early 1870s.

About twenty years later, after a prep school team beat a group of Americans living in Japan, baseball's popularity surged. Japan wanted its own style, one that borrowed from other aspects of its culture. A college coach named Suisha Tobita stressed Bushido, the way of the samurai, virtue-laden and intense. He put players through *shi no renshu*—death training. If they didn't puke and piss blood, they were slacking.

Generations passed down the same tenets, an endowment that practice, repetition, and training ensure success. It's why, after his elbow started hurting in 1981, star pitcher Choji Murata kept throwing, ignoring the advice of his doctors and the wishes of his wife. She told him to stop. He refused, and when excessive throwing didn't cure his issues, he tried acupuncture and massage instead. She told him to go to Los Angeles, meet Frank Jobe, and get Tommy John surgery. He refused.

"A man should pitch until his arm falls off," Murata said.

This is the culture that Shota and Hirokazu Tatsuta—a teenaged boy and his dad from a place with a sign that reads "Welcome to Socks Town"—vowed to fight. Despite shunning the customs that surrounded him, Shota was one of the best amateur pitchers in the country, his fastball sometimes hitting 90 miles per hour, his arm seemingly healthy. Skepticism still accompanied every pitch he threw. It's not like the American way worked, either. All their science and pitch counts and babying amounted to what? More elbow injuries than ever? And *that's* a system worth following? Hirokazu asked himself those questions. He never pretended to know much about biomechanics. He didn't know what valgus stress was. He just knew what an open road looked like and didn't want his son to end up staring at it every day because he refused to question institutional stubbornness.

"I might be the last hope of the family," Shota said. "If I become successful, my family becomes glad at my success, and I can make my family happier."

Rather than leave home for one of the private schools that recruited him, Shota chose to attend Yamato-Koryo High School, a five-minute walk from his home. Hirokazu went to Yamato-Koryo, too, and Shota wanted to do what his father never could: carry the school to its first Koshien.

"I'm sure my father is actually hoping I can achieve his dreams as well," Shota said. "I am pursuing this career for myself and for my father, because he's been with me for all of the time. This is what I am."

I HOPPED OFF THE TRAIN AT Shibuya Station, a gateway to the splendor of Tokyo, to meet one of the country's most famous baseball players. Shibuya spills into the busiest intersection in the world, and at one corner sits a statue of a dog named Hachiko. He was an Akita with a gorgeous golden coat and a droopy left ear. Every day, Hachiko walked from his home to Shibuya Station in Tokyo to meet his master, a professor named Hidesaburo Ueno. In 1925, a cerebral hemorrhage killed Ueno. That did not stop Hachiko. For the next nine years, nine months, and fifteen days, all the way to his death, Hachiko trundled to Shibuya Station at the same time every evening, waiting for Ueno to come off his train, only to turn around and return home when he didn't arrive.

Of the seven Bushido virtues, loyalty may well reign supreme, and I wanted to ask Daisuke Araki whether he remained loyal when the culture that gave him everything also took so much of it away. One glance at Araki and it was easy to see why an entire nation of girls once swooned over him. At fifty, he is still that annoying kind of handsome, effortlessly so, with black hair parted down the middle and a square jaw. He can at least go out in public now with only a mild fear of recognition. When Araki was fifteen, he needed an army of friends to encircle him from female admirers when he stepped outside, as well as from TV cameras and writers, all frothing for a little piece of a boy who just wanted to play baseball.

Daisuke Araki wasn't like *a* Beatle. He was John, Paul, George, *and* Ringo. Of the many stars in the 1984 combined Spring and Summer Koshien contests, perhaps none enraptured Japan like Araki. He pitched in five consecutive Koshien tournaments, the most possible for a high schooler. He stood atop the mound and felt it rumble. This wasn't like the Little League World Series, where he had pitched a few years earlier. Whistles and chants and claps echo at Koshien. Cheerleaders and spirit squads and parents bellow. Sellout crowds of forty-eight thousand fill the stadium daily. People from nearby Kobe and Osaka, people from far-flung Hokkaido and Kyushu, people from everywhere get together to celebrate baseball, which might as well be a celebration of Japan.

"For me, Koshien is a kind of a religious place," Araki said, "I just think, 'Can I put my feet on the mound?' My foot was shaking."

Araki pitched his school, Waseda Jitsugyo, to the Summer Koshien finals in 1980. The invitation-only Spring Koshien welcomed him the next two years, and his school earned two more Summer Koshien berths through regional tournaments. Araki turned into a viral phenomenon before such things existed. Legions of new fans tuned in to watch him pitch that first year, including an eight-months-pregnant Tokyo woman named Yumiko Matsuzaka. Like thousands of other mothers across Japan over the next two years, she would name her son Daisuke.

Eighteen years later, on August 20, 1998, Daisuke Matsuzaka found himself on the mound for a semifinal game at Summer Koshien. Long before the Boston Red Sox spent more than

$100 million on his rights, Matsuzaka was best known for a high school game. He threw seventeen innings that day, willed himself to 250 pitches, a kaibutsu personified. The performance sounds mythical. It is not. Koshien invites it. Bring all of your arms, your strong, your weak, and let them compete. Let courage and respect and sincerity and righteousness and benevolence and honor and loyalty, the Bushido code, guide them. And hope for a year like 2006, when a boy named Masahiro Tanaka reached the Koshien finals and lost after throwing 742 pitches. Yuki Saito, like Araki of Waseda Jitsugyo, was nicknamed the Handkerchief Prince because of the cloth he kept in his back pocket to dab his face. He won Koshien when he struck out Tanaka on his 948th pitch of the tournament.

"I can't say abuse, but that's too much," Araki told me. "Even to Japanese baseball players. That's one reason why Koshien fans get so excited. But this is time to make better for the future. We have already lost a lot of good prospects at Koshien. All of the baseball people think that because we have Koshien, we produce the best pitchers. But now there are some people who have different opinion, like me."

Araki put his coffee down and flipped his palm to reveal the underside of his right arm. A jagged scar cut across his elbow. The pain started in 1988, when he was twenty-four. He met with Japanese doctors. All of them told him it was tendinitis. He rested for a month. His elbow still hurt. So he went to the United States and met with Frank Jobe.

For years, Japanese players refused to acknowledge surgery as an option. There was no fixing what was broken, because those who abide by yakyu aren't supposed to break. Masaharu Mitsui, a pitcher for the Lotte Orions and in 1974 the Rookie of the Year in Japan's Pacific League, ignored the stigma and asked Jobe to save his career with a UCL transplant in 1979. Choji Murata, the pitcher who vowed to let his arm fall off, relented after two years and became the second Japanese player to undergo Tommy John surgery. Daisuke Araki's place in history is a bit more notorious: he was the first Japanese player with two UCL reconstructions, after the first snapped when he tried to return too quickly.

Araki spent six disappointing seasons with the Yakult Swallows before he agreed on surgery in 1988. Between the two procedures, Araki missed nearly four years. He returned in 1992, threw 201 innings over the next five years, and retired at thirty-two. His relationship with Koshien is complicated. He sees the fame, the riches, the legacy, and the opportunity Koshien gives to players from more than four thousand high schools around the country to partake of the same.

Then you look at his elbow. And Matsuzaka's, with its Tommy John scar from when he was thirty. And Tanaka's, with his UCL partially torn and Tommy John inevitable. And Saito's, he of the 948 pitches, with damage in his shoulder threatening to end his career at twenty-seven. And Araki wonders: How can he be loyal to this? How can he reconcile what he loves with a trail of broken elbows?

"We're in a good direction," Araki said. "Generations change. So many high school managers are protecting the pitcher's body and elbow and they worry about them. And having many Japanese baseball players go to the US makes us change. We watch MLB and we get information on pitch counts."

I asked for his favorite Koshien performance, figuring he would name himself. He didn't. "Daisuke against PL," Araki said. He meant Matsuzaka's seventeen-inning, 250-pitch game against PL Gakuen, a powerhouse high school. "I want to protect the Koshien kids," Araki said, "but in this game I completely concentrated on the game. And that's the Koshien character."

The Japanese deify Koshien. Every year, Araki, now a TV commentator, goes back. In the summer of 2014, he was excited to watch one player: Tomohiro Anraku. There was one problem: Anraku and Saibi didn't make it to Koshien.

"His fastball," Araki said, "is not fast enough anymore."

THE NUMBER 772 MEANT NOTHING to the woman sitting amid a crowd of parents at the Saibi High School practice. Long ago, she learned, the only numbers that matter at Koshien flash on the scoreboard. Everything else is immaterial.

"I'm so proud of my son," Yukari Anraku told me, happily recounting how her boy became another kaibutsu. She and Koichi Anraku met at Koshien. They were college students and baseball fans who happened to work at the same concession stand. They fell in love at a baseball tournament and passed it on to their precocious boy. At three, Tomohiro started training to be a pitcher. Every day, he went to a nearby park, where Koichi made him throw strikes, even when he cried because he couldn't. On weekends, practices stretched to three hours. His parents massaged him afterward. "It just seemed like a regular practice between father and son," Tomohiro said, allowing that "it might be too much for a two- or three-year old."

They threw and threw and threw because, in Japanese baseball, "proper" pitching mechanics are paramount. The typical Japanese delivery is slow and methodical, with a gradual arm lift, a hands-above-head pause, a pronounced body turn to face third base, a bowing of the legs during the arm swing, a dip of the torso, and a whirring follow-through. Every little idiosyncrasy is a hallmark of a Japanese pitcher, almost embedded in his DNA. Anraku throws that way. So does Tatsuta. Mechanics, the belief goes, keep a pitcher healthy, impervious to both genetics and overuse. Generations of Japanese pitchers, the story goes, avoided arm problems throwing this way, although no known facts, evidence, or data beyond the anecdotal supports this.

Even though Yukari Anraku believed in her son's mechanics, she admitted: "I'm also worried about what his future is going to be. Injuries." Tomohiro Anraku's elbow started hurting less than six months after his 772 pitches in 2013. He survived Summer Koshien, his fastball creeping as high as 98, and almost immediately went to the early September eighteen-and-under World Cup in Taiwan, where he pitched three times in five days. Over eighteen innings, Anraku didn't give up a run, didn't walk a batter, and struck out twenty-seven against some of the best young talent on the planet. He was the best player in the tournament, better even than Yoan Moncada, the Cuban teenager whom the Boston Red Sox spent $63 million to sign.

During a tournament with Saibi on September 22, Anraku's elbow flared up in the first inning. "I didn't get injured because I was throwing too much," he claimed. "I had some form imbalance. That's why I got injured." Tired legs from the World Cup, he said, led to a mechanical breakdown. News stories in Japan theorized that the ball used at the World Cup was more slippery than a typical Japanese ball, causing Anraku to grip it tighter, which compromised his standard delivery. The number 772 never came up.

Six days after he got hurt and the swelling subsided, Anraku visited Kenshi Sakayama, a doctor who fancies himself a Renaissance man. He makes stunning wood carvings and creates flavor profiles for artisanal ice pops. His office is a nightmare, littered with paperwork, wood shavings, a freezer, autographs, and pictures of him with famous athletes. Sakayama wore his black hair shaved high and tight on the sides and in the back, a white lab coat with the collar popped, khakis, and sneakers.

The first thing Sakayama told me at his office was that for all the national interest in Anraku's elbow, nobody had asked to talk with him. He seemed genuinely offended by this. His cell phone chirped every few minutes. Two ladies wanted to confirm he would meet them for a boozy dinner at an *izakaya*, a Japanese pub, later that night.

Anraku was unconcerned that Sakayama isn't an orthopedist and has never performed a Tommy John surgery. He is a renowned osteosarcoma surgeon, helping those with bone cancer return to a normal life. Still, Anraku brought his million-dollar arm to Sakayama and returned for appointments and MRIs three more times.

"Nobody has seen this," Sakayama said. He sat at a desk chair in front of his computer, pulled up the images of Anraku, and pointed out his curved spine, a result of scoliosis, before clicking on the first picture of his elbow. "Clean bone," Sakayama said, comparing it to an MRI of another teenager whose elbow had sprouted a bone spur that looked like a meat hook. The integrity of the bones in Anraku's elbow seemed of far greater concern to Sakayama than his UCL, even though Masanori Joko said Anraku had sustained an injury similar to Masahiro Tanaka's partially torn ligament.

Sakayama offered no diagnosis on the cause of the injury, though he did say that shortly before it, in an effort to impress some girls, Saibi baseball players one day banged on a nearby drum set. Anraku, the kaibutsu, struck with the greatest ferocity. Perhaps, Sakayama theorized, the elbow pain came from this recklessness born of raging teenage hormones.

"I know about Tommy John surgery, but I don't know much," Anraku said. "I was thinking when I got injured I may have to have surgery. But the people around me said never do surgery while I was a high school student. It's not a good thing. Compared to the adult body, which can get cured faster, people said my elbow can get back within two months."

During Anraku's visits, hospital staff spirited him to a private room. Sakayama wanted to use low-intensity pulsed ultrasound equipment to stimulate the elbow and promote healing, but insurance didn't cover it. So he prescribed rest. Two months wasn't enough. Anraku needed six months off. His absence meant Saibi would not be invited to Spring Koshien in 2014.

When he returned for the games leading up to Summer Koshien, Anraku's fastball topped out at 92. Between his sixteenth and seventeenth birthdays, six miles an hour had disappeared. Without its monster, Saibi lost in the regional tournament.

SHOTA TATSUTA DIDN'T MAKE IT to Koshien, either. In the semifinal of his regional tournament, he allowed eleven runs to the local powerhouse, Chiben Gakuen. Never before had he yielded more than three in a high school game. Tatsuta did not cry, although he had been conflicted about pitching in the regional. The tattered arms of Koshiens past were familiar to all Japanese and lamented by those who refused to buy into the mythology and perpetuate the cycle of overuse. Just a year earlier, Tatsuta, like so many others in Japan, learned about Tomohiro Anraku and marveled.

"When I was watching him throw 772 pitches, I was hoping he wouldn't break his shoulder and arm," Tatsuta said. "I'm sure Anraku is the type of pitcher who does nagekomi all the time, but I wonder—if I were in that situation, I am not sure if I would pitch that many."

Tatsuta's quandary was a fundamental test of his value system, of Koshien's viability, of Japanese baseball's future. Given his potential for fame and riches and legacy and glory, would Tatsuta continue to heed the stories of his father? At the mere mention of Koshien possibly adopting a tiebreaker, Masanori Joko wondered: "Can that game give the audience enough emotional satisfaction? I understand that rule is for the players' health, but it loses excitement. The game won't move people as much as it does now." And now a nation of like-minded baseball fanatics would hear of Tatsuta's reservations and view him as a traitor, someone who dared debase a Japanese institution.

"If my team moved up in the tournament, I would have asked for help from somebody else for the middle of the games," Tatsuta said. "Otherwise, that would eventually be a bad influence to the team itself. If I was overwhelmed, it would've been better if other pitchers pitched for me or for the team."

I couldn't tell if Tatsuta was just one independent-minded kid or the leading edge of change in yakyu, a culture that exalts pain and sacrifice and gets it wrong the same way Major League Baseball once did. Real sacrifice is not throwing and throwing and throwing and maiming a healthy arm for the sake of the team. The Japanese revere yakyu because the Japanese created yakyu.

"In both America and Japan, people do their own thing because they believe that's the right thing," said Yasunori Wakai, the manager at Tatsuta's high school who accepted his plea not to throw every game. "We don't know which one is right, but I respect his choice. . . . Even though I respect that certain style, and I'm offering that choice to him, I grew up with that old culture. So to me, I still think Tatsuta is a bit strange."

It would be unfair to call Wakai the anti-Joko, just as it would be to call Tatsuta the anti-Anraku. Wakai and Tatsuta harbor a healthy respect for tradition, even if Tatsuta believes that prudence is the best path to a healthy arm and Wakai embraces Tatsuta's unorthodox view. They're not proselytizing, not intent on starting a revolution.

When Tatsuta bowed out of a tournament final his junior year, Wakai didn't quarrel. He prides himself on open-mindedness and understanding other cultures, whether it's American baseball or the fashion his son is studying at college in New York. Others weren't as kind: a club coach threatened to kick Tatsuta off the team for refusing to pitch because he wanted to save his arm for 2011's sixteen-and-under World Cup in Mexico. A tongue-lashing from Tatsuta's father forced the coach to capitulate, and Tatsuta went out against some of the world's top competition, throwing 7⅔ innings in the closer's role without allowing an earned run.

"There are some people who understand what I am doing," Tatsuta said. "I may not be right, either, but the biggest thing is I hope I prove that I am right in the future by becoming a pro."

All Tatsuta wanted from Nippon Professional Baseball was a fair opportunity. People could judge him and consider him a fool so long as they considered him at all. Tatsuta worked out at Yamato-Koryo High School daily. He wore bright yellow socks intentionally; he wanted to be seen, to show scouts that his philosophies on pitching never would hinder his work ethic. It was easy at times to forget he was just a seventeen-year-old who goes for a run when he feels disappointed, plays cell phone games in his free time, and doesn't have a girlfriend. Or that Anraku sits on the bus with his Saibi teammates and sings along, because he secretly wants to be a Japanese pop star.

They're still just kids, pawns in the bigger plans of men who think they know best.

INSIDE THE SPACE 11 DARVISH Museum, no detail is too trivial. There is a list of the fourteen different pitches Yu Darvish throws: four-seam fastball, curve, slow curve, power curve, changeup, high-speed changeup, forkball, split-finger fastball, one-seam fastball, two-seam fastball, vertical slider, slider, cut fastball, and sinker. Care to know the circumference of his shoulders? The right is fifty-seven centimeters around, the left fifty-one. You can't miss the two life-sized Darvish replicas. Wax wasn't realistic enough, so silicone artists rendered more accurate versions of Darvish, down to the bulging veins in his neck.

Tucked amid the boutiques and cake shops of Kobe is a white building owned by Farsad Darvish, the father of the Japanese pitcher who has found the most success in Major League Baseball. The Texas Rangers paid more than $111 million for six seasons of Yu Darvish's services. He's a six-foot-five, 228-pound right-handed colossus with a fastball in the mid-90s and an eephus curveball. Darvish personified cool on the mound and off. However much Tomohiro Anraku and Shota Tatsuta disagreed on pitching philosophy, both said they want to be like Darvish.

The perks for Farsad weren't bad, either. On the building's bottom floor, Farsad sells fine Persian art he imports from Iran, his home country. His office occupies the middle floor; he welcomed me in, guided me to a low-slung couch, offered me a cup of tea, and began telling the stories of the room's assorted amulets—a cardboard cutout of Yu, a gold spray-painted version of his glove, a cowboy hat given to him by Rangers ownership. The museum is on the top floor. Some of the biggest stars in Japan erect similar shrines; at one for Ichiro Suzuki, the hitting star who is likely to be the first Japanese player inducted into the Hall of Fame in Cooperstown, the orthodontic retainer he wore is on display.

Because Farsad was different—a Muslim among Shintos and Buddhists, a foreigner in a place that shuns them—he learned to scoff at tradition. He married Ikuyo, a Japanese woman he met at Eckerd College in Florida, and followed her home in 1982. Four years later, they had a boy—birth name Farid Yu Darvishsefat—whom Farsad promised to raise without strict adherence to Japan's social mores. Darvish threw all the time, nagekomi and otherwise, but he never put Koshien on a pedestal. Even when Darvish pitched Tohoku High to the finals in August 2003, he threw a paltry-for-Koshien 505 pitches over five games and let a sidearming teammate absorb the rest. "He always went to his kantoku saying there are other good pitchers, too," Farsad said. "Please use them."

Already an outsider on account of his mixed blood, Darvish did little to ingratiate himself by getting caught smoking a cigarette in a pachinko parlor before his professional debut at eighteen, a grievous sin that earned him a stint in "reeducation." He later posed half naked in a magazine and knocked up a pop star whom he married and divorced. He was beloved nonetheless, because nobody could deny his greatness. His thriving with the Rangers provided Japan with not just a worthy successor to Daisuke Matsuzaka but a usurper.

The influence of Darvish on the current generation of young Japanese pitchers is apparent. Anraku said he started doing more weight training to ape Darvish but couldn't fathom baseball without the extreme nagekomi Darvish derided. At the All-Star Game in 2014, Darvish suggested that Major League Baseball consider switching to a six-man rotation, as in Japan's top leagues, to better protect pitchers. Back home, they applauded, framing his proposition as a tacit approval of how Japan handles arms while ignoring Darvish's implicit criticism. He was hardly a spokesman for yakyu.

That was Daisuke Matsuzaka's province. "When I was a little kid," Anraku said, "my hero was Matsuzaka." He was everyone's kaibutsu, forever the conqueror, because throwing seventeen innings and 250 pitches harkened back to when men were *men*, when Japanese were *Japanese*. It never troubled Matsuzaka to feed the folklore, either, whether it was his nod-and-wink discussion of a mystery pitch he said he wanted to throw called the gyroball or the interminable throwing sessions through which he further distinguished himself.

In 2004, when he joined the Seibu Lions as pitching coach, Daisuke Araki, the former Koshien hero, marveled at how often his namesake threw. Almost every day, even twenty-four hours before his starts, Matsuzaka would throw 150 pitches, sometimes more. "Daisuke always declined, even if the manager or I would say it's time for a change," Araki said. "He'd say 'No, no.'"

The better Matsuzaka got, the more he threw. During spring training a year before he joined the Red Sox, Matsuzaka dug in for ninety minutes one day and threw 333 pitches. Nearly four pitches a minute, never stopping. Like Murata, willing to throw until his arm fell off. Matsuzaka earned his Tommy John scar. Hero at eighteen, dominant at twenty-two, unimpeachable at twenty-six, hurt at thirty, and back in Japan at thirty-four with a few souvenirs: tens of millions of dollars, a World Series ring, and a permanent reminder of the arm's frailties tracing his elbow.

Matsuzaka isn't seen as a cautionary tale in Japan but a triumphant one worthy of emulation. When I asked Anraku about

Matsuzaka and nagekomi, he nodded along in full agreement. "A good arm can't be made without nagekomi, especially for the Japanese players," Anraku said. "Compared to other countries' players physically, Japanese players are different. We believe that the power is different. That's why the Japanese player needs to practice more and train more. That's why nagekomi is very important to build good muscles and good arms."

I heard this over and over, players and coaches attributing dubious practices to nationality. While it is true the average Japanese male is smaller than the average American, Anraku was a leviathan compared with his teammates. The closest thing to a medical study that has compared Japanese and Americans physiologically focused on clogged heart arteries. If the Japanese arm really *is* different, like the legs of the Kalenjin tribe of elite runners in Kenya, that's one thing, but from everything doctors in the United States have seen, their arms are practically the same. "Maybe the joint is a little looser, but it's really no different," said Dr. James Andrews, who performed Tommy John surgery on at least three Japanese pitchers, none more important than the most recent.

Toward the end of the 2014 season, Yu Darvish's elbow started hurting. The MRI showed standard damage, ordinary enough that an insurance company sold the Rangers a policy on the elbow in case of injury. Darvish made it through a typical off-season throwing program in good health and came into spring training feeling strong. One inning into his first start, Darvish tore his UCL. As much as Farsad tried to protect him, as much as he tried to protect himself, Darvish was just like Matsuzaka and the other Japanese players who sought professional glory in the major leagues and wound up scarred.

It reminded me of a conversation with Masanori Joko, the sage of Saibi High School. He was just as curious about American culture as I was about Japanese.

"What is it about America," Joko said, "that makes Japanese pitchers get hurt when they go there?"

He wondered about the American ball and the five-man rotation and the lack of nagekomi and dietary changes and the dirt on the mound and everything except the endless throwing sessions Joko long ago convinced himself weren't just right but necessary.

FOR HIS SIXTY-SEVENTH BIRTHDAY, MASANORI Joko received a gift from his players. In the middle of a large piece of poster board, one of the kids drew a perfect rendering of the most famous outfield fence in Japan. Joko knew it well, though in case anyone else needed help identifying it, two words were looped in English cursive: "Koushien Stadiam." The drawing sat on a table in Joko's office behind a pair of gloves marked "95" and "85," for the ninety-fifth Summer Koshien and eighty-fifth Spring Koshien.

For thirty-three years he'd done this—coach baseball, spread yakyu, sprinkle some of what TV commentators called "Joko Magic"—all because owning a drugstore in his prior life bored him. He left the business he had built to coach his first team, Uwajima Higashi High, which made Koshien in his fifth year and won the spring tournament two years later. Other coaches wore excruciating looks during the high-stakes games. Joko grinned, like he knew something the rest of them didn't. He earned a nickname for it: "Smiling Joko." It was an odd dichotomy, his insistence on enjoyment amid the practice of a century-old style that frowned upon it. From January 3 to December 29, his teams practiced or played every day. The dankest summer afternoons, the most blustery winter days—neither weather nor physical condition nor any excuse, however legitimate, interrupted Joko's lessons. His children swung and threw and ran. They hopped onto rowing machines, yelling on every pull-back to show Joko their dedication, as if two thousand daily meters wasn't evidence enough. Wearing a Saibi jersey compelled a boy to forever seek Joko's approval.

"When my father is not here," Tomohiro Anraku said, "Joko-san is my father."

Koichi Anraku works for a paper company in Tokushima, about a two-and-a-half-hour drive from Saibi, so he entrusted Joko with that role and, by extension, Anraku's arm. With no think tanks advocating pitch limits and only a handful of youth leagues with hard-and-fast usage rules, the coach in Japan serves as gatekeeper. And in a society where age equals status, and winning Koshien magnifies credibility exponentially, Joko's word was bulletproof.

"Everybody listens to the manager," said Kenshi Sakayama, Anraku's doctor. "Culturally, Japan has a relationship between manager and players that managers are not forcing them to do it. But if the manager has to argue, then the only answer from the player is: 'Yes, I am OK.'"

Joko ceded on just one matter with Anraku, and even that was begrudging. He could not understand why Anraku iced his arm after starts. Starting in elementary school, Anraku mummified himself in ice to stem the swelling. This did not compute with Joko; he worried ice halted blood circulation and didn't promote healing. In June 2013, he found a powerful ally: the *American Journal of Sports Medicine* published a study that questioned the efficacy of ice, noting that while it reduced inflammation, it also slowed healing.

If that was wrong—if Americans spent nearly four decades listening to doctors' and trainers' orders to treat inflammation with the famous RICE acronym: rest, ice, compression, and elevation—Joko wondered what else was faulty. Professional players in the United States blew out their elbows at record rates in recent years, and they wanted to call *him* the abuser?

"It's the final game of the Koshien tournament," Joko said. "That's two high schools out of four thousand–something. It's a very honorable thing to be in the final game of that tournament. I can't even put it in words. As a pitcher, it can be a pretty memorable and honorable thing for them. As long as he said he wants to pitch, I want to send him to the mound."

Heading into the 2014 Summer Koshien, Joko wanted to summon his kaibutsu one final time. If that meant 772 pitches or 800 or 949, one more than Yuki Saito's record, Joko would allow Anraku to choose, knowing what the answer would be. Saibi's defeat in the regional tournament made it moot.

"Everybody was sort of relieved that he lost," Sakayama said.

It's cruel to think it's that way, winning and arm health the two ends of yakyu's imbalanced scale. Backward though it may be, the truth is that getting injured may have been the best thing that happened to Tomohiro Anraku. It saved him from even worse.

THE FIRST PATIENT ARRIVED a little before two p.m. The waiting room around him at Mito Kyodo Hospital bustled with noise and activity. He was nervous until the blue door to one of the offices that ringed the room slid open. Dr. Naotaka Mamizuka greeted him with a smile and welcomed him in. Two afternoons a week, Mamizuka takes time off from his work as a spinal surgeon to treat baseball players with hurt arms. Wearing a head-to-toe Adidas getup instead of a lab coat, the athletic-looking Mamizuka projected an aura more coach than doctor. Children from everywhere in Japan travel to see Mamizuka. They are as young as eight. Nearly every one is injured.

For the next four hours, I watched a parade of kids come through the sliding door into a twelve-by-ten-foot hospital room and reveal the true story of yakyu today. The bones in the first patient's arm were not yet fully formed, and the UCL yanked a piece of bone off the inside knob of his elbow, similar to the injury Braedyn Woborny suffered. Mamizuka diagnosed it as an avulsion fracture of the medial epicondyle and said this wasn't the first time. The boy likely broke his elbow once before, did not allow proper healing, and fractured it again. He was ten years old. And his story mirrored that of almost all the nineteen other patients Mamizuka saw that afternoon, a typical Friday other than it happened to be one day before Summer Koshien was set to begin.

"I say to parents: This is not good," Mamizuka said. "Bad training. Bad pitching. Bad coaching."

Millions of Japanese boys play baseball, and studies show the youngest are hurt far more frequently than kids in the United States. During a regional tournament in July 2011, an orthopedist named Tetsuya Matsuura surveyed every participant, ages ten to twelve. While Matsuura was looking for cases of a bone injury called osteochondritis dissecans (OCD), he found something far more interesting: of the more than one thousand players with no signs of OCD, 43.4 percent still reported elbow pain, according to his article in the *Orthopaedic Journal of Sports Medicine*. Another study of youth players in Yamagata, Japan, found that two-thirds of the sixty-three-pitcher sample suffered elbow injuries. By contrast, in a ten-year-long study conducted by Glenn Fleisig at the American Sports Medicine Institute, 25.5 percent of American children in the same age group copped to elbow pain.

Mamizuka once visited ASMI in Birmingham, Alabama, and returned to Mito wishing his life's work of fixing Japanese baseball wasn't the solitary windmill-tilting it's always been. In a few years he turns fifty, and he hopes that his added gravitas will make the baseball power structure start listening to him. For now, a small, dedicated bunch reads his book, *The Baseball Medicine*, and feasts on the Facebook posts in which he politely dismantles Japanese baseball's willful institutional ignorance. In the meantime, he serves as one of a handful of doctors who treat arm injuries. Because the demand for his time is so great, a standard Mamizuka appointment consists of him perusing an MRI—every kid gets one because they cost only $70 at Mito Kyodo, compared with around $1,000 in the United States—and delivering a quick diagnosis before it's another patient's turn.

"Next!" Mamizuka said after the first boy left, and the blue door slid open and in walked Ryusei, an eleven-year-old. His name means "shooting star" in Japanese.

Though the fracture in his elbow had healed—the medial epi-condyle often breaks in cases of so-called Little League elbow, a malady from which kids usually return to play but find themselves at greater risk for future injury—Ryusei's arm still hurt. Mam-izuka pulled up his MRI and clicked at a feverish rate, zooming, panning, explaining. Ryusei's UCL was damaged. Mamizuka couldn't do anything. Unlike some American doctors, he refuses to perform Tommy John surgery on anyone younger than fifteen, and even those cases are infrequent. Just rest, he told Ryusei. This would not be the last boy Mamizuka saw that day whose UCL injury preceded a full set of teeth.

A twelve-year-old needed Tommy John surgery but wouldn't get it. A nine-year-old had an avulsion fracture. An eleven-year-old suffered a broken foot, which Mamizuka worried came from too much running during practice. A nine-year-old, wearing a splint two months after doctors healed his avulsion fracture by inserting a pin into it, was asked by Mamizuka whether he still liked baseball. "Yes," the boy replied. A fifteen-year-old was di-agnosed with OCD. Mamizuka had told him to stop playing at thirteen and let an elbow injury heal. He didn't listen, and the condition turned necrotic. Mamizuka carefully explained to the boy and his mom that doctors would need to transplant bone from the rib or knee to fix the elbow damage.

Every time the door slid open, another heartbreak walked in. I looked at Mamizuka once, in between appointments, and asked if it's like this all the time. "Every week," he said. One of the nine-year-old boys said he had daily four-hour practices and spent most of his weekend days playing, too. If any more evidence was needed that Japanese baseball had institutionalized injuries, just as its American counterpart had, here it was: the eerie sight of chil-dren lining up as though at a buffet to see a man who would say that baseball failed them, not the other way around.

Most came and left with the same advice. Rest your arm. Schedule a follow-up for a few months down the road. And under no circumstances throw. When a high school–aged kid rolled in, his mom in tow with a Louis Vuitton bag in her hand and Crocs on her feet, Mamizuka asked him to pantomime his delivery. Mamizuka shook his head and stood up. He wanted to teach everyone what he taught his son: throw with less than 100 percent force. "Power is bad," Mamizuka said. Naturally, his most famous patient, a twenty-year-old named Shohei Otani, threw a pitch in Japan's 2014 All-Star Game clocked at 101 miles per hour, harder than any Japanese-born player ever had thrown. So far, Otani is perfectly healthy. American executives froth at the possibility Otani could soon join the major leagues and foresee a bidding war for his services likely to exceed $200 million.

Because Mamizuka couldn't do anything about stemming velocity, and because so many refused to listen to his criticisms of nagekomi, he focused with older patients on the one thing he could change: mechanics. He demonstrated the proper way to throw a baseball. "*Ichi, ni, san,*" he said. "*Ichi, ni, san.*" One, two, three. One, two, three. Shift the weight through the pelvis. Rotate the trunk to the right. Swing the arm with purpose. It was rhythmic. *Ichi, ni, san.* One, two, three.

If only it were that easy. Mamizuka had minutes to explain what would take months to perfect. This is how it works when a doctor jams twenty patients into an afternoon. No chitchat. In and out, appointments as short as two minutes. For two more hours, kids showed up. Only one left with a clean bill of health from Mamizuka. MRIs, like radar guns, never lied, and child after child showed signs of damage directly related to baseball.

The last, and most vexing, case of the day was a slight twelve-year-old. He had come in months earlier with an epicondyle fracture. It looked better, as did his UCL. He was a sweet kid, his lisp endearing, his self-awareness more so. He didn't understand how he got hurt. He didn't even throw hard. Mamizuka told him it would be OK. That's what kids needed to hear.

He'd said the same to other kids for years. As the doctor for a national youth team, he did periodic assessments on some of the players. One in particular, the team's closer, intrigued Mamizuka. His name was Shota Tatsuta. Years before Tatsuta made Japan think about its baseball culture, Mamizuka worried what it had done to him already.

"I checked him at the end of [a tournament]," Mamizuka said. "His UCL is a little bit damaged."

THE NATIONAL SPORT OF AN educated, industrial society encourages behavior that endangers children's health. This sounds so primitive until one considers football's popularity in the United States. The sanctimony exasperated plenty inside the Japanese baseball establishment, particularly when elite baseball in Japan and the United States is so similar. For Anthony and Nelson Molina, there are Tomohiro Anraku and Masanori Joko. For Riley and Neil Pint, there are Shota and Hirokazu Tatsuta. For the showcase circuit, there is Koshien. For the nonexistent offseason, there is nagekomi. The radar guns are the same. The monetary incentives exist in both places. The only difference is the United States knows its system is defective and Japan is slowly figuring it out.

To show me the progress Japan is making to change its attitude toward pitching, Farsad Darvish invited me to meet someone. Night had fallen. A late-summer rain fell on Kobe. Farsad took the highway about a half hour to Onijus coffee shop in south Osaka. In the parking lot stood a white-whiskered sixty-seven-year-old man with gingham pants, a striped shirt, and a sport coat accented by mother-of-pearl buttons. Farsad introduced him as "kantoku."

His real name was Asao Yamada, and he was Yu Darvish's middle-school coach. For decades he had coached kids in Habikino, the midsized city outside Osaka where Darvish spent his childhood. Yamada grew up playing baseball himself, often teaming with another talented young player: Masanori Joko. As both went into coaching—Joko full-time, Yamada part-time—they kept in touch. Neither drank sake. Both enjoyed the sauna. They would talk baseball, their philosophies in lockstep, the sanctity of yakyu nonpareil. Though they hadn't seen each other in a while—Yamada said Joko spent some time in a hospital recently—Yamada sympathized with the American scrutiny his old friend endured because of 772.

At an international youth tournament in Phoenix half a decade earlier, Yamada coached the Japanese national team. Day after day, he ran the same pitchers out to the mound. During a lunch with coaches from other countries, Yamada learned they'd bestowed upon him a nickname. "They called me Crazy Yamada," he said.

Time passed, and as much as Yamada wanted to blame the cultural divide for his fellow coaches' perspective, he started to ask himself what supported the Japanese way other than its familiarity. When Darvish's elbow blew out, it complicated matters even more. Yamada's generation was supposed to be the protector of yakyu, and suddenly he wasn't sure whether it was something worth protecting.

"It's very important to win," Yamada said, "but now for me, as I get older, it's very important to see the kids stay healthy."

Yamada coaches a fourteen-year-old boy named Shinji Oishi who throws left-handed and conjures a mirror image of Darvish at the same age. Yamada's instinct is for Oishi to throw and throw and throw, teach those muscles how to feel on a proper delivery, reach for perfection of form. Then he reminds himself: With something as fallible as the arm, perfection exists only in the minds of the stubborn and anachronistic, a myth unworthy of preservation. He would treat Shinji more like Shota Tatsuta than Darvish.

I left the coffeehouse with a smidgen of hope. If someone like Asao Yamada could grow, surely others could. Maybe even Masanori Joko.

"Who is to change this?" Farsad said. "I suppose only time can."

TOMOHIRO ANRAKU SNIFFLED TWICE, SWALLOWED hard to compose himself, and sneaked a look at the speech he clutched with both hands. At Murata Hall in Matsuyama, more than 750 people showed up to honor a beloved figure in the community. And the kid who wanted to play baseball and sing pop songs was asked to eulogize him.

"*Kantoku-san*," Anraku began, sure to include the formal honorific because Masanori Joko would've expected it. Joko had been sick, like Yamada said, living out his final days with bile-duct cancer before dying September 1, 2014. He was sixty-seven.

When Joko started cancer treatment in the fall of 2013, he didn't tell anyone on his team. Joko's final months were blackened by scandal. Before a spring game in 2014, one of Joko's sophomores had insisted a freshman put a dead bug in his mouth or drink kerosene. The boy chose the bug. A month later, a group of sophomores made freshmen fight one another, encouraging them to punch harder and throwing rubber balls at the underclassmen. The Japan High School Baseball Federation, calling the behavior a "deep-rooted problem," suspended Saibi from competing in any games, including Koshien, for a year. Joko went to the hospital a week later and never left.

The mourners wept at the smiling picture of Joko in better days and the three jerseys and the purple flowers and the advice of Joko they remembered, like taking little moments and connecting them to survive in bigger moments. Kantoku was right: This is what real pain felt like. This is what true loss felt like. Nothing—not even 772 pitches—could prepare him for this. "You always considered my condition first, putting your own matters aside," Anraku said. "Even when you were not feeling well, you didn't show that to us. Instead, you always faced us with full force.

Speak when spoken to, greet well, pay attention, be considerate, be thoughtful. Those were the words you always valued from your belief that students shall grow up not only as great baseball players but also great people in an adult society."

Anraku had set three goals with Joko: win Koshien, throw a fastball 160 kilometers per hour (99 miles per hour), and become the first overall pick in the draft. "I wasn't able to make the first two promises," Anraku said, "but I still keep my challenge to make our third promise."

Seven weeks later, with the number two overall pick in the 2014 Nippon Professional Baseball draft, the Tohoku Rakuten Golden Eagles chose Tomohiro Anraku. In the first round, all twelve teams name the one player they covet most. If more than one team chooses the same player, a lottery determines where he goes. Four teams selected Kohei Arihara, a pitcher from Japan's baseball factory, Waseda University. Despite Anraku's elbow issues and velocity dip, Rakuten and the Yakult Swallows both wanted him.

While Anraku prepared for a press conference in his traditional *gakuran* school uniform, Shota Tatsuta went home to watch the draft on TV. He wasn't going to be a first-round pick; he didn't throw hard enough. He probably wouldn't be a second- or third-rounder, either. And at that juncture, he feared teams wouldn't want him because of his baseball beliefs. He watched with his father, and when the Hokkaido Nippon Ham Fighters chose Tatsuta with the eighth pick of the sixth round, they started to cry. He'd made it. They'd made it. The plan worked. Maybe Shota did have some UCL damage, like Mamizuka said, but it had presented with no symptoms for long enough that he could convince one team, which is all he needed.

"There's no right answer," Shota said. "There are many younger kids who hurt their throwing arm, but at the same time there are so many kids who don't get injured no matter how many pitches they throw. It depends on the individual. There's no right answer."

In Masanori Joko's mind, the right answer was Tomohiro Anraku. He willingly embodied the tradition upheld by generations of Japanese baseball players and unwittingly became the face of a debate that spanned the world. On the day Joko was laid to rest, Anraku's face was again the focus as the entire Saibi baseball team gathered outside the hall. The players wore their uniforms, head to toe, and they were clean, just as Joko would have expected before practice. The hearse started to pull away. Joko's children doffed their caps. They said good-bye to their kantoku and the style that went with him, the former gone forever, the latter not far behind.

CHAPTER 12

Changeup

ON THE FIRST NIGHT OF a visit back to his parents' Virginia house in the fall of 2013, Daniel Hudson glanced around the kitchen, saw the bottle of Barefoot Sweet Red Blend, and knew he needed to make a run to the ABC store. One perk of being injured for two years was the chance to try new things, and Hudson and Sara had discovered the joys of good wine, which had the added benefit, of course, of blunting the drudgery of rehab.

When Hudson left for the store, Sara retreated to the bathroom, and set out to eliminate one reason for her nausea that morning. She'd taken pregnancy tests before, and they all turned out the same: one line, many disappointments. As she held the stick this time, she held her breath, too. When a second pink line crept across the surface, she couldn't move. It was five p.m. on November 19, 2013. "You never forget that moment," Sara said, "when your heart stops after you've been trying for two years."

By the time Hudson returned, Sara was catatonic with joy.

"What's wrong?" he said. She showed him the test. Hudson hadn't given up hope for a baby; a few weeks earlier they had scheduled an appointment to talk with a doctor about in vitro fertilization and other potential remedies. His speechlessness awoke Sara from her trance. She jumped up and down. He couldn't remember the last time he smiled like this.

"A lot of news we've gotten recently has been just bad," Hudson said. "This is the first good thing."

Now it made sense why Hudson reacted as well as he did to the Diamondbacks taking him off the roster two weeks later: for the first time in his life, something beyond himself was driving his baseball career. When Hudson shot up between his junior and senior years of high school and his fastball ticked up from 87 to 93, he felt a certain power on the mound, an impregnability that nothing in life could match. He burned for the competition.

Something changed in Hudson after Sara took the pregnancy test—and five more, just to make sure the previous ones weren't lying. His choice was clearer: sit around and feel sorry for himself or become proactive about his faltering career and try to understand how the arm works, why it works that way, and what he could do to make it work for him and his wife and baby. It wasn't that Hudson became more outwardly positive; he was simply reminded of the world outside this bubble he created for himself, one with buckets of rice and hours of sculpting scapulas and Jobes and the godforsaken treadmill he'd worn out as much as it did him. Baseball does a great job of convincing players that's what life is until life proves otherwise.

The baby was due July 21, 2014, just about the date of its father's projected return to baseball after what would be thirteen grueling months of recovery. His own due date depended on his health, of course. The Diamondbacks had built in multiple-week breaks to give Hudson's arm a breather. At the sign of even the tiniest bit of soreness, Hudson shut down his throwing program for a few days.

Hudson's protocol was essentially a slightly more cautious version of the typical twelve-month post–Tommy John surgery plan. In mid-January, back at the Diamondbacks' spring-training complex in Scottsdale, Hudson was throwing for about ten minutes at a time, starting at sixty feet and backing up to ninety. On the other end of the throws was Brad Arnsberg, still the rehab coordinator, still the consummate bullshitter.

"I love war, the old wars," Arnie said to me during his catch with Hudson. "Anything from World War I, World War II, the Korean War, Vietnam. I've read a lot of the Navy SEAL books. I think if I could do it all over again and didn't choose baseball, I always had a big affection for the military and a great respect for it. I'm not saying I could've. Those guys are built out of a different cloth."

Throw. Pop.

"I always had great work habits and pushed my body to the limit," Arnie said. "I did things not a whole lot of other guys did. I might've given it a try. But to say I could've gone through the training. I don't know. It's the mentally tough guys. The ones who can handle the ups and downs. It reminds me a lot of playing baseball. Knock on wood, there's been no setbacks. Every day he's gone with me, it's not like he has a couple steps forward. But he's either treaded water or gained steam. No setbacks."

Throw. Pop.

"And knock on a big piece of wood," Arnie said. "I hate to jinx something like that."

"Couple more," Hudson called out, and after precisely two throws, he rejoined Arnsberg for a pat on the back. "Solid, man," Arnie said.

Hudson proceeded inside to the Diamondbacks' weight room, a massive structure with thirty-foot-tall ceilings and futuristic equipment, and opted for something basic: standing in front of a mirror and cutting short full throws of two-pound medicine balls. Then he loaded a four-ounce baseball into a sock and threw it, making sure to hold on to the sock. He did the same sock drill with a six-ounce ball. All the while, he paid particular attention to his hand in relation to the rest of his arm, slowing himself down when it felt wrong.

As the greatest change in his life beckoned, so did the transformation of his career. After years of protest, Hudson was ready to overhaul the most fundamental thing about himself: how he threw a baseball.

BOREDOM SNUCK UP ON TODD Coffey in interesting ways. During the early stages of his recovery, he took perverse pleasure in getting booted from the youth-league softball games of his daughters, Hannah and Haley, for arguing with the umpires. That got old after the fourth or so ejection, so he moved on to something with the promise of far greater rewards: Dumpster diving.

Over his baseball career, Coffey had made around $7 million. After his second Tommy John surgery, he tightened his budget and started impersonating someone a lot more strapped for cash than he was. He traded original, in-box Nintendo cartridges to earn small profits. He hit swap meets and thrift stores in search of bargains. Coffey even jumped into a trash bin to snatch a particularly lucrative supermarket flyer to use in his latest round of extreme couponing.

"I can't believe I did that," Coffey said. "Actually, yes I can. Hey, it's free money."

Extreme couponing is the art of stacking discount on top of discount and leaving a store with large and often unnecessary amounts of stuff for a pittance. During one such trip, Coffey and Jennifer got $160 worth of hair-care products, toothpaste, and granola bars for thirteen bucks. Another session yielded more than one hundred bottles of Powerade for free. When he wasn't preparing for his next showcase, Coffey scoured the Internet for the best coupons.

"I really need to pitch," he said.

With every week that passed, he achieved a new level of delirium. Coffey wanted another showcase at the end of April. Then he injured his knee when emphasizing lower-half mechanics and trying to get an extra mile per hour from his legs. "I'm there," he said. "I am so close. But I've got to be smart about it. What's an extra week right now? Nothing."

He was approaching the two-year anniversary of his surgery date, a year longer than he wanted, even longer than Dr. ElAttrache anticipated, and Coffey still couldn't stay healthy. Minor though they were in the grand scheme, every twinge and tweak put him further from where he was supposed to be. On May 2, 2014, a former closer named Joel Hanrahan signed for a guaranteed $1 million with the Detroit Tigers less than a year removed from his Tommy John. Coffey was incredulous. Hanrahan's fastball sat around 90 and topped out at 93 in his showcase. Coffey's fastball was parked at 92 before the leg flared up.

He couldn't wait any longer for his second showcase. "Especially after seeing Hanrahan get what he got," Coffey said. He booked a flight to Phoenix for May 4 and gave himself ten days to get used to the mound at Physiotherapy Associates, rid himself of the bad memories from the last showcase, and prepare to win a job. On Coffey's fourth day there, former big league catcher Lou Marson, also rehabbing an injury, caught his bullpen session. "I finally get some big league feedback," Coffey said. "He said, 'If I was you, I'd do my showcase. You hit all your spots. The ball was heavy and hard. I wouldn't want to face you.'"

Coffey set the showcase for May 14. Another performance like the first one and his career was over. This frightened him; Coffey didn't spend much time thinking about his future after baseball, because baseball still dominated his present. He had neither the patience nor the desire to coach. Front-office and scouting work sounded fun, as did the agent side of the game, but only a privileged few get to stay in baseball, leaving the rest to explore alternative interests. One business idea stuck with Coffey.

"A legit go-kart track," he said. "Take Dave and Buster's, and add electric go-karts inside. Add alcohol to it, too. I'd do it somewhere in the Midwest. You're freezing. You're always cold. Everything has to be indoors. When people go out in the Midwest, they want to be out two to three hours. Adult go-karts, kid go-karts, food. One-stop shop. With the alcohol, everyone purchases everything on a card. If you've had too much to drink, they'll know and you won't be allowed to race."

Before he entered the semidrunk go-karting business, Coffey needed to prove to himself this return to pitching wasn't some flight of fancy. He said it himself nearly two years earlier: he didn't want to be the guy whose lack of self-awareness left him hanging on long past his time. He was certain he wasn't. Someone would see what he saw. They always did. When that happened, he would pitch his way back into the major leagues. Once there, he'd finally get to do something ten years in the making.

"Every rookie who comes up, I tell him before his first outing, do your warm-ups and do a three-sixty," he said. "Look around the stadium. You'll never get the chance to do it again. You have only one debut. You deserve to be selfish. Take your ten seconds and get back to work."

Coffey hadn't done that on April 19, 2005. It was a Tuesday. After seven years clawing through the minor leagues, not listening to the teammates who laughed at him or the scouts who ignored him or the people who told him to lose weight, he joined the Reds in Cincinnati. His manager, Dave Miley, called on him to start the sixth inning against Derrek Lee, the best hitter in the National League that season. Coffey was too young to treasure the moment, too frightened to do anything but throw sinkers and hope for ground balls. After Lee welcomed him to the major leagues by whacking a single, Michael Barrett continued the hospitality with a home run, and so began the run he refused to let end.

He had to make it back, if only so he could have that feeling once more. His arm new, his career reborn, these two years worth something.

"I'm gonna run in from the bullpen," Coffey said. "I'm gonna do my three-sixty, and I'm gonna take my ten seconds. Maybe even more."

THE ARM IS NOT JUST the arm. It is, as the anthropologist Neil Roach said, "everything from the feet to the fingers." The St. Louis Cardinals were one of the few teams that understood this. A few years ago, they hired Paul Davis, a former college baseball player and coach working toward his doctorate in leadership studies. Davis spent years trying to wrap his head around the mysteries of the arm. He struck up a friendship with Brent Strom, the Buzz Aldrin of Tommy John surgery. Strom, then the Cardinals' minor league pitching coordinator, recommended Davis to the organization.

In 2012, they hired Davis and two years later gave him his dream job and a most unique title: coordinator of pitching analytics. The Cardinals wanted Davis to apply his knowledge to the twin problems of keeping their pitchers healthy and steering clear of ones susceptible to injury. He read more than 150 academic papers from around the world that covered every aspect of the throwing motion. He used himself as a guinea pig to test what he learned, a fifty-year-old man trying to re-create the motions of someone half his age.

Davis studied video of four pitchers in the Cardinals organization—starters Shelby Miller and Joe Kelly, relievers Trevor Rosenthal and Mitchell Boggs—and focused on a single measurement: the position of the back ankle during a pitch. Davis subscribed to the theory of triple extension—the ankle, knee, and hip extending were critical to an efficient pitching motion. Everything started with the foot. He paused the video, zoomed in, and studied the ankle's dorsiflexion, or how far it extended.

Rosenthal had the best ankle mobility of the group. He's the only one of the four still with St. Louis.

"If you start incorrectly, it's just going to be a snowball," Davis said. "You'll see guys who come to a set and their first move they get their pelvis in a bad position, which is reflected in their ankle, and the very first movement they make, they're screwed. I can say that's a bad delivery and he's got bad arm action, and the analytics guys will tell me that I can't say when he's going to break. And they're right. What I can say is this guy has a riskier delivery. It's like insurance. If you're in a flood zone, there's more risk there."

While Daniel Hudson preferred not to turn himself into a laboratory experiment, he refused to play innocent bystander again. If others wanted to stare at Hudson's ankles, they could. Ken Crenshaw, the Diamondbacks' trainer, instead devised a program for Hudson to shorten his arm swing behind his body and get his hand on top of the ball, so he could pull down on it rather than fling it off the sides of his fingers. Essentially, it was what Brad Arnsberg wanted to do the first time around.

"I've been thinking about it," Hudson said. "A surgery that has an eighty to eighty-five percent success rate, where guys get back to their previous level or better, didn't work for me. So am I going to just do it again the same way or try something different? Once I had surgery again, I'm like, 'I gotta fix something. Something's gotta change if I really want to pitch for ten, twelve, fifteen more years. I've got to figure something out to stay healthy.' I basically had to reteach myself how to throw."

Remaking Daniel Hudson into Greg Maddux was not going to happen. Bad habits can be learned in a matter of hours. Hudson spent nearly a quarter century repeating his. He couldn't just deprogram it at the snap of Crank's or Arnie's fingers. Only a few cells in the human body contain more than one nucleus. Muscle cells are among them, and the body's ability to recruit nuclei to allow it to learn and retain movement patterns—to create muscle memory—is one of human beings' great wonders. It allows us to walk and talk. Every movement we make comes from the symbiosis of muscles and the brain. Even when muscles shrink—as happens following Tommy John surgery—the nuclei survive in the atrophied fibers and, after rebuilding, they're anxious to reenact what they knew before. If Hudson tried to start from scratch, his body would rebel. He'd never have pristine mechanics. He just wanted lesser degrees of bad.

Hudson first looked at video of pitchers he respected. Diamondbacks video coordinator Allen Campbell queued up a lot of Justin Verlander, the Detroit Tigers' bell cow whose arm had survived eight straight two-hundred-plus-inning seasons with fastballs in the upper 90s. Hudson also watched Yu Darvish and Hiroki Kuroda, because he figured Japanese pitchers threw frequently and stayed healthy. Hudson zeroed in on their pitching hand in relation to their legs and the rest of their body, pausing and rewinding, pausing and rewinding, before split-screening his iPad to compare their deliveries with his.

"And it's like, 'Jesus Christ,'" Hudson said. "Because you don't realize until you watch it slowed down." He saw how far back he reached, like his arm was being pulled in the wrong direction by some delivery devil. "I always knew how long my arm actually was," Hudson said. "You wouldn't send a video of my mechanics to a six-year-old kid learning how to pitch. I never really had pitching lessons growing up. That's what came naturally." And it worked, which is what's so bittersweet. If Hudson threw like Maddux or Nolan Ryan or any other mechanical paragon, he might not wear a scar across his elbow. He also might never have played past high school.

Hudson resigned himself to changing his mechanics because it was the easiest potential solution. Nobody could tell him whether his old ligament and new tendon were structurally weak, the result of some bad genetic luck. And while usage might have worn down his original ligament, his second, with its low odometer, went just the same. Flaws hid even among the seemingly flawless. Verlander missed the first two months of the 2015 season with arm issues and lost four miles per hour from his peak fastball, and Darvish's UCL soon blew.

What Hudson gleaned from watching translated almost immediately into an adjustment. During his throwing sessions before spring training, Hudson's arm took a less circuitous route to its loaded position. He would never throw over the top, but his hand position at release looked closer to the ideal. Crank gave him breathing exercises to build up his core. Inside the trainer's room, Crank ordered a half-dozen Diamondbacks to blow up balloons in a specific fashion that maximized their breathing. The tiniest movement patterns mattered. Hudson worked his internal oblique, the muscle that abuts the chest cavity, with nothing more than a light stretch done so much it became a part of his routine and muscle memory.

"Mechanically, the first time, I don't think he saw the need to change," Crank said. "He figured he'd get it repaired and be good. He's done a tremendous job changing where he was. I'll let you know in a year or two if it works."

Hudson tested his new delivery with Arnie on flat ground, where he could focus on its individual pieces and try to overwrite the memory embedded in his muscular and cranial hard drives. Standing ten inches up on a mound, atop the world, with someone sixty feet, six inches away, swinging a bat designed to punish pitchers who second-guessed themselves—that posed the great challenge. "We gave him one time where we kind of said, 'All right, do it your way, Huddy,' and it was pretty damn good," Arnie said. "He was ready to go back to the big leagues basically. And he blew out. Well, now we do this. Because it seemed like after one Tommy John, you might have to change."

During Hudson's rehab in 2013 and 2014, four more Diamondbacks pitchers blew out: relievers Matt Reynolds and David Hernández, and starters Bronson Arroyo and Patrick Corbin. Arroyo was the epitome of durability, a fourteen-year career without a disabled-list stint. Corbin was a mirror image of Hudson when he blew out: a twenty-four-year-old left-hander coming off a breakout second season. The injuries torpedoed Arizona and threatened the jobs of Kevin Towers and Kirk Gibson. Arizona found itself so hard-hit that a support group met daily in the trainer's room. Hudson, Reynolds, Hernández, and Corbin called themselves the UCL Club, and they spent far more time together than any would've liked, particularly Hudson, given the role that came naturally to him. "He's like the president," Reynolds said. "Grandmaster. You have questions, you go to Huddy. He knows all."

This made Hudson cringe; he preferred doling out advice on throwing changeups or approaching hitters. This was his lot, and he felt a duty to share his wisdom regarding how to deal with various Tommy John maladies, like differentiating between soreness and pain. "You get the sore days," Hudson said, "and you're like, 'Oh, no, am I broken again?' And then you come back the next day and it's fine."

UCL clubs popped up around the league, preaching that coming back from a torn elbow ligament takes far more than twelve steps. "What makes Tommy John scary is the amount of time," said Pittsburgh Pirates starter Charlie Morton, like Hudson a client of Andrew Lowenthal's and a 2012 Tommy John recipient. "The concept of a year. Being out a year, rehabbing for a whole year—that concept is overwhelming." Together Hudson and his hobbled teammates worked, laughed, struggled, and looked forward to their expulsion from membership in the UCL Club. It wasn't ideal, but it beat the loneliness of having to do it all by yourself.

SILENCE AND TODD COFFEY RARELY share the same space. There is always something to talk about, a story to relay, a question to ask, a laugh to elicit. If the shoulder internally rotates at 8,000 degrees per second, Coffey's mouth moves at least 7,999.

At three p.m. on May 14, 2014, an hour before his second showcase, Coffey vegged out inside Physiotherapy Associates in Phoenix, same as he'd done every day for more than a week. His easy smile in the days leading up to the showcase had changed into a grim countenance. Nothing—not kind words from his wife or pep talks from his agent—affected it.

"He's just extremely nervous," Jennifer said. "He's like, 'What if I throw eighty?' I'm like, 'I don't think you're going to throw eighty.'"

"If he throws eighty, I'm gonna kill him," said Rick Thurman, his agent. "That's what'll happen. He could run up to the plate faster than eighty miles per hour."

Only eight teams RSVP'd for the showcase, which meant nearly three-quarters of Coffey's potential market wanted nothing to do with him even before he threw a single pitch. Of course, it was unrealistic to have expected more after his showing four months earlier. In any case, he had willed himself to a major league career before, and he could do it again, even if under tougher circumstances.

Following a treatment on his arm using a handgun-shaped Deep Muscle Stimulator and a liberal application of Hot Cheese, Coffey slipped out the side exit of Physiotherapy, walked onto the practice field, and started a soft toss, same as he had four months earlier. His arm felt great—legitimately so, and not as the product of a wish. Manual therapy and rest had cured his leg ailment, too, leaving him without excuses. The radar gun would be his judge and jury.

Scouts from ten teams actually showed. There were contenders like St. Louis and Baltimore, also-rans like Houston and Miami. Seattle wanted depth for its young bullpen and Atlanta backfill in case of further injuries. Detroit sent two sets of eyes: Scott Reid, its scouting chieftain, and his son, Brian, a Tigers area scout. Thurman engaged the group, emphasizing that Coffey's first showcase was to show he was healthy while this one better represented what he would take into a game.

"The first time was fine," Thurman said, "but the second time is important because we want to show the progress."

"And now he needs to get some innings," Scott Reid added. "Did he just get out here today?"

"He's been here for about a week and a half," Thurman said.

Reid nodded and jotted a few notes. As other scouts did the same, Coffey finished his warm-ups and crept through the netting and back to the mound filled with bad memories. Jennifer stood in a different spot this time, closer to the scouts and their radar guns. The first number would tell the story. If it started with an eight, he might as well start studying up on go-karts. If it started with nine, he would probably have a contract signed within a week. A couple of miles an hour: the difference between needing a wealth manager and Dumpster diving.

All the scouts poised their guns. Coffey fired a sinker. Every gun read the same two digits: 91

The next pitch came in at 92. Coffey threw fourteen more sinkers, all of them 91 or 92. The sixteenth pitch had heavy, late movement at 92. "That's gonna be hard to hit," Brian Reid said. The twenty-fourth pitch was his best of the day, a hard sinker the catcher struggled to handle. Coffey threw one more pitch, a tight slider, and stepped off the mound. As the scouts put away their guns, Coffey ambled over to Jennifer and Thurman.

"Felt good," Coffey said.

"Looked good," Thurman said. "Nothing was under 91."

Coffey grinned, his arm once again an ally. The scout from Houston asked a few questions about his readiness. Others listened in. Coffey radiated confidence. "I've got to face some hitters," he said. "All I've faced is high school kids, and that's not a challenge."

The scouts packed up their radar guns and notebooks, thanked Coffey, and walked toward their cars. One hung around: Mike Fetters, the right-hand man of Kevin Towers and a longtime friend of Thurman, dating back to their days as pitchers at Pepperdine University. Fetters spent sixteen major league seasons as a relief pitcher and underwent Tommy John surgery at thirty-eight years old. He returned ten months later, fearful nobody would want a forty-year-old reliever, and lasted twenty-three appearances before retiring. He knew what a day like this meant. Fetters had postponed a lesson with some Phoenix-area kids at Physiotherapy to watch the showcase.

With a handful of quality big league relievers, plus Daniel Hudson nearing a return, Fetters didn't think the Diamondbacks were a fit. He promised to pass along a report to Towers, anyway. "I've got to get going," Fetters said. "Got some young kids in there. Got to develop some young Todd Coffeys."

Once Fetters left, Coffey started to wonder whether there would be more teams like Arizona, happy enough with their bullpens to pass on him. "We're gonna get calls," Thurman reassured him. "You'll be fine, Todd." Coffey wanted to know where he might end up. "Braves," Thurman said. "But don't be surprised if Seattle makes a strong push. Their guy was here. I know him pretty well. He's brother-in-laws with my next-door neighbor."

"I can't handle much more of this waiting," Coffey said, and he wouldn't have to. Over the next few days, he would know which teams were feigning interest and which were serious, which were offering the best opportunities and the most money, which uniform he would wear when he sprinted in and finally did his 360.

Coffey and Jennifer jumped into their rental car, hooked a left out of the parking lot, and headed to the hotel, their first stop on his way back to the major leagues. He talked the whole ride.

AROUND THE SEVENTH MONTH OF her pregnancy, when the rigors of carrying a child during a Phoenix summer started to take a toll on her psyche as well as her body, Sara Hudson just wanted a little old-fashioned romance.

"Dan," Sara said, "how come you never stare at my eyes?"

"Because," Daniel Hudson said, "your jugs are huge right now."

She playfully slugged him and laughed. Romance might be missing, but Hudson's sense of humor—one of the reasons Sara fell in love with him in the first place—had returned after going AWOL for a couple of years. He tore his UCL the first time while they were still newlyweds, but their marriage had been tested by his being home twenty hours a day. The second surgery had solidified it. "You can't do anything," Sara said of the first post-op period. "You can't go bowling. You can't go golfing. You can't do anything physically active. So we go from not seeing each other at all to me washing his balls. This is the shit that you save for eighty years old."

Gone, finally, was the tension of uncertainty. Sara could laugh again at Hudson's overreactions, like when a dab of butter from a mishandled bagel ended up on his shirt and he went on an obscene minute-long rant. He rejoined her more fully in the marriage. "It's not about you anymore," Sara said. "You've got a kid on the way to feed. And a bitchy, pregnant wife."

Hudson took the one-day-at-a-time vow by which so many other athletes profess to live. It's a throwaway cliché for someone who hasn't slaved through the same rehab for two consecutive years. For Hudson, it was literal. If he felt anything in his arm, he stopped throwing immediately. No sense in pushing himself when his pace already more than halved Doug Brocail's return time. Between his cardio work and his improved breathing from the techniques and stretches Crank taught him, Hudson felt better than he had in years. He even stopped playing his avatar in the baseball video game, faux glory unnecessary when the real stuff was that much closer.

"I guess I'm just being smarter about it," Hudson said. "I can't mentally do this again. I'm to the point now where if this shit doesn't work this time, I'm basically done. I'm going to ride this one out until it goes again. And hopefully it doesn't. Maybe I have that thought in my mind, and I'm trying to get my body and mind stronger for this run."

Normalcy returned as Hudson's life got crazier. He and Sara looked after the neighbors' kids as practice. They found time to go to a weekly trivia contest at a local bar with friends. On the ride home one night, Hudson started talking about how excited he was, how great his arm felt that day throwing changeups off flat ground.

"I don't know what the fuck he's talking about," Sara said. "I know nothing about baseball. But to see his face light up excited me. I think he's so Zen about it this time because he feels really good. He's really confident with his doctor, the fact that he's with the same training staff he loves. I just think he feels really, really good." In mid-July, after Sara had spent all week calling the hospital to push up her elective induction, it finally found room to squeeze her in. She and Hudson ran home and packed their wares. By midnight, the Pitocin drip started. The contractions came on strong, and when Sara asked for an epidural, the anesthesiologist was assisting with a C-section and couldn't come for an hour. "That, honestly, was the most helpless feeling of my life," Hudson said. "You can't do anything except sit there and watch her go through this pain. Literally the only thing I could do was hold her hand. Every forty-five seconds to a minute, she's squeezing the shit out of it."

Once the drugs hit, Sara and Hudson snuck in an hour of sleep. When they woke up around five thirty a.m. on July 17, Hudson said he wanted to jump in the shower. Sara told him to hurry up. "I thought she was kidding around," Hudson said. She wasn't. Three minutes of pushing, and out came Baylor Rae Hudson, 20¾ inches long, 7 pounds, 4.4 ounces, the most beautiful girl Daniel Hudson ever had seen. He held her and everything else vanished.

"You just think about the shit we've gone through for the past two years," Hudson said. "I don't want to say it was worth it, but you forget about it for a while."

This was a crucial juncture in his rehab, and he paid it no

mind. His elbow, the object of his attention and affection for far too long, could wait. Hudson first needed to learn how to hold Baylor when feeding her and inure himself to nights filled with sleeplessness. The mystery of the swaddle confounded him. "It looks so easy," he said. "Why can't I do that?"

Being a dad suited Hudson well. Everything his elbow had taught him—the discipline, the diligence, the prioritizing—seemed to prepare him for this. Hudson developed a guardedness to keep him from planning too far ahead. Even when something was good, it couldn't be too good. "Everything's kind of looking up right now," Hudson said. "I don't know if something bad is supposed to happen."

TODD COFFEY, CEASELESSLY UPBEAT, DIDN'T know what to do and started to panic. Choices are supposed to be good things, rich with possibility. Coffey worried he was making the wrong one.

He had convinced himself he would return from his Tommy John surgery within a year, and that didn't happen, and then a 1.5-centimeter intruder squatted in his elbow, and that waylaid his plans, and then he insisted on throwing in his first showcase, and that bombed, and now two teams with almost the exact same offers wanted him.

Coffey cared about only one thing: "Fastest to the big leagues is all that matters." But he had no idea whether his path was clearer with the Atlanta Braves or the Seattle Mariners. Both teams contacted Rick Thurman almost immediately after Coffey's showcase and said they were preparing contract offers. The first official offer arrived in Thurman's in-box from Braves assistant GM Bruce Manno. The terms were straightforward: Start at Triple-A Gwinnett, in the Atlanta area, and make $15,000 a month. A promotion to the major leagues bumps the salary to a prorated $750,000, with performance bonuses for appearances starting around thirty games.

The next afternoon, Seattle assistant GM Jeff Kingston sent Thurman a more thorough proposal, even though the minor league and major league salaries were the same. The Mariners gave Coffey out clauses—dates he could opt out of the contract and become a free agent for any reason—on June 30 and July 31. Kingston outlined the pitchers currently in the Mariners' bullpen as well as their arms at Triple-A, separated into pitchers on the forty-man roster and nonroster players. The pitchers on the forty-man could be called up at any time, whereas a nonroster player—as Coffey would be in Seattle and Atlanta—must overachieve to merit an eventual roster spot.

"The nonrosters [sic] guys have been ok but none have been lights out," Kingston wrote. "Todd could easily put himself at the top of the list if he comes in and pitches the way he has when healthy."

This sounded like what he wanted, and doubts about Atlanta lingered. "If you look at the Braves bullpen," Coffey said, "it just looks . . . stacked." Craig Kimbrel was the best closer in baseball. Two other Braves relievers sported ERAs in the twos. Rookie David Hale was in the midst of a scoreless streak that would span all of May. Setup man Jordan Walden soon would return from the disabled list.

Six hundred eighty-seven days after his UCL blew out, Todd Coffey signed with the Seattle Mariners. "Is this the right choice?" he asked. Only if someone on the Mariners' roster got injured, a cruel fate he knew all too well.

On May 21, 2014, Coffey packed a suitcase, placed his glove into its special suitcase, and decamped to Phoenix. His first day at the Mariners' spring-training complex in Peoria, Arizona, included X-rays on his elbow and shoulder; both checked out fine. When he put on a nameless, numberless jersey, it felt better than a Savile Row suit. "To put a uniform on. To finally feel like a baseball player again," Coffey said. "That felt awesome."

Later that week, Coffey drove to the stadium at six a.m. for his first game. He beat up an elliptical machine for forty minutes, did ab work, and strengthened his arm with rubber tubing. He faced rookie-ball kids from the Cincinnati Reds. He was one of them once, young and not very good, and he looked every bit the big leaguer comparatively. The first hitter struck out on three pitches. The next two broke their bats on sinkers that tore in at 94 miles per hour. The adrenaline of a game increased his velocity, which held steady in his next outing two days later, when he pitched two perfect innings and broke four bats against kids from the Milwaukee Brewers.

"Bet you money before the season's out I'll hit 88 on a slider again," Coffey said. "And I guarantee I'll hit 96 before the season's over. Here's the thing. My arm's only going to get stronger when I throw more. I told Dr. ElAttrache how my first game was. And he said you're going to gain one to two the next month, month and a half, just from throwing hard in games."

On May 29, Coffey left for Tacoma, Washington, home of the Mariners' Triple-A affiliate. The Mariners vowed to ease him in. No back-to-back games for a couple of weeks. One inning at a time. All building up to his first opt-out on June 30. Coffey hoped his arm would make it moot, that Seattle would see him fit for the big leagues and bring him thirty-five minutes up Interstate 5 to Safeco Field.

"If in a month they don't have a spot for me and I'm pitching good, I know quite a few other teams," Coffey said. "It's all in my hands. Finally. It's all been on how quick my arm gets better. I don't have any second guesses. I think the opportunity to get to the big leagues with the Braves would have been a lot longer."

Coffey pitched his first game for Tacoma on May 31. That day, in Atlanta, the Braves promoted Shae Simmons, a hard-throwing twenty-three-year-old from Double-A Mississippi. One Braves official, asked why the team chose Simmons when they could have kept him off the major league roster for at least another year, said: "Because Todd Coffey signed somewhere else."

CHAPTER 13

The Swamp of Possible Solutions

WITH A PROBLEM THIS ACUTE, with this much money at stake, I figured doctors, biomechanists, and others from the academic world would find themselves at the cutting edge of research into how to save the arm. Instead, I found a swamp. All you need to be a pitching guru is a cell phone to take videos, some cursory web-design knowledge, and search-engine optimization skills. The arm-care business is massive and potentially worth billions, and some of its most visible names and voices know more about marketing than science. It's easy to take advantage of parents who listen to anyone promising to keep their son healthy, even if it means throwing plastic bucket lids and wearing thick, duct-taped wrist weights.

Dr. Mike Marshall, once the best reliever in baseball and the 1974 National League Cy Young winner, actually does live near a swamp, in tiny Zephyrhills, Florida, where I first met him in 2007 at his pitching compound. It was a ratty old place, though the faith that emanated from it was infectious. About a dozen young men used to pay ten dollars a day for on-site housing and another ten dollars to learn how to throw a baseball from Marshall, whom everyone at the facility called Doc. They believed in him, despite baseball's overwhelming skepticism toward his methods.

Today, Marshall is seventy-three years old, his body slowing, all the way down to the atrophied muscle between his thumb and index finger. His 106 games and 208⅓ innings pitched during the 1974 season for the Los Angeles Dodgers remain records for relievers, each less likely to be broken than Joe DiMaggio's hitting streak. Barely five feet eight, Marshall had pain in his right throwing shoulder following his rookie season in 1967. He wanted to understand why, so he used high-speed video to analyze his delivery well before doing so became standard practice, spent his offseasons at Michigan State earning a doctorate in exercise physiology, and built a philosophy that has endured for almost half a century.

Marshall took the pitching delivery and blew it up. What he spawned was so unorthodox an approach, so far afield from what baseball pitchers were supposed to look like, that no matter how biomechanically sound—no matter how many injuries it may have prevented—nobody would ever adopt it.

Even Marshall admits that the delivery won't win any awards for aesthetics. It starts with feet parallel and belt buckle facing the catcher. A right-hander starts his arms together above his head, then drops his pitching arm straight down. As he brings it up directly behind him—"Pendulum-swinging," as Marshall calls it, "eliminates Tommy John surgery"—the pitcher steps with his left foot to about 10 o'clock. He wills his pitching arm straight up, with zero external rotation, then starts to heavily pronate it, using the forearm muscles to turn the ball over as he half jumps off his back leg and whips his body around to face first base.

Baseball misfits ended up training with Doc. This was last-resort-type stuff for the injured, whom he promised to nurse back to health, and the velocity-deficient, to whom he promised another ten miles per hour. In the mornings, before their throwing sessions, the students strapped ten-, twenty-, even thirty-pound cuffs onto their wrists to practice pronating and build their arm muscles. They threw with six-pound iron balls. Marshall even made them throw footballs and weighted lids from four-gallon drums to simulate the release of the curveball he wanted to teach them.

His best students were a flameout named Jeff Sparks, who used a Marshall-style delivery, and a longtime reliever named Rudy Seanez, who threw traditionally and spent only a short portion of his career under Marshall's tutelage. Otherwise, it was kids looking to play low-level college ball or maybe get recruited to go somewhere bigger or land in independent ball. In 2008, Tommy John, one of Marshall's old friends from his Dodgers days and then the manager of the Atlantic League's Bridgeport Bluefish, invited two of Doc's best pitchers to spring training.

"There wasn't any harm in bringing them in," John said. "Kinesiologically, physiologically, it's probably correct. But you would need fifty years of everybody throwing like that to get into the game. It's so different from what's done that baseball establishment won't allow it. So every kid would have to throw like Mike wants them to."

No Marshall-style pitcher ever sat at 95 miles per hour and wowed scouts. Nobody who already threw 95 was willing to completely subvert his game in an effort to validate some mad scientist. So after years of publicly criticizing conventional pitching motions, Marshall took what amounted to the Pepsi Challenge in 2008: he brought his four best pitchers to Birmingham and had Glenn Fleisig run his typical biomechanical testing on them to see how their objective markers compared with the traditional method.

The results: Marshall's method "produced similar shoulder and elbow torques, but significantly less ball velocity" than "elite traditional pitchers." Compared with others throwing at the same velocity, the Marshall pitchers' joints were far more stressed. Marshall took exception to Fleisig's findings, using his blog to drop an almost nine thousand–word refutation of the study's methodology, which ended: "That is all I can think of, for now."

Over the next four years, self-styled pitching gurus hawked their methods on the web while Doc's site looked like an old Geocities page. None of his competitors boasted a doctorate like Marshall. Few bothered with legitimate research. All they needed to do was trick Google's algorithms into thinking they were experts. That's a game Marshall refused to play, and in 2012 he shut down his academy, the frustration of rejection too strong. Marshall still believes he can end all pitching injuries. It's just that nobody will listen to him.

I swung by Zephyrhills again in 2013 to see the fallout from two decades of proselytizing to skeptics. As he sipped a drink on his patio, Marshall lifted his right arm, revealing a scar that ran along the inside of his elbow. I didn't think he had ever needed surgery. He started to explain the one drawback to a pitching motion with excessive pronation: it can wear out the ulnar nerve. The atrophy between his thumb and index finger happened because of it. The solution, Marshall explained, was simple: when a pitcher showed professional potential, he would go in for surgery to transpose the ulnar nerve.

It took a second to process what Marshall was saying: in order to pitch in a fashion that he believes helps avoid Tommy John surgery, he suggested a pitcher undergo another kind of surgery— one that, with even slight complications, could leave a person permanently disabled.

"It's ironic, I guess," Marshall said. "But I've said since even back in the sixties that the ulnar nerve is the contraindication, and we have to recognize that. We're going to move the nerve on the inside, and it'll never have a problem. But that's trivial. When I went in and had the surgery, I was in for less than a half hour and was able to go to dinner and a movie with my wife that night."

Never, right up to the end, would he settle on anything less than the full Marshall delivery. There was no compromise in Doc. It made him who he was. And wasn't.

"If you're a guru on anything, I think you need to be careful," said Brent Strom, the Astros' pitching coach. "Because what you'll have is gurus clashing with each other. I think if we keep in mind that we don't fall into the trap that 'my mind is made up, don't confuse me with the facts,' I think we're better off. Because we're going to continue to evolve and see what works best.

"There's a lot of charlatans out there."

OVER THE COURSE OF THREE years, I encountered plenty of people who believed they could help solve the scourge of Tommy John surgery, and one of the most vociferous was named Dr. Tommy John.

He was born Thomas Edward John III on September 27, 1977, almost three years to the day after his father's procedure, the eldest son of Sally and Tommy John, whose second career meant little Tommy got to hang out with Don Mattingly, Rickey Henderson, and other New York Yankees luminaries. He was a standout high schooler in Minnesota, played college ball at Furman, and parlayed a health and exercise science degree into a job as a personal trainer. Over time, as he worked toward his doctor of chiropractic, John started to champion his ability—anyone's ability, really—to avoid the surgery named after his father. "That's the big thing," he said. "I want to prevent the cutting."

The pitching subculture on the Internet works like this: Academic types commission studies and use data to construct hypotheses and test, test, test. Mechanics wonks believe in the purity of the perfect throw, their faith rooted in kinesiological principles.

Charlatans theorize and yell the loudest, research and physiology be damned. The discussions, debates, and disagreements in online forums grow heated, a sign of how imperative the issue is to baseball as well as the levels of self-importance and delusion that percolate throughout the subculture.

Tommy John III is far from a big name. Scott Kazmir and Barry Zito parlayed time at Ron Wolforth's Texas Baseball Ranch into revitalized major league careers and helped turn it into a cash cow. Much of what Wolforth teaches—the value of tempo, the use of weighted balls, mechanical efficiencies, and the importance of intent to throw, or getting in a ready position early and with a purpose—came from a man named Paul Nyman. He quit baseball for years, like Marshall frustrated that others got the attention he felt due him. Nyman didn't want to be Nikola Tesla, the genius bound to be appreciated only after he's gone.

Nobody could say for certain who in the swamp was right. For years, Alan Jaeger, a yoga-practicing Taoist, has tried to convince me the key to arm health is in extreme long toss, whereby pitchers throw baseballs on an arc up to four hundred feet to build arm strength. When I asked for evidence, he provided data he keeps. When I told him it's biased, he chuckled and said I'll see that he's right someday. Paul Davis, the Cardinals' pitching analytics coordinator, suggested I call an Arkansas-based CPA named Lloyd Lee. "He's the smartest person in the world when it comes to the arm," Davis said, and I scoffed for a moment before remembering that the smartest person in the world when it came to baseball statistics was a security guard at a pork-and-beans factory. Once Bill James got a voice, he changed the game.

So I figured it couldn't hurt to hear out Tommy John III. He brought a bit of everything to his philosophy, minus the pretense of most who built their businesses around teaching proper throwing mechanics. John wanted to heal. Much of his work existed in the alternative-medicine space he occupies, without significant clinical research to support his theories. He believed in brain-body symbiosis and how something as simple as cross-crawl patterning—moving the arms and legs in the same fashion as babies—was integral in creating the sort of healthy movement patterns he sought.

He sounded like a quack, the very last person who could save an arm, especially when I asked how he did it. "What I do is a form of direct current therapy," he said. "It's electricity." He uses a machine called the ARPwave, a small, portable device with a power switch, a knob, and two output cords with pads that sit on the skin. ARP stands for Accelerated Recovery Performance, and the ARPwave purports to use electrical current to shock muscles into high-velocity contractions that strengthen them. Some call it a scam, others a miracle device.

When John suggested the therapy to a high school junior named Jared Martin, the seventeen-year-old blanched. Martin was a catcher at Dunwoody High, about twenty miles outside Atlanta, and John was the school's conditioning coach. When Martin's elbow started hurting, he saw an orthopedic surgeon in Atlanta who recommended Tommy John surgery. His parents sought a second opinion, taking Martin to Birmingham to visit James Andrews. He diagnosed a partially torn UCL and told Martin he could try rest and rehab or get the surgery and miss a year.

Martin agreed to try John's protocol. John ran the pad along Martin's arm, searching for "hot spots," or areas of particular weakness. He targeted muscles in the flexor-pronator mass, turned on the machine, and watched Martin writhe.

"It felt like I was getting electrocuted," Martin said. "He would hit a spot down on my forearm, nowhere near the UCL, and I'd have the most unbelievable pain. He'd say, 'Here's the hot spot.' I can't even describe the pain I felt when he hit the hot spot. I told him I didn't know if I could do it. He was sitting there by my side the whole time, motivating me."

Two or three times a week, John used the ARPwave on

Martin. The elbow pain lessened. A rehab plan mapped out by John complemented the ARPwave sessions, and after four months Martin's arm felt good enough to visit the orthopedic surgeon in Atlanta for a follow-up appointment. The results of an imaging test shocked even Martin: the damage to his UCL was gone. John believed that by strengthening the muscles around the UCL and allowing inflammation to promote healing, he fixed it without so much as touching a scalpel.

"The doctors [in Atlanta] had no idea what happened," Martin said. "It was magic. No one believes me."

He wants to believe it was the machine. Not the time off. Not the rest. Not the other rehab exercises. There are no studies on the efficacy of the ARPwave, nothing to back up its claims aside from unverifiable anecdotes and cases with no control to isolate what really promoted the most healing. Other electrical-stimulation devices regularly adorn pitchers' arms in clubhouses after outings to encourage blood flow. Never had I heard anyone suggest it can mend the UCL, and the idea of a ligament healing on account of the muscles around it growing stronger does not compute.

"I really think that if the ligament healed, it healed by the natural processes of the body," said Dr. Chris McKenzie, a physical therapist who trains baseball players in the Philadelphia area. "[ARPwave] is no different than most stim machines. Nothing I have learned, and nothing that any reliable medical professional would say, would show that it can fix a ligament. There's no evidence out there to support that. It's pretty much just complete crap."

In 2014, ARPwave sent a unit to McKenzie, which he tested on two people with soreness on the inside of their elbow. He jumped on a Skype call with an ARPwave protocol specialist who gave specific directions on where to place the electrodes. After the session, the patients were asked if they felt any better. One said no. The other said a little bit. Then, after the Skype call hung up, the patient confessed to McKenzie that he felt nothing except pain. He just didn't want to hurt the ARPwave specialist's feelings.

Whatever caused the healing mattered not to Martin. He could play baseball. After a stint in junior college, he joined the University of South Carolina baseball team, one of the country's finest programs, without another visit to an orthopedist. "It's gotten sore every now and again," Martin said, "but I've never really had bad arm pain since." If ever anyone asks, Martin plays evangelist for the ARPwave. "I still try to tell people," he said, "and they don't believe me and have Tommy John surgery right away."

One rehab clinic in Dallas claims to have saved more than forty kids from Tommy John surgery using the ARPwave, and Dr. John swears by it. He also makes rehabilitating adults crawl on the floor and believes the body can be trained to withstand between seven hundred and nine hundred throws every day. He sounds like the classic charlatan until Jared Martin flips the narrative and provides the sort of triumph rare for baseball today: a partially torn UCL that didn't necessitate Tommy John surgery.

I don't know if the ARPwave is just another machine that leeches thousands of dollars out of patients or one that can replace platelet-rich plasma therapy as the go-to method to help damaged but still intact UCLs. For his varying philosophies, Dr. Tommy John is unquestionably right about one thing: he believes the human body is a sublime creation capable of the seemingly impossible. That idea comes from wisdom passed along by his father. Tommy John's curiosity and courage live on not just in the scars of elbows across the sport he loves but in the mind of a son who tries to do the same thing as another doctor he knew well: help people.

TWICE A WEEK FOR SEVERAL years, an eighty-eight-year-old man with a full head of white hair, tinted eyeglasses, and a welcom-

ing smile used to pull up in a car to the Kerlan-Jobe Orthopaedic Clinic. Frank Jobe couldn't stay away from the building with
his name on it. He parked himself on a bench near the facility's
front entrance and said hello to everyone who walked by before
retreating to the lunchroom, where he regaled his dining com-
panions with stories.

One of Jobe's favorites involved the trespassers in his backyard
in Brentwood. They'd come for more than twenty years, arriv-
ing at all hours of the night with metal detectors and flashlights
and magnifying glasses, hunting and snooping and skulking along
the ground. None ever found the prize: a murder weapon. Jobe's
house happened to back up to 360 N. Rockingham Ave., the address of O. J. Simpson.

Doctors sat rapt listening to Jobe the raconteur, almost as good
as Jobe the orthopedist. To them, he was a demigod because of
Tommy John surgery, today still the crowning achievement in all
of sports medicine. It was the big bang of the arm, the moment
that gave life to limbs without any, and the appreciation of Jobe
from medical offices to clubhouses multiplied even after he retired from active practice at eighty-three.

Every biomechanics obsessive wants to do for baseball's future
what Jobe did for its past. During retirement, the credit due Jobe
finally started to find him. Before a game at Dodger Stadium
in 2012, Tommy John stood on the mound, ready to throw out
the first pitch, when he signaled for a new pitcher. Over walked
Jobe, still John's closer decades later. "Thank you, Dr. Jobe," John
said. A year later, they saw one another again in Cooperstown,
New York, home of the National Baseball Hall of Fame, which
honored Jobe's career during induction weekend. John sat in the
audience that day.

"We did a little surgery, but the man did all the hard work,"
Jobe said in his speech. "His tenacity and unique intelligence enabled us to develop the rehab program that has lasted the test of
time. We all worked together and as a result, Tommy returned

and played fourteen years without missing a start and he won 164 games after returning from his surgery."

This was the Frank and Tommy show, both of them modest and deferential to the end. As confusion about the arm endangered baseball, they were proof that progress is not a dead end. Every day, Todd Coffey and Daniel Hudson and thousands of other pitchers from high school to the major leagues were performing a series of strengthening exercises developed by Jobe and physical therapist Diane Radovich Moynes. Officially, they're called the Thrower's Ten, but everyone knows them by another name: "Jobes."

Mostly they focus on the shoulder, and it was Jobe's obsession with strengthening it that helped revolutionize the maintenance and care of the arm. The unintended consequence, of course, left baseball in its current place. "We do such a good job with the shoulder," Jobe said, "that it ends up hurting the elbow."

John's left shoulder never bothered him until a few years back, when pain from arthritis seared through it. Before he went in for an MRI, John's agent, Kim Berger, wondered if the technician might pan down. No one ever had seen an image of the most famous elbow in the world. John picked two still pictures, mounted them side-by-side, added photos of himself and Jobe, and sent Jobe a hundred copies to sign. Today, they sell for $1,295 a pop. The proceeds, John said, go to the Let's Do It Foundation, named after the words he once uttered in his most desperate moment. "If I had any idea it would've been this big," John said, "I would've trademarked the surgery and had all those SOBs pay me."

Unless Tommy John's son or anyone else invents a more successful procedure, he will have to settle for the unpaid prestige of having a more lasting influence on baseball than most players in Cooperstown. It's a burdensome honor, too, since the last two words baseball players the world over ever want to hear themselves utter are "Tommy John."

The stigma doesn't do justice to the miracle it was, one that Tommy John and Frank Jobe celebrated whenever possible. Chance brought the two together in January 2014 at the Humana Challenge, a golf tournament in California that John attended as a fan and Jobe as emeritus physician for the PGA Tour. A mutual acquaintance told Jobe that John was in town, and Jobe relayed a message: "You'd better get your butt up here." John rushed up to the rehabilitation trailer and gave his old friend a hug. Jobe looked frail to John. They spoke for ninety minutes, traded stories, mostly the same ones they'd laughed about for years. When John said good-bye, he made sure to take a mental snapshot of his old friend.

Six weeks later, on March 10, 2014, Frank Jobe died. Nearly every obituary included Tommy John's name in the first paragraph.

"We're going to be identified together for the rest of our lives," Jobe once told me, and though John's name will live on for time immemorial, Jobe remains a constant source of inspiration in a place that matters even more: the part of the swamp that eschews the marketing for the sort of pure, fact-based science Jobe himself practiced.

FROM THE THIRTY-FIRST FLOOR OF 245 Park Avenue, the world looks like one giant possibility. Major League Baseball's offices sit almost smack-dab in the middle of Manhattan, surrounded by progress and innovation, but baseball is a reactionary business, as was never more evident than during a conference call in the spring of 2014, when, from his office in Milwaukee, commissioner Bud Selig demanded action on the elbow issue: "I want you to do something about it," he said.

Over the previous few weeks, Selig and his eventual successor, Rob Manfred, heard from Atlanta Braves president John Schuerholz, whose opinion Selig held in the highest regard. Over a four-

day span in March, Schuerholz saw 40 percent of his rotation vanish due to Tommy John surgery. Kris Medlen underwent a second Tommy John, just three and a half years after his first. Brandon Beachy hadn't thrown a single pitch between his first Tommy John and the revision twenty-one months later. Schuerholz, the architect of the Braves dynasty led by two paragons of durability, Greg Maddux and Tom Glavine, called upon Selig and Manfred to use baseball's resources and figure out how to stop it.

Chris Marinak had been girding for this moment for five years. Marinak is Major League Baseball's senior vice president of league economics and strategy. He is thirty-five, tall, with an executive's head of hair and a mind to match. After he graduated from the University of Virginia, Marinak spent four years at Capital One working as a data-analytics manager before grabbing an MBA at Harvard and joining baseball's labor-relations department. He earned a reputation as someone who could be trusted on big projects, and this particular one was a doozy: he wanted to create a massive database of standardized health records that extended from the major leagues to the lowest level of the minors. Marinak understood the best chance baseball had at preventing injuries was stopping them before they happened, and the quickest path involved towers of data and the possibilities inside them.

Starting in 2009, Marinak oversaw the construction of baseball's Health and Injury Tracking System, or HITS, an electronic medical records system that logs everything from icing an arm or swallowing an Aleve to full MRIs or biomechanical analyses. Teams used to keep medical data on paper. When a deal was in the works, teams would FedEx reams of records to their trade partner. Now it would be as easy as a click.

Marinak's aspirations for the system were far bigger than convenience. He wanted to truly comprehend complicated injuries. At its finest, HITS could help answer a question Marinak has been asking himself since he was a teenager: Why does this happen? Playing elite baseball as a kid, Marinak's elbow hurt. Doctors di-

agnosed a bone spur when he was fourteen and told him to keep
pitching. The discomfort was a constant companion, all the way
through his four years pitching at UVa. He considered surgery but
thought better. "Sitting out for a year with no guarantee of return
seemed like a lot to sacrifice, especially if you weren't on track to
make millions in the future," Marinak said. "I pitched through
it, but it definitely held me back at points pitching through pain."

The pain only heightened his curiosity. Surely others hurt in
the same areas he did. What were their symptoms? Or their usage
patterns? Or the angle of their shoulder at maximum external
rotation? These were all measurable with a visit to the trainer,
some good bookkeeping, or a biomechanical analysis. And with
240 minor league teams on top of the 30 in the major leagues,
that would be more than three thousand pitching samples a year.
Some would flame out, but plenty would last multiple years,
giving Major League Baseball a longitudinal set of data. With
that, the possibilities were endless, the knowledge limitless.

When devising HITS, Marinak called Dr. Keshia Pollack, an
associate professor at the Johns Hopkins Center for Injury Research and Policy. Pollack was an epidemiologist, sniffing out patterns that lead to disease or injury. She would study everything
from military vehicle crashes to obesity in the African American
community, and Marinak asked her to consider diversifying her
scope of practice by studying a multibillion-dollar industry and
helping fix it.

Involving epidemiologists to assess the arm was vital. No individual team had cracked the injury code. Marinak's time in data
analytics taught him that the right people can move mountains
with numbers. Major League Baseball was the perfect subject
to study. Once the union signed off—the prospect of baseball
using the data or findings to punish players financially was out-
weighed by the potential benefits of finding a solution to arm
issues—Pollack and her colleague Dr. Frank Curriero had a seven
thousand–subject population.

Even one year's worth of data immediately changed the way baseball operated. In the program's pilot season, Marinak and his team focused on concussions. Though football's concussion issues dwarf those of Major League Baseball, Marinak figured any head trauma warrants a better understanding. Baseball tracked 190 concussions that season between the major and minor leagues and found that roughly half of the cases returned in seven days or fewer. Rather than force teams to place players with mild brain injuries on the fifteen-day disabled list or return them to action prematurely, Major League Baseball created the seven-day disabled list for concussions in 2011.

"This is probably one of the richest data sets I've experienced in my public health career here," said Curriero, who joined Pollack on the baseball project in 2012. "I would always err on the side of wanting more information than less. You just need to suspend the time and effort to go through it."

After suggesting the concussion DL, Pollack and Curriero studied the most common injury in baseball—the strained hamstring—and found the vast majority occur within the season's first six weeks. Teams instituted protocols during spring training to promote hamstring health, and the number of injuries fell immediately. That, Pollack said, is the objective: "Take data, change policy, and make the environment safer." While Curriero, a biostatistician by training, specializes in mapping data and finding geographic cues—do hamstring strains really happen more in cold-weather cities?—Pollack takes macro approaches in how to promote secure and healthy workplaces, a goal that sounds better suited for a widget plant than a field in which the average worker makes more than $4 million a year.

What made HITS tantalizing was its ability to transform data into change. So many potential advances in the knowledge of the arm were purely theoretical, rooted more in belief than science, and here Marinak was hoarding a mother lode of fact. It was a fact, for example, that right before Daniel Hudson flew to Jacksonville for the rehab start after his first surgery, Ken Crenshaw's note in HITS said: "Feeling good this a.m., played catch with no issues. Flying to Jacksonville to make rehab start with Mobile. Seven innings, 80 to 85 pitches."

I looked over Marinak's shoulder in his office at 245 Park as he scrolled through Hudson's file. It was about a month after his second surgery, and there were already 272 notes related to his elbow alone. The ones with yellow flags came from Crenshaw's almost-daily updates and the blue flags from diagnostic tests. Green flags indicated doctors' reports, like the one Dr. Michael Lee filed after Hudson's second blowout.

"Unfortunately, showed a complete proximal tear of his UCL graft," Lee wrote. "The chance of him returning to play is high but is not guaranteed. Somewhere between 75 and 80 percent. Recovery time will be extensive, up to one year or longer as well, and there is no guarantee."

Marinak shook his head. Pitchers never lose sympathy for their brethren.

"The question is, 'What do you then do with that?'" he said. "You have to have some sort of hypothesis, like, OK, guys are pitching too much in the minor leagues or pitching too much from year to year or not doing the right training program or you don't have the right mechanics." None of this will reveal itself anytime soon, surely not like the concussion DL conclusion. With another decade's worth of data, Marinak figures, complemented by the right sorts of studies, maybe baseball will find an answer or two. And once that reveals itself, it will take time, baseball being baseball, to implement any changes.

He typed in 841.1—the medical code for an ulnar collateral ligament sprain—and clicked Run. Marinak exported the data to Excel, opened the file, and started reading numbers.

Six hundred fifty-eight. That was the number of players across all levels of professional baseball from the beginning of 2010 to the middle of 2013 with UCL sprains—ligament tears of any kind, from slight to full. The number of days lost on the disabled list to UCL sprains—145,824—averaged 221 per player. Hundreds of millions of dollars in salary, and even more in surplus value, vanished.

When Bud Selig and John Schuerholz and so many others in baseball wanted solutions now, Marinak told them the truth: They're not coming, not for a while. Finding hope in this environment requires optimism on the level of Todd Coffey. "I think it's more about creating the community," Marinak said. "Creating the people to come together to find the insight."

Before spring training in 2015, Major League Baseball and the MLB Players Association agreed to a landmark project: For the next five years, the New York Yankees, the New York Mets, and three other teams would participate in a study of all their pitchers from the 2014 draft class. They would undergo biomechanical analysis, reveal as much detail as possible about their history in youth baseball, and serve as a pilot program for vast data-gathering that soon enough could be standard across the sport.

The class of 2014 study allows Pollack and Currrero to watch in real time the ascent and breakdown of players. It fills in the context that the trove of HITS data lacks. Combine the two—a wide swath of well-documented subjects and a smaller, intensely followed group—and Pollack is not shy with her intentions.

"What I'm comfortable saying," she said, "is that I would be confident we can make significant positive public health progress into this injury." Translation: if she can't fix UCLs tearing everywhere, she can at very least provide better ideas as to why they're tearing. The ball is then back in Major League Baseball and Marinak's court. He plays policymaker, and his answer to Bud Selig's plea to fix the elbow started not with major league players but with players at the lowest levels possible.

On November 11, 2014, Major League Baseball launched Pitch Smart, a website dedicated to educating coaches, parents, and children about the dangers lurking within the arm. The slick production includes sections offering an age-appropriate pitch-count chart, a Tommy John FAQ, and a list of taboos. Almost all of the recommendations stemmed from a 2012 study from ASMI's Glenn Fleisig published in the journal *Sports Health*. Almost everything on the website points to usage. Regularly pitching while fatigued left kids thirty-six times more susceptible to arm injuries. Children who throw more than one hundred innings a year are three and a half times likelier to get hurt. Even though no studies concluded definitively that preteen curveballs were bad for the arm, Dr. James Andrews urged in a video on the Pitch Smart website, "Don't throw a curveball until you shave." Andrews's folksy chestnuts were everywhere on the site, and they appealed intentionally to an underappreciated group: moms. "Sometimes," Andrews wrote, "the only person they will complain to about having a painful shoulder or painful elbow is their mother."

By targeting the youth system, baseball was issuing a warning that over the next decade it intends to reappropriate the sport at all levels. "So many of these youth organizations are very much mom-and-pop-type places," Marinak said. "That's where we need to start educating and convincing them this is good for present and future. And that's not even to consider these travel-ball-type teams."

Perfect Game, the fulcrum of the showcase circuit, pledged to follow the Pitch Smart pitch-count recommendations almost immediately. Its commitment gave Major League Baseball the use of the recognizable PG logo, the one Perfect Game wanted to be as ubiquitous as Nike's. The league, hopeful that Pitch Smart could evolve from a slick PSA into an influential program, needed all the support it could get, even if it came from a company with a hand in the problem.

"There's a lot of catching up to do," Marinak said. Baseball's $10 billion industry can't allow Perfect Game's $15 million business to continue threatening it. It needs educated, forward-thinking scientists to build a culture of knowledge instead of a culture of fear. Because that's exactly what the charlatans use to ensnare their prey.

LATE AT NIGHT, WHEN THE rest of his family was asleep, Ed Harvey surfed the Internet looking for tips and tricks to teach the kids he coached at Fitch High School in Groton, Connecticut. One night, trawling a message board, he stumbled upon a poster named Chris O'Leary, who ran his own website dedicated to hitting and pitching mechanics. Harvey clicked, liked what he saw, and navigated to a link that said: "Baseball Pitcher Evaluations." For twenty dollars, O'Leary would give a thumbs-up, thumbs-down analysis. For forty dollars, he offered a detailed write-up. And for a hundred dollars, the deluxe: a frame-by-frame breakdown of a pitcher's delivery.

Ed Harvey reached out and said he wanted the works. His son, Matt, was about to start his freshman season at the University of North Carolina. He turned down $1 million from the Los Angeles Angels, who had drafted him six months earlier. Harvey refused to sign for anything less than $2 million and resolved to bet on himself. Ed just wanted to ensure his son wasn't gambling on an arm that might break sooner than he figured.

Just like Neil Pint and Nelson Molina and Hirokazu Tatsuta, Ed Harvey took an active role in his son's career. Matt started only once a week. Never threw more than 120 pitches. Ed couldn't help that his son threw 98 miles per hour at seventeen years old. It was so effortless, so smooth, that injury issues rarely concerned him. Still, he wanted to hear it from someone else. On January 17, 2008, an email from O'Leary arrived in his in-box.

Dear Mr. Harvey,

I reviewed the tape of Matt that you sent me. In general, I really like what I see.

When I am looking at pro prospects, I evaluate their pitching mechanics for their similarity to Greg Maddux at a similar age. I use a 2–8 scale where 8 is a clone of Greg Maddux and 2 is a clone of Mark Prior.

I would put Matt at a 7, which is very good (and relatively rare).

Matt also has a lot of Roger Clemens in him, which is good. If you compare the clips of Matt to the breakdown of Roger Clemens that I have in my Proper Pitching Mechanics essays . . . you will see a lot of similarities.

After his analysis, which covered ten categories and was almost wholly complimentary, O'Leary offered a "LEGAL DISCLAIMER":

When reading the above, please keep in mind that I am not guaranteeing your son's future health or success. Instead, what I am giving you is an educated guess. Also, keep in mind that I have no formal medical training, so you should consult with a doctor before deciding to act upon any of the recommendations that I make.

O'Leary is not a doctor, kinesiologist, or biomechanist. He has no educational credentials that might lend his insights some authority. The closest he came to the medical profession, he admits, was a summer job with his attorney father going over medical files for an asbestos lawsuit. O'Leary is, on the other hand, a damn good salesman, and Ed Harvey could've seen that for himself on the website. Right next to his link for pitching evaluations was one for a book O'Leary wrote called *Elevator Pitch Essentials*, about selling someone on an idea in less than two minutes.

The ascent of Chris O'Leary as one of the most influential voices in pitching mechanics happened because he sold the baseball world a damn fine elevator pitch. Amid Glenn Fleisig's burdensome academia, Mike Marshall's jargon-loaded instruction, and Tom House's teacher-to-the-stars reputation, O'Leary came across as comparatively relatable, a self-taught guy with an awfully compelling message.

"He did a good job of promoting himself," said Paul Nyman, the Tesla of the arm. "Chris is representative of picking the low fruit. The low fruit was, 'I'm going to tell you how not to get injured.' Immediately, people are going to say, 'Whoa, let me hear what this guy is saying.' Chris O'Leary is a perfect example of what self-promotion will do."

Frustrated like Mike Marshall, Nyman stepped away from baseball for five years, only to resurface in April 2013 on the website of a pitching coach named Lantz Wheeler. Nyman wanted to set the record straight on a term he coined: "Inverted W." In trying to break down pitchers' deliveries into three distinct categories, Nyman described one group as hanging their pitching arms in an inverted fashion before bringing them up to form a W with its glove-side arm. It was a benign motion. Over the previous six years, Chris O'Leary had taken the phrase "Inverted W," twisted it into a Godzilla-like monster worthy of fright, and built his business on the back of such fear.

The rebranding of the Inverted W was O'Leary's masterstroke. He was just another Marshall adherent, parroting Doc's teachings on his website, until he one day noticed a common point in the delivery of some pitchers. Both their elbows came above the top of their shoulders mid delivery. Their arms formed an M shape—or, as O'Leary started calling it, an Inverted W. He found a number of his Inverted W pitchers who suffered from arm troubles and began evangelizing that it led to injuries. Even if O'Leary couldn't prove causation, correlation was enough, and his definition stuck.

The problem: no evidence existed that the motion itself blew out elbows or injured shoulders. In 2015, the *Orthopaedic Journal of Sports Medicine* published a study by Wiemi Douoguih, the

Washington Nationals' team doctor, that looked at the deliveries of 250 pitchers and broke them into groups: Inverted W and non–Inverted W. Of the roughly one-third of the pitchers surveyed who threw with the Inverted W, 30 percent had arm surgeries. Of those with non–Inverted W deliveries, 27 percent underwent surgery. The difference was negligible.

O'Leary argued that the findings didn't invalidate his theories. He said the Inverted W in and of itself wasn't troublesome but caused a timing problem in which pitchers' arms lagged behind when their torsos started to rotate. Indeed, Douoguih's study showed a statistically significant difference in surgery rates among those with early rotation. It did not show that Inverted W pitchers were any likelier to exhibit the tendency than the other group.

The greatest obstacle in the guru business is science; besides Glenn Fleisig, few in the biomechanical community bother with it. Research—real research—is difficult, expensive, and time-consuming, and it doesn't make money, which ultimately drives so much of what happens in biomechanics. Nyman called the biomechanical world "a swamp, quicksand, a horror show," and he's right.

Which makes Lloyd Lee's humility so refreshing. Lee is the CPA. Next to nobody knows who he is. He believes he understands the pitching arm as well as anybody, even if his elocution could use some work. "I don't have a PhD in kinesiology," he said. "A lot of times when I'm talking, people want to correct my pronunciation of words. And all I've done is read the word. And I don't look it up and see the phonetics in the dictionary."

Lee can't say whether he'll change the game. Just that he wants to. For nearly a decade, he has honed his theories in a ten-page abstract with the intention of expanding it into a book that Paul Davis and the Cardinals can use as a research primer. "Everything I've got just about contradicts everyone else," Lee said. His grand theory would indeed turn everything baseball knows upside down. Lee believes pitchers who extend their elbows and delay the internal rotation of the shoulder until after releasing the ball not only generate more power but stay healthier. While it violates the principles of the kinetic chain—everything is supposed to move inside out, or proximal-to-distal, instead of outside in, like the elbow extending before the shoulder rotating—a 2011 study from Dr. Masaya Hirashima at the University of Tokyo supports Lee's theory and suggests that it merits a deeper look.

"I don't have the peer-tested science," Lee said. "But there's places to jump logically, and I could wait until I'm a hundred years old to test it, or I can take what I've got practically to see that it works and logically see and throw it out there and let guys try it. They can prove it to be bullshit. I'm not scared of anybody proving me wrong so much as I am wanting it to be done in a fair way."

Fairness is a difficult standard in biomechanical studies. The Douoguih study on the Inverted W had its flaws. The survivorship bias of examining just major league pitchers and the use of the naked eye to categorize them instead of kinematic data were two obvious ones. Considering what little data on the Inverted W existed before, it was a myth-busting start.

O'Leary was used to people questioning him, so he shrugged it off. Every day, those who disagreed with him on Twitter needled him and tried to goad him into fights by pointing out inconsistencies in his analysis. He responded on May 15, 2015, just three weeks after Douoguih's study, with defiance. "I'm too busy leading the field to worry about following (most) people," O'Leary wrote, but he couldn't gloss over his mistakes with hubris alone. His analysis of Matt Harvey, the almost-perfect pitcher, missed badly. The New York Mets drafted Harvey with the seventh overall pick in the 2010 draft. By 2013, he was one of the best pitchers in the major leagues. Then his UCL blew.

"The way he throws, I never thought he'd get hurt," Ed Harvey told me. "He's got about the cleanest delivery going, in my opinion. The ball comes out of his hand really freely. He's usually on time."

O'Leary blamed the miss on a new theory: premature pronation. He said Harvey changed his delivery since high school and was pointing the ball to center field upon foot strike. This, O'Leary claimed, was unnatural. Nolan Ryan's and Tom Seaver's and Mariano Rivera's and other pitchers' palms pointed toward third base. He didn't offer as examples all the pitchers—and there were plenty—who pointed the ball toward second base and stayed healthy.

"This is admittedly a theory," O'Leary said, and I suggested it wasn't a very good one. One of the great mysteries of the arm is how the forearm muscles work when a pitch is thrown, and for O'Leary to suggest he had any clue what was happening to them because a pitcher held a ball in a particular position was a leap Evel Knievel wouldn't dare make.

It was a mistake in the same vein as with the Inverted W. O'Leary liked to say that he had changed, that his understanding of pitching had grown and he focused more on the timing than the brand name. The phrase Inverted W still screams out from every corner of his website, though, and O'Leary never divorced himself from it. When those in baseball find religion, they're loath to give it up.

"People will criticize me for stuff because I'm changing things and making all these exceptions after the fact," O'Leary said. "I'm just trying to be scientific about it."

ALMOST IMMEDIATELY AFTER DR. JEFFREY Dugas arrived to practice at the Andrews Sports Medicine and Orthopaedic Center in 1999, the incidence of kids seeking Tommy John surgeries started to grow. In 1994, Dr. James Andrews didn't repair one UCL in a child. Over the next four years, the number maxed out at 11 percent of his yearly surgeries. In 1999, Dugas's first year, it jumped to 18 percent. By 2003, kids accounted for a quarter of Tommy John surgeries. And nearly a third in 2008. No longer does ASMI keep exact numbers, with Andrews splitting time between Birmingham and his Florida clinic, but he estimated he cuts one hundred youth elbows a year.

"I was there right as that explosion started to happen," Dugas said. "And it made you think: Holy cow, this isn't a good thing." More and more kids who visited Birmingham were doing so with only mild UCL damage. Kids like Braedyn Woborny, the Kansas teenager who didn't need Tommy John surgery, were everywhere.

Dugas wanted to find a repair that wouldn't necessitate the yearlong grind of Tommy John recovery. He started to consider a handful of factors. When other ligaments around the body partially tear off bones, the healing process takes around two to three months. The UCL should be no different. In early Tommy John research, doctors attempted to reattach a partially torn ligament. It failed miserably.

At the same time, Dugas couldn't ignore new research from a familiar ally of arm surgery: the ankle, the same joint that first inspired Dr. Frank Jobe. In recent years, doctors had used suture tape, a relatively new product, to help fix ankle instability inside the body. One study, from a foot and ankle surgeon named Nicholas Bevilacqua, showed how the tape—made of long, invisible-to-the-eye strands of the plastic polyethylene wrapped in a braided polyethylene-and-polyester jacket—helped stabilize damaged ankle ligaments not responding to treatment.

Dugas theorized that he could insert anchors, which look like small screws and hold the suture tape in place, into the humerus and ulna, eliminating the need to drill through kids' still-fragile bones. Once he reattached the partially torn ligament to the bone, the tape would heal into the ligament and serve as a reinforcement. Even better, the medical-equipment company Arthrex offered a three-millimeter-wide, one-millimeter-thick tape dipped in Type-I bovine collagen, a material extracted from the hides of cows that promotes quicker healing. Unlike the current preferred treatment for a partial tear, platelet-rich plasma (PRP)—in which blood is spun in a centrifuge to extract growth factors, then re-injected into the elbow to boost tissue repair—Dugas's surgery would mend the ligament and aid in its regrowth.

The first tests came in a room at ASMI whose sign outside belies the activity inside: SKILLS LAB. I first met Dugas there in August 2011. He was holding a leg chopped off on one end at the femur and the other just below the knee. Before he started to cut the skin off the knee joint, Dugas paused for a moment to thank the woman to whom it once belonged. He did not know her name or anything else about her, aside from the basic information that accompanied her knee. She had stood five feet four and had weighed only eighty pounds when she died of cancer at sixty-nine.

New joints arrive at ASMI all the time, and they're taken to the freezer in the skills lab until they're needed for a test. The elbow fascinated Dugas. He applied in 1999 for a fellowship under Andrews because of a deep interest in baseball medicine. Dugas was hired full-time in 2000 and, along with Dr. Lyle Cain, became one of Andrews's handpicked heirs to a sports-medicine empire. Before Andrews abdicated, they would spend thousands of hours in the skills lab, dissecting joints and readying them for testing.

After resecting the skin, Dugas sliced his scalpel through the leg muscles and peeled them away, exposing the woman's bone. He was studying the meniscus, the C-shaped piece of cartilage that serves as the knee's shock absorber, and needed a clear view of the joint. It was a hinge, much like the elbow, with the anterior cruciate ligament playing a similar stabilizing role as the UCL. Dugas was testing the force on the knee joint and the point at which the meniscus would tear. He feathered a paper-thin, five-thousand-dollar sensor inside the joint and onto the meniscus to measure it. He prepared the monstrous automated vise that would apply pressure until the joint no longer held. He glanced to his left and asked how the cement was looking.

Glenn Fleisig stood in front of a bowl, mixing a paste that

would harden around the two ends of the knee joint and hold it in place inside the machine. Nobody has meant more to the mainstreaming of baseball biomechanics than Fleisig, a mechanical engineer by trade and now ASMI's research director. A majority of the most influential academic papers regarding the pitching arm bear Fleisig's name. He is the reason pitch counts exist in Little League, the man who told us curveballs might not be as dangerous for kids as once thought, the driving force behind the study of how to best protect children from arm injuries.

Dozens of major leaguers have visited Fleisig at ASMI, too, and stepped into his eighty-five-foot-long, thirty-foot-wide laboratory carpeted with artificial turf and studded with eight high-speed cameras all focused on the pitching mound toward the back of the room. This is ASMI's biomechanics lab, a place where technology meets wonder. Fleisig uses the lab to analyze pitchers' form as well as the force on their joints. Children—elite travel-ball kids, mediocre sons of rich fathers, and everyone in between—travel from around the country to consult with Fleisig.

Some professional players swore by it. Roger Clemens, Barry Zito, C. C. Sabathia, Cliff Lee, and Zack Greinke—Cy Young winners all—have stripped off their shirts and allowed Fleisig to attach twenty-three reflective markers to predetermined points on their torsos. A computer program digitizes the markers into a Minecraft-like screen with nothing in it but blocks of three-dimensional emptiness interrupted by nearly two dozen tiny dots that resemble the shape of a human being when they move. When then-Brewers pitching coach Rick Peterson, a longtime partner of ASMI's, asked Todd Coffey one spring to strap on motion-capture technology and throw at 70 percent effort, Coffey scoffed. "I threw it one hundred percent effort because I knew it threw off his data," Coffey said. Daniel Hudson's stance on biomechanical analysis was even starker. "I've got enough people telling me what I do wrong right now," he said. "I don't need more scientists to look at me and tell me that I suck."

Turning the pitcher into a stick figure allows Fleisig to measure joint angles, arm velocity, timing, joint forces, torque, and dozens of other factors. The cameras shoot video of the pitcher throwing at 450 frames per second, slow enough that Fleisig can point out potential mechanical flaws and offer suggestions. Earlier that day, Fleisig had broken down the film with a ten-year-old boy whose father brought him to ASMI to make sure his elbow wasn't in danger of blowing out because of his pitching mechanics.

Fleisig enjoys the early evenings in the skills lab with Dugas because they give him a greater sense of what might be, and the tests on the suture tape were promising enough that Dugas needed to find a test subject. He wanted an Alabama-based kid entering his senior year with a partially torn UCL whose choices—do something radical or don't play again—made experimental surgery seem like the best option. In late July 2013, he found his subject: a five-foot-nine, 160-pound left-handed pitcher. He and his mother drove to Birmingham from southern Alabama and listened to Dugas's pitch. He saved the best part for the end. If everything went according to plan, the kid would return to the mound in six months, maybe sooner. Without a fresh tendon undergoing ligamentization or drill holes needing to heal, Dugas estimated the recovery time on his modified Tommy John surgery would be cut in half.

After a couple more conversations, the kid told Dugas he wanted the surgery. On August 8, 2013, one of the most revolutionary baseball procedures since the original Tommy John surgery took place in Birmingham. There were no complications. The patient rehabbed with Dr. Kevin Wilk, ASMI's director of rehabilitative research and a widely respected sports physical therapist. As Dugas had predicted, the ligament healed around the three-month mark. At five and a half months, the patient's full velocity returned. He pitched his entire senior year in high school with no problems. His fifty-plus innings went so well a local junior college recruited him, and he pitched there for a full season without incident.

Upon the patient's healthy return, Dugas started to use the procedure on others. He fixed a javelin thrower, two wrestlers, and a gymnast. By January 2015, he had repaired twenty-seven UCLs with his modified Tommy John, and not one had run into complications. Even Andrews, who taught his students to avoid making grand, overarching statements, acknowledged to Dugas that he was impressed.

The first batch of one-year follow-ups visited Birmingham in the spring of 2015, and their elbows looked clean, their ligaments back at full strength. "It's too early to wave the victory flag and think we've changed the world," Dugas said. "I think we need a couple years to really see what the spectrum of outcome is going to be. I know there's going to be a failure. And I want to know who those people are. I haven't seen them yet. It's been great. But I'm not egomaniacal enough to think there won't be some."

Barring too many failures, the plan is to scale up into the minor and major leagues. While his ideal patient in professional baseball is a midthirties pitcher looking for one last hurrah, or a late-round draft pick on whom a team didn't spend much money, Dugas knows frontline major leaguers will be more likely to offer themselves up as test cases. Just think: if a player with slight elbow damage can grind through the end of the season, he can undergo surgery October 1 and be ready by opening day with a fresh elbow. Zero days lost, compared with the average of 221 that the HITS database showed with classic Tommy John surgery. It's not the ultimate solution—nothing involving a scar can be—but it's quite an appealing alternative.

The procedure wouldn't work for everyone. When a ligament tears in the middle and not off the bone, the collagen tape can't tie it back together. And because no elite, hard-throwing pitcher has undergone the surgery yet, Dugas can't vouch for its success at the upper reaches of the major leagues.

"Will it work in a high-level pro? I don't know," Dugas said. "But in college and high school kids, it seems to be working great."

Baseball wants to believe. It's a trait cultivated over more than a century. It's why players wear lucky underwear and take B12 shots, why they believed pulling teeth would fix the arm, and why Todd Coffey's glove travels in a suitcase. If anything shows the slightest sign of efficacy, real or imagined, it is immediately embraced. The charlatans make their money off this ethos while the others toil in their labs, test their hypotheses, effect real change.

Jeffrey Dugas, it turns out, believed in something, too. It was nothing novel, nothing revolutionary. In the baseball world, it's not necessarily cool to believe in science. Dugas did anyway. And in the swamp he found a beautiful pearl.

CHAPTER 14

Dog Days

At least once every January or February, Casey McEvoy wakes up in a panic. In his nightmare, he can't find his baseball spikes. He is supposed to long toss before a game, and he realizes he's not ready, and the dread washes over him, startling him back to reality.

"I haven't pitched in fourteen years now," McEvoy said.

Why this recurring dream comes on the eve of every spring training McEvoy still doesn't quite understand. Maybe it takes more than a decade and a half of inactivity to sever the relationship between brain and body. In his parallel world, it's 1998 all over again on his rookie-ball team full of aspiring major leaguers: Adam Dunn, Austin Kearns, B. J. Ryan, Corky Miller, Bobby Madritsch, and, most unexpected of all, Todd Coffey. McEvoy followed all their careers and took bemused interest in Coffey's. The Big Nasty—that's what everyone on that team in Billings, Montana, called him—made it.

"And I always remember how lucky I am," Coffey said, "because Casey McEvoy didn't. I never want to be Casey McEvoy."

McEvoy represented the worst possible scenario for Coffey. Which sounds unfair, considering McEvoy lives a rather enviable life these days. He's the assistant controller at a big bank in Cincinnati. Has an MBA and a master of accounting. Two boys who play baseball. And a physical-therapist-assistant wife whom he met while trying to come back from Tommy John surgery. Coffey knows only the McEvoy whose career ended when his elbow gave out, one of the 20 percent never heard from again, the cautionary tale.

In April 2000, McEvoy, like Coffey a lower-level right-hander in the Cincinnati Reds organization, blew out his elbow. Coffey babied his rehab. McEvoy rushed back, a sixteenth-round draft pick out of college who didn't want to get overshadowed by newer, younger pitchers from the next draft class. By the ninth month, he was pumping fastballs at 94 and snapping off sliders like he could pitch the next day. Then his elbow fractured, the UCL pulled away, and he headed back to school to learn about 10-Qs and 10-Ks and the minutiae of SEC filings.

"I think about him a lot," Coffey said. "That's my greatest fear. Just not making it. You do this work, you put in the time, and it doesn't happen."

Everything Coffey did initially in Tacoma looked promising. Seattle wanted him to pitch back-to-back days. Coffey went June 13 and June 14. He started racking up saves and plowing through innings in a dozen pitches, sometimes fewer. On June 28, Coffey pitched in both games of a doubleheader. "Never done that before," he said. "Guess that shows them the arm is good."

In the meantime, Seattle's relief pitchers—a mixture of the unproven and mediocre—posted the best bullpen ERA in baseball during June at 1.64. Nobody got hurt, either, which left Coffey stuck in Tacoma. His agent, Rick Thurman, called Jeff Kingston, the Mariners' assistant general manager. Coffey would not exercise his first opt-out clause at the end of June, but he wanted a verbal commitment from Kingston that if another team wanted Coffey to pitch in the major leagues, he could leave. Seattle agreed. "How many pitchers have an opt-out at any time?" Coffey said June 30. "It's a win-win. It gives us more time now. Rick's going to call around to teams, talk to teams today, and then hopefully he'll hear back from them this afternoon."

Three days later, Thurman hadn't heard a word of interest from around the league. "A little surprised that no team has jumped on me yet," Coffey said. "Confusing more. Every team we talk to says, 'OK, we didn't know that.' Yesterday they found out I'm available. So they have to go through their whole process." Coffey ignored the slights and lowered his ERA to 1.29 with a scoreless inning July 8. He checked with the person charting his pitches that night, and his sinker ranged from 94 to 96 miles per hour. At 11:45 that night, Coffey sent Dr. Neal ElAttrache a text message.

I know it's late. Sorry for being so late. Just wanted to let you know I was 94–96 sinkers.

His phone buzzed a few minutes later with ElAttrache's reply.

Never too late to hear from you. Especially with that news. Awesome job.

Coffey's ERA lived in the low ones throughout July. He threw a two-inning stint, pitched three times in four days, four times in six days, five times in eight days. "I'm wondering why nobody has come knocking," he said. That included Atlanta, which in addition to Shae Simmons called up Pedro Beato and Juan Jaime and Ryan Buchter and Gus Schlosser—none of them with anywhere near the experience or success of Coffey. The Braves preferred to give their own guys a chance before someone who had already spurned them.

The Mariners' bullpen kept cruising in July, almost as strong as the previous month, healthy as ever. Coffey hoped they would trade one or more of their relief pitchers. They didn't. Thurman hunted for major league interest elsewhere. No teams bit. On July 31, Coffey's contract gave him a second opportunity to opt out. He stayed with Seattle, a decision that shifted control of his rights to the Mariners for the remainder of the season.

As much as Coffey tried not to panic, the frustration of life at Triple-A mounted. On August 14, Coffey sprinted in to hammer down a save in a 7–6 game. The second batter hit a game-tying home run. It was Coffey's second blown save in a week. The next batter dribbled a ball to first base, and the umpire called the runner safe over Coffey's protest.

"How do you not get that?" Coffey screamed. "You have one fucking job in this whole damn game, and you fucked that up."

The umpire didn't eject Coffey; he called a balk during the next at bat. In Coffey's entire major league career, all 1,910 batters, he had not once been called for a balk.

"You're fucking stupid," Coffey said.

He wanted to get tossed from the game; the umpire still didn't oblige. After recording the final two outs to send the game into extra innings, Coffey walked off the field, turned toward the umpire, and said: "You're fucking terrible. Fuck you, motherfucker." That did the trick. Coffey was thrown out, and he responded by helicoptering two folding chairs onto the field.

Triple-A was purgatory, and for what sin Coffey was there he didn't know. He believed he was a major league pitcher. His ERA backed up that idea. Scouts saw a different guy, and they were the ultimate arbiters. There is little upside in going to a general manager and suggesting someone like Coffey—older, bad body, only two pitches—when the baseball landscape is littered with similar pitchers. A veteran reliever named David Aardsma put up almost identical numbers as Coffey for the Cardinals' Triple-A affiliate, and no one was calling him, either.

"I feel trapped," Coffey said. "Very much so. Frustrated.

Trapped. It is what it is. I understand teams are like, 'We've seen this guy. Do we want to bring him in during a tight game in the playoff push?' I can somewhat understand that. But then I see what kind of slop they're throwing out there."

There was no slop in Seattle, whose bullpen continued its superlative performance and pristine health through August. In its fight for a playoff spot, Seattle still could've used the benefit of an expanded roster in September to rest its arms and give someone like Coffey the opportunity to devour innings, and that kept Coffey's faith intact. He just needed someone else to believe in him like he did himself.

"I think Seattle will call me up in September," Coffey said. "I really do."

BEFORE THE REHABILITATION FROM HIS second Tommy John surgery started, Daniel Hudson had wondered about the first pitch he would throw in a game. He'd grown more introspective over the course of the year-plus it had taken him to get here, back on top of a mound, albeit one in front of no fans in a rookie-league game populated with Latin American teenagers getting their first taste of the United States. The last two times he pitched in games that counted were the two worst moments of his life.

"I've been thinking a lot about what am I going to feel like when I'm close to back again," Hudson said. "How am I going to be mentally ready to throw a pitch as hard as I can when I know what happened last time? When I get on the mound for the first time, how am I going to put this out of my mind?"

Every so often, some new thought or comparison poisoned his mind. All the Tommy John surgeries in March and April, the ones that brought about the word "epidemic," spooked him, even if those pitchers looked at Hudson like he was the unluckiest of all. There was the text from Jarrod Parker, his old Diamondbacks teammate and one of six pitchers in need of a revision, seeking advice. The Diamondbacks overhauled their rehab protocol for Patrick Corbin, specifically to avoid a repeat of Hudson's injury. Other teams in baseball slowed theirs because of the number of revisions, too. Corbin didn't touch a ball until six months post-op—two months later than Hudson did following his first surgery.

Hudson was in no hurry the second time, either. Through July and into August, Tuesdays and Fridays were heavy throw days, Wednesdays and Sundays off, and the other three low-intensity, mechanics-intensive sessions with Brad Arnsberg. The language of Arnie made sense to Hudson by now, its wisdom buried underneath the bullshitting. Pitchers need to talk with other pitchers, and at his nadir, Hudson sought someone who understood his apprehension and hang-ups, who could laugh when Hudson received an email from the Diamondbacks urging him to RSVP for the alumni game in August. Between Arnie and Crank, the Diamondbacks forged a strong sense of how to handle Hudson as he prepared to return to the major leagues.

On August 5, 2014, he was scheduled to throw one inning against the Cincinnati Reds' rookie-league team. All he needed to do was survive four rookie-ball games and two more at Triple-A, and he'd be back in the big leagues in less than a month. The Diamondbacks planned to use him as a relief pitcher, easing him back one inning at a time. Depending on how his arm felt, perhaps they would consider letting him start in 2015. Even that was presumptive. Leading into that first game, the doubts crept in. Hudson didn't just ask himself whether the ligament would blow again. He wondered why it wouldn't.

"Once I got out there in the bullpen and threw my eight pitches, I said, 'If it happens, it happens,'" he said. "It was surprisingly easier than I thought it would be to put it out of my mind. Just the natural adrenaline you get when you're playing. Especially when you haven't played in a year. Those juices get going, and it takes over. You don't have time to think about anything else."

His arm held together. One inning, a couple of hits, a run, and two strikeouts. None of the numbers mattered. Just that he left the game in one piece and didn't feel sore when he woke up in the middle of the night to feed Baylor. Hudson usually took the midnight or two a.m. shift, lugging himself out of bed and into her nursery and trying to comprehend the dynamics of the slow-flow nipple. "It's so crazy. I can drink a twelve-ounce beer in a minute," he said, "and this child takes an hour to eat four ounces of water with powder in it."

On August 21, two days after his final rookie-league game, Hudson awoke at five thirty in the morning, trudged downstairs, and smashed the big toe of his right foot against a doorjamb. He screamed in pain. Hudson's arm failed him twice. Some cruel voodoo artist now decided to stick a pin in his foot.

"Who else would this happen to?" he asked.

Hudson reported the pain as 9.5 of 10. He figured he broke something, but an X-ray came back negative. The soreness on the instep and arch eased the next day, diminished again the day after that, and dissipated leading up to August 24. Hudson threw in the bullpen that day to stay on schedule, prompting Crank to pull him aside afterward. "I'm gonna give you a bit of a dad speech," he said, and he went on to warn Hudson about pushing too hard. The big toe had an ignominious place in baseball lore. Even though Dizzy Dean threw more than 1,500 innings between the ages of twenty-two and twenty-six, legend says that Earl Averill's line drive off the big toe of the twenty-seven-year-old Dean in the 1937 All-Star Game forced him to change his mechanics and led to career-ending arm troubles.

Hudson listened to the dad speech and agreed with Crank. "Too close to fuck it up over a toe and five MLB outings," Hudson said. His final two rehab games were scheduled with Triple-A Reno. Rehabbing pitchers will often go to Double-A instead. Mobile's schedule conspired against that. "They're going to be in Jacksonville at the end of August," Hudson said. He did not want to see that city again.

So he threw two scoreless outings for Reno. And three days

after the second, on September 1, the transaction shot across the wire: "Arizona Diamondbacks activated RHP Daniel Hudson from the 60-day disabled list."

ABOUT A MILE FROM CHENEY Stadium in Tacoma, Todd Coffey found an empty lot. He parked his car and sat. He wanted to be alone. His mind was racing. He needed to understand what just happened. For three months, Coffey had been one of the best relief pitchers in the Pacific Coast League. He couldn't forget the words typed by the Seattle Mariners' assistant GM three months earlier when he signed: "Todd could easily put himself at the top of the list if he comes in and pitches the way he has when healthy." He did pitch that way. He was healthy. And it still wasn't enough.

"I don't get it," he said. "I did everything I could."

On August 26, a week before the Triple-A season ended, the Mariners told Coffey that he would not join the team in September when rosters expanded. Most of his teammates milled about the clubhouse, oblivious to the news. A right-handed relief prospect named Carson Smith, whom Coffey tried to mentor, had gotten called up, and that angered him even more. As everyone slipped on their uniforms, Coffey asked permission to leave. He needed to clear his head.

"All day today, I go from moments of being pissed off, and then moments of being like, what the fuck," Coffey said. "This season is a complete waste."

Convincing him otherwise was futile, no matter how hard Jennifer or Rick Thurman tried. In a comeback defined by setbacks, none deflated Coffey like this one. He had talked himself into believing that sprinting into a major league game and doing a 360 was his fate, that his good work in Triple-A would matter, that the low moments these past two-plus years since his second Tommy John surgery existed for a reason.

All the buckets of rice, for nothing.

"I figured, you know, playoff push, they're going to want veterans," Coffey said. "They're not going to throw a young kid out there to get his ass handed to him. That, and the way I've been pitching."

The bone-chip surgery, for naught.

"The shit that I've jumped through to get here," Coffey said. "And the fact that talking to Rick today, he was like, 'You should be in the big leagues somewhere.'"

Rescuing himself from the showcase debacle, for this.

"The biggest kick in the balls was they had somebody from the front office here today," Coffey said. "He comes up to me to shake my hand. 'We appreciate everything you're doing this season on and off the field.'"

Putting up a 1.83 ERA, for an opportunity that may never have existed in the first place.

"I need an explanation," Coffey said. "That's what I asked Rick. Did they give a reason why, or did they say they're not gonna do it? That's my thing. I need a reason. I don't know why. I just need a reason. That's what I can't figure out. I've shown I can pitch multiple innings. I've gone multiple days in a row. I just need a reason."

He didn't realize that since he had arrived in Tacoma in late May, Carson Smith actually had pitched better than him. Lower ERA. More strikeouts. Fewer walks. Fewer home runs. All of the categories were close, but Smith had a future with the Mariners. He was a big kid, too, six feet six, with a fastball in the low to mid-90s and a slider in the mid-80s. At twenty-four, Smith was just ninety-five days older than Coffey had been when he'd made his major league debut. A younger version of himself had stolen Coffey's future.

Every pitcher of his ilk—good enough to kick around the big leagues for a decade but just one year at a time—comes with a sell-by date that moves closer with every injury. What used to be good enough no longer sufficed. Impressing scouts wasn't adequate. Coffey needed to flabbergast them, and even if he did touch 96 on occasion, more than fifty major league relief pitchers in 2014 averaged that velocity, and another hundred hit it at least once. Two hundred fifty relievers sat at 93 miles per hour or better. Nearly every bullpen could stock itself full of guys whose objective measurements rivaled Coffey's. The baseball world Coffey believed in—full of slop, with a place for him—did not exist.

He hoped another team would show interest. Thurman considered Pittsburgh a possibility. Coffey loved the idea of going to Detroit, which was one-half game behind Seattle for the second wild-card spot. Joel Hanrahan, the reliever coming off Tommy John to whom the Tigers gave a million dollars, never threw a pitch for them. They needed bullpen help. "What I want to do," Coffey said, "is go to Detroit and shove it up Seattle's ass. I want it to come down to where I pitch and cost them the playoffs."

Because he did not take his opt-outs, Coffey's mobility now hinged on the Mariners' willingness to let him go. And that almost surely would depend on whether a market developed. Thurman wasn't terribly optimistic. For thirty years, he had represented luminaries like Trevor Hoffman and Tim Lincecum. Thurman was a former minor pitcher himself who retired due to a bad arm, so he appreciated life on the fringes and tried to convince executives that Coffey wasn't just another past-his-prime veteran. "I feel terrible, too," Thurman said. "I almost feel like I failed. When I believe in someone, I don't miss too often. And I totally believe in where he's at. It's not him. He's done his end. I'm just keeping my fingers crossed something happens. He's worked so hard. He deserves to be there."

Deserve or not, he wasn't. Purgatory had turned out to be hell. This was even worse than how Coffey imagined Casey McEvoy's existence: living on the cusp but not there, blue-balled to the point of emotional detachment. At around one a.m. on the night he found out, on the drive back to the Seattle apartment he rented, figuring it was just a matter of time until the Mariners summoned him, Coffey said he wasn't sure he could return to the Tacoma Rainiers. "I can't give anything," he said. "My heart is not in this now. I don't know."

The next day, Coffey arrived at his usual time. He cleared out his locker because it was Tacoma's last home game of the season. In the ninth inning, Rainiers manager Roy Howell called on him. He channeled his rage into what he loved doing most, what he never would let go, and he struck out the side. Coffey hit the road with the Rainiers through their final game September 1, still puzzled, still without an explanation.

When he sought clarity after the season, he found even more confusion. "The Mariners will not release me," Coffey said on September 3. Two days earlier, Thurman had called Jeff Kingston, the Mariners' assistant GM, and asked for Seattle to let Coffey go, just in case another team wanted him as insurance for the final month. According to Thurman, Mariners GM Jack Zduriencik said no because he feared Coffey would go to another team fighting Seattle for a playoff spot.

"I don't think that's accurate at all," Zduriencik told me. Among the most polarizing GMs in baseball, Zduriencik had a mixed reputation among players, former coworkers, adversaries, and agents. Coffey believed he could trust Zduriencik. By September 3, he had assigned Zduriencik a new middle name. "Jack Fucking Zduriencik is the reason I'm not in the big leagues right now," Coffey said.

Thurman eventually called Zduriencik and read him the riot act, saying, "Don't tell me you're going to limit him to not playing for a team that would directly be in conflict with you guys."

Zduriencik denied it. "You don't want to hold anybody hostage for any reason whatsoever," he told me. "But if we didn't invite any particular player from the minor leagues to join our big league club, it was because we thought we had better options. We brought players to the big leagues that we thought could help us. Case closed. Carson Smith in our opinion deserved to be called to the big leagues. Case closed. Not because of somebody else. Only because of him. And that would've been the case with every guy. If we didn't call someone to the big leagues, we didn't think they were going to help us to the degree that we wanted them to."

While Zduriencik's passive-aggressive tone wouldn't win him any congeniality contests—the only time he referred to Coffey by name was when he said, "I'm really not sure why this conversation is in regards to Todd Coffey"—he brought up a good point: "I don't think I got a phone call about him." Other teams' interest in him was at best minimal, at worst nonexistent.

Coffey said Kansas City had inquired, but Royals GM Dayton Moore told me, "Nobody felt that he was an upgrade over what we currently have in the major leagues." The Pirates asked, too, but only for depth purposes. They wouldn't give a forty-man-roster spot to Coffey. He needed one great report, written by a scout willing to go back to his GM and urge him to sign a thirty-three-year-old on his second Tommy John recovery, and that simply did not exist.

"I am not just brokenhearted, but absolutely upset," Coffey said. "I have done everything I can for this team. Helped them out on and off the field. I stayed there because of their word. If I knew they weren't going to honor it, I would've taken my out."

When he landed back in Seattle, Coffey jumped in the car with Jennifer and Declan, who was approaching his second birthday. Off they went through Montana, the first leg of the forty hours it would take to return to Rutherfordton. *Toy Story 3* and *Alvin and the Chipmunks*, the two movies that would silence Declan, played on a loop. Around six p.m. on September 3, as Coffey closed in on Mount Rushmore, his cell phone rang. The Mariners had granted his release.

As Coffey drove into the dusk, the baseball world continued on without him. There were games to be played. The baseball world kept turning, rebalancing itself. One man gone, another one back.

IN HIS DREAMS, DANIEL HUDSON stood on the pitcher's mound. He was back in the major leagues. His delivery felt perfect: short arm path, hand on top, good balance through deceleration. The ball left his fingers as intended, but on the way to the plate, it lost all momentum. As it fell to the grass, Hudson snapped awake.

His mind was often an even greater enemy at times than his arm. Nothing, not even his subconscious, could sabotage Hudson now. On the 799th day since he had last thrown a major league pitch, he took an escalator up three levels from the ground floor of the Omni San Diego, walked thirty steps across a breezeway, and slinked past a half-asleep security guard at the gate that connects the hotel and Petco Park, home of the San Diego Padres. I walked alongside Hudson as he entered his first major league ballpark in more than two years. He surveyed the field, familiar with all its features but one. "I've never been in the bullpen," he said. If Hudson was going to throw in San Diego, it would be on September 3, the final night in town for his parents, Sam and Kris, who had flown in from Virginia to celebrate the occasion with Sara and Baylor.

He was starting to feel like a big leaguer again. Earlier in the week, his catcher, Miguel Montero, and outfielder Cody Ross told Hudson he'd been gone so long he'd have to participate during dress-up hazing for rookies. He told them to fuck off. Despite the September doldrums—Arizona was nineteen and a half games out of first place—occasional laughter pierced the quiet of the Diamondbacks' clubhouse. Hudson was splayed out on a couch, reading a story on his phone, when a fart of unknown origin reverberated off the clubhouse's low ceilings. Ross accused Diamondbacks manager Kirk Gibson, whose denial couldn't have been more vehement. "I wouldn't lie about that," Gibson said. "I'd be proud." The culprit remained at large.

Hudson missed this. The most puerile elements of life in baseball were among the most appealing. Even before he threw a pitch, he was back, and his return energized the clubhouse. Hudson would never be the face of the Diamondbacks, a responsibility foisted on first baseman Paul Goldschmidt, but few players on the

Diamondbacks' roster commanded the respect Hudson did, and his return would be a winning moment in a lost season.

"I love Huddy," Diamondbacks trainer Ken Crenshaw said. "He's a great guy. A great worker. You just pull for him. You want to see him get back and pitch so he can have some comfort in his mind."

Sam, Kris, and Sara certainly weren't comfortable midway through the game. They figured Hudson had no shot at getting in as Diamondbacks starter Josh Collmenter needed just fifty pitches through four innings and Andrew Cashner, the Padres' starter, matched him pitch for pitch in a 1–1 game. The lack of offense was routine for the Padres, who would finish the season with a .226 batting average, the worst team average in baseball since 1972. Arizona, which had scored the fewest runs in the National League during August, didn't want to insert Hudson in a close game. "He ain't ever getting in with our offense," quipped Diamondbacks' starter Wade Miley the night before.

In section 114, row 39, Hudson's family waited. Dumb videos played between innings. The ballpark had all the charm of a mortuary, its upper deck empty and the masochists in the lower one content to witness two bad teams living down to expectations. Sam sat with interlocked fingers, waiting for a reason to unfasten them and clap. Kris slung an arm over his shoulder and patted his back. "You realize how late our nights are gonna be if he stays in this role?" she said.

Baylor wore a pink dress that covered a baseball shirt. Earlier in the day, a stranger mistook her for a boy, so Sara went to her cache of headbands and picked one with a pink, rhinestoned bow. Modern motherhood fit her well: she held Baylor in her left arm, a baby bottle in her left hand, and a phone blowing up with text messages in her right hand.

"I just want him to get in to get it over with," she said.

"I'm nervous," Sam said.

"Not yet," Kris said.

In the fifth inning, a pair of dim fielding plays allowed the Diamondbacks to score three runs. Sara smirked as the Padres threw a ball into left field during a rundown, saying, "We'll take an inning like this." Sam rocked side to side. "All right," Sara said. "Keep fucking up. We need all the help we can get." Baylor slept.

Collmenter cruised through the bottom of the inning on ten pitches. A complete game was well within his reach. More than four hundred feet away, in the bullpen, Hudson silently rooted for a long inning. "I felt bad doing it," Hudson later admitted. "Nobody wants that. I would never root for him to get lit up. Guy just foul seven pitches off."

Sara's mom, her dog trainer, and her neighbors kept texting, asking for updates and pitch counts. After a leadoff single in the bottom of the sixth, the Diamondbacks' bullpen stirred. Instead of squinting to see the uniform number, Sara glanced at the pitcher's legs. "I know those thighs anywhere," she said. "Thunder thighs." It was Hudson.

Almost immediately, Collmenter induced a double-play ground ball. Hudson sat back down, his teammates apparently determined to keep him waiting until day eight hundred. "Gibby and I are gonna have some words," Sara joked about manager Kirk Gibson. She was frustrated, Baylor was crying, and Kris was releasing nervous energy by scratching Sam's back. Meanwhile, Hudson's brother, Dylan, kept sending Kris text messages, saying things like: "Are they gonna put him in? He looks bored as shit."

Then it happened. This wasn't a false alarm like the previous night, when Kris mistook Diamondbacks closer Addison Reed's number 43 for Hudson's 41. This time, after the Diamondbacks scored an insurance run to go up 5–1, the top of the eighth inning would belong to Hudson.

The bullpen gate swung open and he ran down the stairs and toward the mound. It felt a lot farther than he remembered. "You've Lost That Lovin' Feeling" blasted through the stadium's sound system. He jacked up his pants before climbing the mound slowly. He did not do a 360. He just wanted to savor that feeling again, the one that climbing the world's biggest ten-inch mountain gave you.

"Your attention, please. Now pitching for the Diamondbacks: Daniel Hudson."

The commercial break ended and ESPN's national broadcast of the game cut to Hudson standing on the mound as play-by-play man Pedro Gomez gave a CliffsNotes version of his story, catcher Jordan Pacheco laid down the sign, and Hudson nodded. Kris zoomed in with her iPhone to take a blurry picture, which couldn't have looked more beautiful to her, even if it did capture a rather dreadful pitch, 94 miles per hour but bouncing in front of home plate before it reached pinch hitter Abraham Almonte.

Kris looked at Sara and smiled. Sam reclasped his hands. Baylor stopped crying. Kris and Sam started. At third base, Cliff Pennington shot Hudson a quizzical look. He noticed Hudson shaking his arm after the spiked fastball. Hudson indicated to Pennington that he was fine; his elbow was caught on his sleeve, and he was trying to loosen it. To prove it, his second pitch to Almonte was a called strike and lit up the radar gun at 95.

"There it is," Kris said.

Hudson threw eleven more pitches. Diamondbacks shortstop Didi Gregorius saved a hit with a diving play. Yangervis Solarte screamed a line drive right at left fielder Alfredo Marté. A weak groundout to second base by Alexi Amarista ended the inning. Three up, three down. Hudson walked into a dugout full of hugs and congratulations and tears.

The Diamondbacks won, 6–1, and when the clubhouse doors swung open, the media swarmed around Hudson. Three months earlier, he had started scripting out what he would say upon his return. As presumptuous as it was, this felt like his chance to thank everyone: Crank and Arnie, Gibby and KT, doctors and trainers, friends and family. Then his mind went blank. It filled back up not with gratitude but with the rawest, most honest reaction he could muster.

"Even if I go out tomorrow and it blows again playing catch, it was worth it, just to try again," Hudson said. "It's been a long road. Thankfully today came."

Baseball marveled at Hudson's return. Kris Medlen and Cory Luebke and Brandon Beachy and Jarrod Parker and all the others coming back from quick-turnaround revisions saw hope. Doug Brocail welcomed another member to the club. Hudson's 1-in-300 elbow—the one Dr. James Andrews said had failed like only a handful he'd seen—was good enough to retire major league hitters again.

"The dude is special for doing what he did," said Wade Miley, the Diamondbacks pitcher. "He was a week away from being back in the big leagues last year. This dude busted his ass last year."

"We've had a lot of Tommy John guys," Trevor Cahill, another pitcher, said. "And he hasn't said a single bad thing during his rehab, about it sucking, about not wanting to do it. Not one."

"He just did it," Miley said. "This was one of the cooler things I've been a part of in baseball. We went to the playoffs in 2011. That was cool. But this—this is incredible."

In a nearby locker sat Montero, the only Diamondback with more tenure than Hudson. "I get goose bumps talking about Huddy," Montero said. "Because he's great. He always came with the right attitude. He hated it. Of course he hated it. Everyone hates being on the disabled list. Not getting to do what he loves to do. Not being able to contribute. Knowing that he could contribute to the team if he were just healthy."

Montero parked himself in front of a video monitor. He wanted to see Hudson's stuff on film. The delivery looked slightly different, though not the sort of radical departure Hudson had dreamed of, muscle memory being what it is. What Montero really wanted to study was Hudson's stuff, how the fastball, changeup, and slider all interplayed. Harmoniously, it turned out, each pitch playing off the other, like the Huddy of three years earlier. "That was awesome," Montero said.

When the crowd in the clubhouse dispersed, Hudson turned off his camera-friendly face and tried to unpack his night. Congratulatory text messages blew up his phone. Diamondbacks president Derrick Hall said: "Really proud of you. I was emotional. You were awesome, kid." Hudson's brother, Dylan, wrote: "So proud of you. All the mountains you've had to climb over and how you came back strong just makes me so proud to be your brother. You were great tonight. So proud brotha."

Hudson stole a nip of vodka from Cahill's secret stash—"I prefer whiskey," he said, "but I'll take what I can get"—mixed it with orange Powerade, and leaned back in his chair. All his teammates were gone. The clubhouse was his alone until Gibson jumped out from the manager's office for a quick debriefing.

"How'd it feel today?" Gibson said.

"Felt good," Hudson said. "I've got to figure something out. I hadn't thrown since four. I don't know if I need to play catch in the third. It took me a little while to get [ready] on the mound."

"A little blood flow going out there?" Gibson said.

"Yeah, a little bit of a chub," Hudson said.

"Good job, Huddy," Gibson said.

Gibson understood. He hit one of the most famous home runs in baseball history, the one-armed, dead-legged walk-off shot against Dennis Eckersley in the game one of the 1988 World Series that inspired a million fist pumps and helped win the Dodgers their sixth World Series.

"I'm riding this shit," Hudson said. "This one's going, and that's it. I'm not doing this again." The last stage of Hudson's career had just started with three outs in San Diego. If something bad was supposed to happen, it could wait.

CHAPTER 15

The New Frontier

THE RADAR GUN DOESN'T LIE. I learned this long ago, never to forget it, even when the numbers didn't seem real. I was standing in a warehouse in middle-of-nowhere Washington state, watching someone named Casey Weathers, a guy whose elbow had no right to be pushing the limits of human performance, throw a baseball harder than any I'd ever seen.

105.8.

When the numbers first flashed, nobody said anything. They were too high. Granted, this wasn't a normal or legal throw—Weathers took a seven-step running start, muscled into a crow hop, and launched the ball as hard as he could into a net—but still, the fastest anyone had flung a five-ounce baseball off a mound was then-Cincinnati Reds closer Aroldis Chapman at 105.1 miles per hour. Weathers left that nearly a mile in his rearview.

Standing behind the net that mid–November 2014 day was Kyle Boddy, the owner of Driveline Baseball and the man ultimately responsible for these numbers. Which, truth be told, he could barely believe himself. Even though Boddy trained and nurtured baseball pitchers for a living, he had never seen anyone do with a regulation-sized baseball what Casey Weathers had just done.

"I don't know that I believe this," Boddy said, and he poised the radar gun once more, as Weathers kicked into gear for another rip.

105.3.

About fifteen feet to the side, Trevor Bauer, a starting pitcher with the Cleveland Indians, trained a camera on Weathers that captured video at 240 frames per second, necessary for Bauer to study how Weathers's arm worked. These drills were Bauer's domain. He'd long held the Driveline record for fastest five-ounce throw.

"I guess I'm behind now," Bauer said.

"Don't worry," Boddy said. "Nobody else on the planet throws as hard as you two."

105.8.

Weathers had just done it again. It was an ugly day in Puy-allup, Washington, home of Jon Lester and Driveline. Weathers wore a gray T-shirt, black shorts, and neon orange shoes, Bauer gray sweatpants and a navy hoodie, and Boddy his customary uniform of a black Driveline Baseball T-shirt, gray sweatpants, and old Nikes. Others milled about the complex, as they often do at Driveline. Fourteen-year-olds mingle with major leaguers. Loud noises emanate from a combination office-laboratory upstairs. Boddy rents the space, so the run of the facility isn't exactly his, even if he and the Driveline crew walk around here—and everywhere, really—like they own the place.

"I'm the most skeptical guy that does this shit for a living," Boddy reiterated. Every day he used a tuning fork to calibrate his radar gun, and it continued to spit out numbers that boggled his mind. For the last half decade Boddy had lived to see someone have a day like Casey Weathers was having.

Boddy seemed to ignore the core principles of the arm. It is made of bones and muscles and tendons and ligaments, all of which are fragile; when any piece of the arm is strained or stressed beyond its limit, it breaks. Boddy believed his training allowed pitchers to throw hard and stay healthy, and he saw Driveline as baseball's Bonneville Salt Flats.

"Let's do some crazy shit," he said, picking up a four-ounce ball.

If Weathers could throw a five-ounce ball 105.8 miles per hour, Boddy wanted to see what he could do with a baseball with the same circumference but an ounce lighter. The first four-ounce ball Weathers threw lit up the gun with a new number: 115.3 miles per hour. The throws with three-ounce balls topped 118. With a two-ounce ball, Weathers nearly hit 120 miles per hour.

The unlikeliest part of it all actually had nothing to do with the numbers or the science behind throwing what amounted to feathers, and everything to do with the guy behind it. When Weathers arrived in Puyallup for the first time seven months earlier, he was a complete wreck, barely touching 92 miles per hour on his maximum-velocity crow-hop throws, acting like someone scared of his elbow, which was a rather warranted fear.

Weathers wasn't the typical player to seek help at a facility like Driveline. He had pedigree: a distinguished college career as Vanderbilt University's closer, the number seven overall pick in the draft by Colorado in 2007, a nearly $2 million signing bonus, bronze medal from the 2008 Olympics. Two months after the Beijing Games ended, Weathers tore his UCL during an Arizona Fall League game. The fallout was a mess. Weathers didn't throw until seven months post-op. Platelet-rich plasma treatment in his elbow failed to help. A bone spur started to hook off one of the tunnels drilled into his arm. When he returned twenty months after surgery, Weathers couldn't throw strikes. The Rockies released him. He signed with the Cubs in 2012, walked fifty-three batters in thirty-four innings, and lost the will to lie to himself anymore.

"One thing I never wanted to do in my whole life," Weathers told me, "was make excuses and say, 'Well, I've walked eleven guys per nine in the last three years, I'm basically a bust at this point in my career, and it's not my fault, it's your fault. It's the doctor who did the surgery. It's my elbow's fault.' Making excuses is just not something I enjoy doing."

Surgery cleared out the bone spur. It also left Weathers damaged goods, the sort on whom no team dared take a chance, not with him barely hitting 90 off a mound. Weathers needed a facility to help rebuild him, and his old Vanderbilt teammate Caleb Cotham, a New York Yankees organizational player whose overhaul at Driveline turned him into a big leaguer, recommended he read up on Boddy. His website is a font of information and myth busting, and after receiving an email from Weathers on March 27, 2014, Boddy invited him to Puyallup.

The first step was to reprogram Weathers's brain as much as his arm. No longer would professional baseball's take-it-easy standard apply. Weathers would subsist on a diet of underweight and overweight baseballs, the product of research Boddy did in his homemade biomechanics lab and reinforced by a paper from University of Hawaii professor Dr. Coop DeRenne that showed training with weighted balls had a significant effect on velocity gains. Throwing weighted balls, a controversial practice that only recently gained traction with major league teams, was at the heart of Boddy's training. When a pitcher throws an overweight ball— Boddy disciples use balls up to 11 ounces—his arm slows down to handle the added mass and increased force on the shoulder and elbow. Boddy believed the body desired to get stronger, and this sort of adaptation built speed and strength while allowing humans to throw overweight balls safely. Underweight balls encouraged throwers to reach peak force, a onetime stressor that complemented the slow build of overweight balls. Throwing anything below five ounces calls upon the shoulder muscles in charge of deceleration even more than regular-weight balls, rounding out the best-of-both-worlds training Boddy aims to employ.

Weathers bought in. Within a month, he constantly hit 95 off a mound and went from zero prospects to an offer from the Tampa Bay Rays. He shipped out to the low minor leagues and couldn't throw strikes, but his arm didn't hurt for the first time in six years. So back he came to Driveline for the winter, took a six-month lease on a place fifteen minutes away in Tacoma, and resolved to learn how to throw strikes. He wanted one more shot. It didn't feel foolhardy, not when the training at Driveline helped his mashed-potatoes elbow feel right again, especially not when the ball came out of his hand the way it did.

"There's no way you should believe that a guy with a destroyed elbow threw 105.8 multiple times," Boddy said. "There's no reason to believe it."

THE FIRST TIME I SPOKE with Boddy, he told me I was going to see someone throw a baseball 106 miles per hour. I called him a liar and figured he was just another velocity-crazed parasite. Boddy, much to my surprise, didn't turtle away or snap back defensively.

"The people that are my enemies or whatever have a point," he said. "Velocities have never been higher, and those guys sort of tend to get hurt more. It's kind of close cut. I get it. From a pure biomechanical standpoint, of course torque is incredibly high, right? And so that should lead to injuries. But nobody focuses on the kinesiology of it."

Over his seven years studying baseball, Boddy has constantly run studies to test his ideas, challenge himself, and learn more about whether he really can churn out pitchers who throw hard and stay healthy. Boddy was wrong about one thing: He wasn't the most skeptical guy in the pitching arm business. That was me. I'd seen Daniel Hudson's arm blow up a second time and Todd

Coffey's take him nowhere good. I'd heard a guy named Tommy John say he's going to make Tommy John surgery obsolete with electric pulses. I'd witnessed kids risking arm injuries across my own country and in another halfway around the world. I'd watched a team pay $155 million for an arm that might require surgery. Nobody was more skeptical than I, and now I'd seen a guy with a chronically bad elbow throw 105.8 miles per hour and declare himself healthier than ever.

"His arm was killing him for four years," Boddy said. "Now it doesn't, and he can train as hard as he wants and maybe make something out of himself. That's way more fun. The problem is no one gives a fuck unless they've had elbow problems, because they just assume it'll never happen to them. You can't sell people preventive medicine. I think the American healthcare system and the rise of antivaccination people is proof enough of that, and baseball people are at least one order of magnitude dumber than the average American citizen."

Boddy's active dislike of the baseball establishment brought him here. In many ways, Boddy is a slightly more sociable, far less peremptory Mike Marshall. The name Driveline was cribbed from a favorite Marshall phrase. On the back of Boddy's Driveline T-shirts is another Marshall axiom: "Rest Is Atrophy." Those are for sale on Driveline's website, $24.95 a pop. While Marshall erred in alienating the public and never building a viable business, Boddy sells T-shirts, weighted baseballs, medicine-ball sets, and Alan Jaeger's tubing bands, and makes a tidy-enough profit that kids who want to train at Driveline pay only a nominal one hundred dollars a month.

I walked into the upstairs portion of the facility and was greeted by a wall with inch-thick mats backed by two-by-four reinforcements every foot or so. Driveline students whipped medicine balls into the padding with reverse throws, like a tennis backhand, to strengthen the three rotator cuff muscles that contract during the deceleration portion of the delivery. On the adjacent wall, there was visible electric piping. The place looked more like a meth lab than a science lab.

Boddy's desk, which he shares with the CEO he hired, a former waste-management operations manager named Mike Rathwell, was a disaster covered by weighted balls, batteries, two printers, and a PC missing a side panel, its guts exposed. A few feet away, Weathers had dropped a weight on the ground after a grueling set and destroyed the plywood in the floor, leaving a gaping hole beneath the carpet. Rather than fix it, Boddy covered it with a mat and told everyone to avoid the manhole. Of the stack of books on top of a drawer, one was Boddy's much-thumbed copy of *Gray's Anatomy* and two were in Japanese, written by Kazushi Tezuka and Ryutaro Himeno, the theorists behind the mysterious gyroball pitch. The body mobility bible *Becoming a Supple Leopard* had yet to be cracked. "I am not a supple leopard," Boddy said. "I think I'm going to celebrate with some pizza tonight."

Boddy claimed moments like Weathers's 105.8 as his own victories. They validated his decision to leave behind his previous career as a nerd-for-hire and pursue Driveline full-time in 2012. Until then, he had worked exposing security flaws at the gambling operation PokerStars, played cards and bet sports himself, spent a year at Microsoft, and jumped around in data-science jobs. He was depressed and suffering from anxiety attacks, convinced that he was missing his baseball calling. The game had been his passion since his Cleveland childhood. Boddy's father worked as an electrician and his mom stayed at home. Boddy was a bad ballplayer, more knowledgeable than skilled. He spent his senior year in high school taking classes at a nearby community college and turned down opportunities at more challenging schools because he couldn't afford them. Instead, he took a full scholarship to Baldwin Wallace University in Berea, Ohio, but eventually dropped out.

Driveline Mechanics, the blog Boddy started in 2008, relied significantly on the theories of Mike Marshall and Chris O'Leary.

Parroting others' work didn't satisfy him, so he set out to create something that seemed impossible: a biomechanics lab, just like Glenn Fleisig had at ASMI. "It's just math, man," Boddy said. "I'm Asian. I got into MIT. I can do this."

At a dilapidated warehouse in Seattle, Boddy installed four high-speed cameras and enlisted the help of a research assistant for Jesus Dapena, one of the earliest baseball biomechanics experts, to walk him through the rest. As Boddy moved into bigger, better spaces, the lab grew as well: EMG sensors, force plates, inertial measurement units, and even a contraption made from a Nintendo Wiimote that aimed to measure elbow torque. Working out at Driveline meant being part of a running experiment. Never in professional baseball had any team done this. The most active research that teams do on players involves a biomechanical analysis at ASMI or another lab. As former Boston Red Sox general manager Ben Cherington said, "We don't want to turn them into guinea pigs. If there was a parallel universe somewhere with baseball player clones and there was no human attached to it, you could do whatever you want."

Cherington's science fiction is Boddy's science. He wants to marry velocity with health, and his simple, reasonable proposal is an extension of the epidemiological study Major League Baseball is undertaking. "You take all first-year pitchers and measure everything," Boddy said. "Maybe you even spring for MRIs on everyone to do a cool research project. Then you track specific metrics at all levels every two to four weeks and see where things go from there. When there are large deviations, experiment with recovery techniques. See which ones work well and which ones don't. Discard the shit, keep the good stuff. Constantly iterate."

For three years, I'd waited to hear someone say this. Teams operated more than $600 million in the black during the 2014 season, according to a Forbes analysis, and money spent on injury research amounted to nothing. Moreover, the union would instantaneously object to major league players being used as guinea pigs, even if the greater good was obvious. In the minor leagues, where the union has no say, teams still didn't bother with substantive research.

"They don't do it because trainers aren't paid shit, strength-and-conditioning coaches at the minor league level are totally unqualified to do any of this stuff, and, well, it's never been done before in baseball," Boddy said. "And since it's never been done, why start it now?"

Major League Baseball's and the MLB Players Association's agreement to the study on the 2014 draft class of pitchers is the closest they've come to following Boddy's suggestions. Not even the Houston Astros, baseball's avant-garde franchise, for which Boddy consulted, were ready to try it. And it's not like they're categorically averse to new ideas. The Astros have instituted the long toss for all their minor league teams, piggy-backed their young pitching—two starters throw in every game, like Toronto did with Noah Syndergaard, Aaron Sanchez, and Justin Nicolino—and hired Bill Firkus, a Cal-Berkeley MBA, as director of sports medicine and performance. While Boddy's weighted-ball program proliferated throughout college baseball—starting with Vanderbilt and Oregon State, two national championship–caliber programs—as well as in high schools around the country, major league teams retreated to their fiefdoms. This left Boddy with few allies and forced him to dig into the deepest corners of the Internet, seeking intellectual equals to help grow Driveline. Trevor Bauer was one, and he was a good one to have, because he was every bit as smart as Boddy and even more curious. On the day of 105.8, he came to Driveline with his father, Warren, a chemical engineer who helped make Bauer a major leaguer. And amid discussions about health and mechanics and physics, Warren piped up during a lull in the conversation.

"Kyle, Trevor and I had a question for you," Warren said. "Do you think you can teach command?"

DURING LUNCH PERIOD IN HIGH school, Trevor Bauer used to escape to room J2, which kids called the Physics Palace. Martin Kirby, a renowned teacher at Hart High, thirty miles north-west of Los Angeles, presided over it with great majesty. As a sophomore, Bauer took AP Physics with Kirby, and it intro-duced him to a new world, one with force and momentum and everything else that went into throwing a baseball. Kirby spoke Bauer's language far better than any of his peers. "I didn't have a whole lot of friends in high school," Bauer said. "I'd go in, and I'd play chess in his classroom. Or talk to him about quantum physics at lunch just so I didn't feel awkward out there standing alone, again."

Kids used to laugh at Bauer for wearing baseball pants to Meadows Elementary School. He spent his teenage years as an oxymoron: the elite-athlete outcast. He was too smart for his own good, too dedicated to the craft of throwing a baseball to hone his social skills. When Bauer wanted an ultraheavy ball for training, he drilled holes into softballs and pounded lead fishing sinkers into them with a hammer. Little did those around him understand how hard he had to work to overcome genetics. Even now, after maniacal training, Bauer's vertical leap is barely thirty inches and he runs a bit like a mule. As a freshman, his fastball was in the mid-70s, fifteen miles per hour less than the Anthony Molinas of the world.

"Trevor was never an elite arm," Warren Bauer said. "Trevor made himself an elite arm. There's a difference."

Bauer's long-term plan irritated his coaches. Bauer's high school coach sent him note after note telling him he would amount to nothing if he refused to follow the standard, mapped-out protocol for pitchers. Every day after school, Bauer rode to nearby tennis courts on his bike with a bucket of baseballs on each handlebar and a heavy rope around his neck. His three-hour workout included a long-toss session into the fence surrounding the courts. One morning, police officers showed up at his coach's office, asking about a kid named Trevor. It turned out that a tennis instructor had called the cops on him. "The fence deformed a little bit," Bauer said, "so I was a vandal." When Bauer's coach was through berating him in front of the team, Bauer said, "Sorry my parents didn't raise me to be blindly allegiant."

Bauer framed the coach's most obnoxious letter, glanced at it for motivation, came to be one of the best players in Los Angeles as a junior, and graduated a semester early as a high school senior so he could enroll at UCLA as a seventeen-year-old. Six weeks later, he was closing games for the Bruins.

Bauer's routine irked his college coaches, too, but nobody questioned it. He estimates that he threw 360 days a year, the rare American to embrace nagekomi. He struck up a friendship with Alan Jaeger, the long-toss guru, and became its greatest acolyte, throwing balls four hundred feet and beginning his innings with a running crow-hop throw, many of which soared to the backstop. By his junior season at UCLA, he was the best pitcher in the nation, a six-foot-one, 175-pound anomaly, a mite next to his six-foot-four, 220-pound teammate Gerrit Cole, who was born to throw 100 miles per hour.

Bauer is exhibit one in favor of sport specialization, the exception to the rules against year-round baseball and year-round throwing and everything else I'd come to believe. He was a freak of intelligence, self-awareness, and dedication. Bauer's body gave him 80 miles per hour. He discovered the last 20 himself.

"I'm an argument in favor of development, that it's possible subpar genetics can get to the level I'm at," Bauer said. "People could be a lot more like me than you see if they did it as long as I've done it. It's one of the reasons I have such a clean throwing pattern and arm action and don't have pain when I throw. I throw all the time."

Bauer built himself into a pitching machine with help from around the country. He spent weeks at a time at Ron Wolforth's

Texas Baseball Ranch. Every offseason, he visited Dr. Marcus El-
liott, who took his Harvard Medical School degree and devoted
himself to athletic performance and injury prevention. Alan
Jaeger counted him among his most dedicated students. And for
two years he had gone to Driveline because Kyle Boddy made
him think.

The issue of command was a particularly good brainteaser.
Control—throwing strikes consistently—was difficult enough.
Command is the ability to locate those pitches. It is considered
unteachable. Pound strike-throwing into a guy's head enough and
he probably can get the ball over the plate. Command, the belief
goes, is as inborn as eye color, and no matter how hard he tried,
Bauer hadn't found it. He struggled with it after Arizona drafted
him third overall in 2011. He wasn't much better after a trade to
Cleveland prior to the 2013 season. Bauer refused to believe he
couldn't master it, and his father wanted to know whether Boddy
had any ideas to complement the offseason plan they were about
to hatch.

Bauer wanted to expand upon a randomized-training program from the previous offseason. He would throw either a
four-, a five-, or a six-ounce ball, different every time, and the
varying weights would help him gain better proprioception, the
subconscious feedback that allows muscles to repeat movements
and organize the body. That wasn't enough for Bauer. Baseball is
imperfect. Some mounds are slanted one way, some another. Days
are hot or cold, sunny or gloomy. Pitching in the first inning is
an entirely different animal than going in in the eighth after one
hundred pitches. The variables in a game are infinite, Bauer figured, so if his training were the same it could theoretically help
him command pitches in any type of environment.

"I throw a pitch, and before the next one I do twenty single-
leg squats with my right leg," Bauer said. "Now I go to throw
the pitch, this [leg] is partially fatigued. I still have to try to hit
that at sixty feet, so that's going to be different, but still trying to

execute the pitch. So you teach your body to be able to, if this is slightly fatigued."

Bauer didn't stop with the squats. He wanted to "destabilize the system." After throwing a six-ounce cutter, he would do some sort of rotational drill. Then he would throw another six-ounce cutter before reaching randomly for a four-, five-, or six-ounce ball to throw. One more six-ounce cutter preceded the final flourish. Bauer would take a ball and shoot into a bucket, like he was playing hoops, or kick a soccer ball, or swing a bat, or jump. And finally he would grab a four-ounce ball and try to cut it to the same spot he had with the six-ounce ball.

"The more you change up the system of how your body has to move, the more natural your body actually looks to solve that trick," Bauer said. "Your body is a great problem solver, so you're going to solve that equation a lot better."

Nearly every day Bauer followed this routine with his fastball and cutter, the two pitches he wanted to throw for strikes. Boddy had predicted six months earlier that Bauer would come into the 2015 season sitting 100 miles per hour. Had he scrapped the experiment and focused on velocity, Bauer probably could've. An extra couple of miles per hour for a guy who sat 94 off the mound wasn't going to change his life nearly as much as command would.

"I've gone through a lot of changes to be able to actually execute, make it all better," Bauer said. "It's taken a couple years, and I've become a head case and a bust and all the different stuff in between."

Performance determines reputation, and Bauer understood that his career ERA of 4.44 going into the 2015 season gave him little leeway. He was lucky to be with the Indians, an organization deep in pitching minds—Eric Binder, with whom Bauer had worked at the Texas Baseball Ranch, was the team's assistant director for player development—and willing to let him experiment. If one of the 750 Major League Baseball players in the world wanted to use training modalities rooted in decades of obscure studies to defeat the impossible, the Indians wouldn't argue. It would be a far easier sell if he cut a point or two off that ERA. If the command training worked, he would, and it might help him move closer to achieving another dream.

"*ESPN the Magazine*'s Body Issue," Bauer said. "Five years. That's my goal. The Body Issue in five years. You want to hear my life plan? In five years, be on the body cover, and that's going to buy me enough notoriety that in six years I can find the most attractive gold-medalist track athlete from the 2020 Games."

Though he had grown up since his trade from Arizona and had found comfort and camaraderie in the Indians' clubhouse, on occasion Bauer lapsed back into the weird kid who hung with the physics teacher during lunch. Stumping for eugenics qualified as one of those times, and yet he was as serious as could be: the curious side of Bauer wondered what a structured intersection of nature and nurture could produce.

"My kid is going to be raised in an environment that loves growth mind-set and work ethic," Bauer said. "And by the time he's fifteen, he's going to be throwing a hundred."

Genetics being what they are, he was reminded, it's about as likely he would father a girl.

"If it's a she," Bauer said, "she'll be number one in the world in something."

MICROCHIPS, AS MUCH AS MUSCLES, contain the keys to unlocking the secrets of pitching arms. Moore's law says computing power doubles every two years, which for baseball means the future is nigh. It may already be here. In Philadelphia, a company called KinaTrax built a platform that it says can capture motion data without markers. If KinaTrax's technology works as advertised, it means that the twenty-three reflective pads Glenn Fleisig sticks on pitchers at ASMI, or the full-body motion-capture suits athletes wear to help map out movement for video games, could soon be obsolete. The implications are enormous. The two great drawbacks of Fleisig's biomechanical testing are the unnatural feeling of being marked up and the sterile feeling of throwing off a portable mound inside a laboratory. KinaTrax purports to capture the same kinematic data as Fleisig's and other indoor labs but in natural environments like Tropicana Field, where in 2015 the Tampa Bay Rays became the first major league team to install a system.

KinaTrax is essentially a high-powered multi-camera version of the Xbox Kinect, the first mass-consumer motion-capture product. Its eight cameras shoot 200 to 300 frames per second and use telephoto lenses accurate up to three hundred feet. Every pitch takes up more than ten gigabytes of data, which gets uploaded into the cloud and is available for retrieval the next day.

mThrow, a compression sleeve with an embedded sensor that claims to capture live data and send it to a smartphone app via Bluetooth, says it can provide a more immediate pitch-data fix. For two years, Motus Global, a Long Island–based biomechanics company that caters to baseball, football, tennis, golf, lacrosse, and track athletes, has poured money into the sleeve in hopes that it becomes standard on not only big league pitchers whose arms are worth millions but also Little League pitchers who want to avoid injury. mThrow is a clean, simple device. A packing-peanut-sized sensor slips into the sleeve and is placed in the nook of the elbow where the UCL ties together the upper and lower arms. After every pitch, the app registers the newton meters of force on the elbow, the angle of the forearm at release, the shoulder's range of motion, the speed of the forearm, and the number of pitches thrown. The question, as with KinaTrax, is whether it actually does what it claims to do. Motus has the exclusive right and ability to download mThrow's data, a fact that bothered Kyle Boddy.

"I did what any mad Asian would do," Boddy said. "I impersonated the Motus servers using software, intercepted the 'phone calls home' [that] the unit and my phone make to Motus, and figured out exactly how to get the data I want." Boddy analyzed the data and came away doubting its accuracy. Compared with the Wiimote contraption he built in 2011 that measured the same things, Boddy said, the mThrow wasn't the revolutionary solution Motus claimed, as did *Popular Science* magazine, which trumpeted: "This Sleeve Will Help Save Pitchers' Arms."

The mThrow was a fine first step, Boddy thought—certainly better than nothing—but it needed complementary pieces. The sleeve gave no advice about how to correct bad mechanics or what to do if the torque on a pitcher's arm jumped too high. Numbers are just numbers without context, and even the numbers themselves depended on the position of the sensor, which could slip without a pitcher noticing.

"The measurements are still wildly incorrect," Boddy said. "Do I have to do everything in this fucking industry to get things done? Is everyone that incompetent?"

Given Boddy's bouts of egotism, the email he sent me February 13, 2015, felt uncharacteristic. He linked to two papers written by Dr. James Buffi and said he was close to hiring him:

It's actual genius-level material that goes beyond the inverse dynamics of what ASMI does. It could be exceedingly revolutionary. Fortunately for me, he's read my site and he thinks that I'm the only guy who understands how to train pitchers. Works for me.

Never before had I seen him lavish praise on a peer without caveat. And to call Buffi a peer was a stretch. He was a postdoctoral fellow at Northwestern University, biding his time for a few more months after finishing his research on the muscles in the forearm and their effect on the UCL. After hours of scouring the Internet for his intellectual and scientific equal, Boddy had found one.

Buffi, who grew up in Smithfield, Rhode Island, playing baseball, was always one of the smallest kids—he stands just five feet six today—and wanted to learn how to throw as fast as his taller teammates. Buffi's parents bought him a Tom House book on mechanics. "That's when I realized how complex the pitching motion really was," he said. After graduating from Notre Dame, Buffi went to Northwestern to study the forearm muscles in hopes of making better prosthetic limbs. He stumbled across medical literature relating to baseball, got hooked, and received permission from his advisor and PhD committee to write his dissertation about the forearm muscles' impact on the throwing motion. Buffi's goal was to figure out exactly how much the muscles contribute to protecting the UCL and how it varies from pitcher to pitcher, and to do so, he used a method rarely applied to baseball.

Almost every biomechanics lab, including ASMI's, uses a process for measuring force on joints called inverse dynamics. It starts by figuring out the total loads on joints, then works backward and assigns the amount of force to individual joints, including the valgus torque on the elbow. Buffi specialized in musculoskeletal modeling, in which he loaded motion-capture data of a college pitcher throwing a pitch into a computerized version of the human body created by his advisor. He used the model to simulate the force on each of the four forearm muscles that make up the flexor-pronator mass. This was called forward dynamics, and while in the biomechanical world it's nothing new—researchers have used it to analyze walking patterns for years—the gait is a far simpler pattern than the throwing motion.

"One of the things Kyle said when we were talking, which really struck a chord with me, was that compared to where technology is, baseball science is like back in the 1970s and '80s," Buffi said. "When I follow Kyle's stuff, he's fairly close to the present. When I started looking into baseball research, I was like, 'Oh, my goodness. I can do anything I want and it's going to be novel and awesome.' This whole field is wide open."

Prior research had focused on the flexor-pronator muscles. One of Mike Marshall's grand theories held that the pronator teres, the largest muscle of the four, helped protect the UCL. A study overseen by Dr. Frank Jobe in 1996 using EMG sensors said the flexor-pronator muscles "do not supplant the role of the medial collateral ligament during the fastball pitch," a conclusion that another paper eight years later would dispute. In that study, Dr. Christopher Ahmad, now the team doctor for the New York Yankees, wrote, "The flexor-pronator mass dynamically stabilizes the elbow against valgus torque." Translation: valgus torque, the injurious force believed to rip apart elbow ligaments, could be lessened with better use of the forearm muscles. Of particular importance was the flexor carpi ulnaris, a muscle that Jobe's study said covered the UCL during 120 degrees, or nearly two-thirds, of shoulder rotation.

Buffi's initial research confirmed the importance of the flexor muscles. Perhaps they were what enabled R. A. Dickey to pitch without a UCL. Maybe they explained why some pitchers stayed healthy and others didn't. To further test his hypothesis, Buffi worked with researchers at Massachusetts General Hospital's biomechanics lab, which captured the throwing motions of twenty college pitchers with markers as well as ground-force data collected with force plates. Buffi's optimization algorithm fit the markers in the model as close as possible to those on the real pitchers. "The goal," Buffi said, "is to get the model to move in exactly the same way the real pitcher moves."

Of the twenty pitchers, thirteen had no previous major arm injuries and seven did. Blinded to the results, Buffi correctly identified six of the seven injured pitchers and twelve of the thirteen without injuries based solely on the model's data. Buffi then used inverse dynamics, the standard method, to assess all twenty pitchers. It could not tell the difference between who had been injured and who hadn't.

This was just the beginning of his research, too, and that's what excited Buffi the most. "I'm optimistic it will also be predictive," he said, and if it were—if a simple biomechanical analysis fed into his model really could portend danger—the implications would be huge. Same with the knowledge Buffi could glean from other pitches. Motion-capture data is almost always restricted to pitchers throwing fastballs only. Baseball, meanwhile, is littered with theories on the adverse effect of other pitches on the elbow.

Bill James long wondered whether sinkerballers are more injury-prone. Sliders are anecdotally death to elbows. Split-fingered fastballs fell out of favor because of concern that they led to arm troubles. Cutters and curveballs and screwballs at one time or another have all been Public Arm Enemy Number One.

Perhaps Buffi's model could establish a stronger relationship between particular pitches—or even the particular grips on pitches—and health. Boddy wanted to try that and a million other things with it: test different strengthening exercises on each individual forearm muscle to find a proper way to train the flexor-pronator mass; run Driveline clients' biomechanical profiles through the model to sniff out red flags; and maybe even produce a proper compression sleeve whose engine would put the mThrow to shame. If Buffi consulted with Driveline, or even joined full-time, it would ensure the world could see his research.

"If you work for a team, nothing gets out," Buffi said. "Everything stays in-house. I'd really like to help as many people as I can. I've never been trained as a clinician or in therapy, so I need to work with someone in science who can translate the findings into something that can train pitchers."

Drawbacks to forward dynamics do exist, and Buffi's findings weren't an automatic change to how we view the arm. "Parsing the individual contributions of muscles and stresses experienced by ligaments and tendons is very difficult," said Neil Roach, the biological anthropologist who used inverse dynamics for his study on the evolution of prehistoric throwing. "Forward dynamics is a potential way around this problem, but it requires some major assumptions and can be quite error-prone. I think a combination of the two methods is advisable. This allows us to cross-check any errors in both models and further parse total joint contributions into the constituent parts."

Still, it was different. And though baseball frowns upon things that are different, that's what made it such a potential gold mine. Roach read through Buffi's work and was impressed. Mike Marshall called Buffi and wondered if he could run one of his pitchers through the model. When Buffi wrote a series of articles outlining his methodology and results for Driveline's website, baseball took notice.

"I don't want to say I can fix elbow injuries, but I think I can compensate for the thing that I found with training," Buffi said. "It's a really, really hard problem to solve. Hopefully I'm making some good steps toward solving it."

IN THE MIDDLE OF JANUARY 2015, Casey Weathers was throwing only 90 miles per hour off the mound. Every day, he came into Driveline Baseball's rickety gym, and every day he stared at the radar board on the wall and wondered what the hell happened to his arm. It felt fine. He was still healthy. The arm that threw a ball 105.8 miles per hour simply vanished.

"I suck," Weathers muttered, and Kyle Boddy would nod along, still confident his grand plan was unfolding at just the right pace. A month earlier, Weathers agreed to a minor league deal with the Cleveland Indians. He would report to Goodyear, Arizona, for spring training just like Trevor Bauer, and he'd bring with him stories of playing test subject for Bauer's and Boddy's mad-scientist routine. Weathers was doing command training, too, a variation on Bauer's but taxing nevertheless.

Depending on the day, Weathers would throw anywhere from twenty-five to sixty pitches at a seventeen-by-seventeen-inch black pad that serves as a strike-zone proxy and looks like the back of a chair. Bauer first used it at the Texas Baseball Ranch, and the thud when the ball hit the pad was a nugget of positive reinforcement for a job well done. Weathers wanted to make the drill even harder. Rather than aiming for a specific area—low and away, high and inside, middle-out—he spaced dime-sized colored dots a centimeter or two apart from each other and aimed for one minute spot. Often he was close enough that a miss didn't feel as much like a miss might have otherwise.

Weathers started at fifty-four feet with only five-ounce balls. Once he started hitting his target on 75 percent of his throws, he moved back to sixty feet, six inches, and added weighted balls to the mix. Five throws at six ounces, five at four ounces, with mixed intent—sometimes 80 percent, sometimes max effort, always chopped up.

"We want them to hate their workouts," Boddy said. "Well, not really, but the training has that effect. Like, throw a four-ounce ball at 80 percent of perceived maximum effort to a low target, then your next throw is a regular baseball as hard as possible to a high target. That's impossible to do. But over time it absolutely helps because you don't get trapped in 'throw a pitch, miss, complain, throw a pitch, hit, great, who cares.' They actually have to think every rep through."

As February dawned and Boddy tapered down the intensity of Weathers's workouts, his velocity returned alongside his command. He was sitting at 92, touching 95, and banging his low-and-away strikes 70 percent of the time. The plan was working.

"I knew it would," Boddy said. "I took the foot off the abuse meter. It's not physical. A guy like Casey has no problem with the physical stuff, but they've generally never been mentally challenged or psychologically challenged in that way. It's very tedious, boring work that they're bad at. Not only is this boring, it's really hard and it sucks."

How it would translate a few weeks down the road Boddy didn't know. If Weathers and Bauer threw strikes, maybe he was on to something. If they didn't, he'd try his best to understand the limitations of the training and apply the pieces that did work, adding new components.

"I haven't solved shit," Boddy said. "I think I have a good

idea how to get people throwing harder and how to get guys healthy who were written off. But not everyone. Two kids have had elbow injuries, severe ones, while training here. There were extenuating circumstances, of course, but that's weaseling and cheating to hide behind that. It's the truth. Kids have been hurt under my watch, and more will."

I grew to appreciate Boddy because, for all of his arrogance, he refused to present failures as exceptions. One was an elite high school kid whom he couldn't convince to throw less in high school and on the showcase circuit. He underwent Tommy John surgery as a junior. The other dove for a ball at first base, hurt his elbow, and kept pitching. He suffered an avulsion fracture, like so many of the kids in Japan, and wound up needing surgery. A longtime adherent of year-round throwing, Boddy has peeled back his offseason program in recent winters as an acknowledgment of its potential harm.

He wanted so badly to fix what was wrong with professional baseball's approach to the arm. Boddy tried to appeal to the rational side of baseball's front offices with a blog post entitled "Making the Sabermetric Argument for Increasing Fastball Velocity." In it, he argued that a player whose fastball jumped from 86 miles per hour to 90 would be worth around an extra marginal win per season because of the likelihood the extra velocity would lop off some home runs and add some strikeouts. It behooved teams to encourage their pitchers to throw harder and hope the training protocols he employed could help keep them healthy.

"This can be done to Todd Coffey," Boddy said. "This can be done to Scott Kazmir. This can be done. . . . I'm asking you to believe that someone who was good, who has been failed by player development, like Casey Weathers, could again be possibly worth something to the organization. Casey Weathers is worth a lot to an organization even if he never throws a pitch in Major League Baseball because it's an amazing, not story, but validated experiment, that this can be done."

While Boddy chafed at the Astros' unwillingness to implement more of his training methods—he even had the backing of Brent Strom, their big league pitching coach, who ran in the same hipster-pitching-coach circles—he found a new favorite team in a familiar place: Cleveland, where he grew up rooting for the Indians. Bauer and Eric Binder vouched for him. Mickey Callaway, Cleveland's pitching coach, visited Driveline in the offseason before 2015 to understand what Boddy did. Others in the organization liked his work. Weathers was a testament, as was Nick Hagadone, the Indians' hard-throwing left-handed reliever who trained with Boddy and emerged with a new cut fastball. If Buffi joined the staff, which Boddy expected, Driveline only would get better.

And maybe at some point, as with the sabermetric revolution, major league teams would no longer be able to ignore the world of arm health. Perhaps it would take a standard-bearer, someone waving a bright flag of major league success, to speed up the process.

"If Trevor wins the Cy Young, it makes a big difference," Warren Bauer said. "The difference isn't going to be any change, but it's going to put a question out there."

Trevor Bauer didn't come to Indians camp in the spring of 2015 in *ESPN* Body Issue shape, but he looked nonetheless like a new pitcher. One of his new toys was a drone he built during the offseason that Major League Baseball banned him from flying around the Indians' facility. The other was a new pitch nobody knew existed.

The laminar-flow fastball was the brainchild of Trevor Bauer. Other pitchers threw it. They just didn't realize how or why it moved like it did. A video on YouTube featuring an Australian professor named Rod Cross discusses the idea of laminar and turbulent flow. Laminar flow is when air goes over an object smoothly. Turbulent air, as every airline passenger understands, is rough. Cross showed how with the right grip and proper axis of spin, a pitcher could throw a ball with a large smooth patch on one side and a rough seam on the other, and the turbulence would cause the ball to move almost twice as much as standard spinning-ball physics would suggest.

Bauer felt comfortable enough with the laminar-flow fastball that he unleashed it during his wildly successful spring training. Over 27⅔ innings in exhibition games, Bauer walked one batter and struck out twenty-six. His stuff was as good as ever. His command of it was better than he could've imagined.

On the other side of the Indians' complex, Casey Weathers kept throwing strikes and was assigned to Class A Lynchburg. At twenty-nine, he was seven years older than the average player in the league, and in order to validate his position in the Indians' organization, he needed to show one of two things: exquisite command or monster velocity. Weathers walked two in his first game with Lynchburg and two more in his second, and his fastball sat around 93. It started ticking up, and he didn't walk anybody in half of his next ten games, and the velocity went a little higher, and the outs were coming, the ERA dropping. And on May 24, 2015, the same day Weathers walked two batters, the same day he hung a slider that got tattooed for a three-run home run, he did something that before going to Driveline never could've happened.

The guy with the mashed-potatoes elbow hit 100 miles per hour off the mound.

I USUALLY AGREED WITH KYLE BODDY and his analysis of why baseball keeps regressing while ostensibly trying to keep arms healthy, but one thing he said struck me as terribly pessimistic: "I think we are about twenty-five years away from having the same type of revolution that *Moneyball* struck."

What I see doesn't look nearly as grim. Soon enough, the mThrow sleeve will seem comically oversized. Maybe Motus creates the mSticker, a disposable adhesive affixed to the elbow that wirelessly sends every sliver of biometric data imaginable to a computer. Perhaps it's a molecule-sized device injected into the elbow or fastened via minimally invasive surgery that allows for twenty-four-hour monitoring. Biohacking isn't just for sci-fi movies. Offer pitchers unparalleled knowledge about their most vital equipment and plenty will ask for a pen and the dotted line.

The nanotechnology revolution will arrive well before the next quarter century has come and gone and bring with it entirely new ways to treat injuries. The repair of a torn UCL without surgery? Not out of the question. The growth of stronger ligaments in laboratories using stem cells? Quite possible.

For today, we already have KinaTrax, or whatever markerless motion-capture company eventually corners the marker. We have ASMI's Throw Like a Pro app, which keeps track of pitchers and offers educational videos. We have the potential prospect of Jeffrey Dugas's modified Tommy John surgery to halve the recovery time.

Lurking on the periphery of this landscape are individuals like James Buffi, hoping somebody notices their work. If his model really could help predict injuries, Kyle Boddy said, "he could be Dr. Frank Jobe." Boddy wasn't the only one paying attention. Buffi heard from Matt Arnold, the Tampa Bay Rays' director of pro scouting. The Rays are one of baseball's most progressive organizations, employing a disproportionate number of analysts and data crunchers for a team with such a low payroll. For years, they avoided pitching injuries, emphasizing one of the best shoulder-strengthening programs in the industry. Then their young star Matt Moore needed Tommy John surgery. And so did his replacement atop the rotation, Alex Cobb. Even without a breakthrough, Buffi wouldn't make enough money for there to be any downside to the Rays' hiring him.

Another call frightened Boddy far more than Tampa Bay's: a man named Doug Fearing, the director of research and development for the Los Angeles Dodgers, wanted to speak with Buffi about his findings. The Dodgers were run by Andrew Friedman, the hyperintelligent president of baseball operations who had just left the Rays after a decade-long run of success. In Los Angeles, no budget bound Friedman. The Dodgers had just started an $8 billion local-television contract that allowed their annual payrolls to threaten $300 million. Even better, Friedman and general manager Farhan Zaidi were allowing Fearing to build baseball's biggest, best think tank. They were seeking experts in quantitative psychology and applied mathematics. One of Buffi's friends from Northwestern's PhD program, a data scientist named Megan Schroeder, already was working with the Dodgers as an analyst. She raved to Buffi about the Dodgers' new front-office brain trust.

Boddy's chief concern was that the Dodgers would steal Buffi and his work for their organization alone, further setting back the cause of all baseball pitchers.

"He's gonna work for the Dodgers," Trevor Bauer told Boddy.

"What makes you say that?" Boddy said.

"When you were twenty-nine and I met you," Bauer said, "would you have worked for Ron Wolforth or for the Indians?"

"Ah, fuck you," Boddy said.

"Exactly," Bauer said.

In June 2015, Buffi accepted a job with the Dodgers about three months after he told me he didn't want to work for a team.

"I did believe that," Buffi said. "But when I came back from the Dodgers, I was so impressed by the people they had on board. They were talking such a big game about research and creating a premier baseball think tank and hiring the smartest minds in baseball. And they have Andrew and Farhan and Doug."

Buffi wasn't a hypocrite. He was a realist. Working for the Dodgers provided an incredible opportunity to continue his research. He had endless money, an available pool of test subjects inside the Dodgers' farm system, and the chance to learn from some of the finest minds in the sport. If he wanted to track the arm using inertial measurement units—a sensor used more often to guide airplanes, spaceships, and missiles—track it he could. Buffi could buy all the joint-angle-measuring electrogoniometers his heart desired.

The Dodgers would be happy to provide whatever it took to perfect his model, especially if it did what he thought it could. As he completed his research, Buffi used his model to develop a radical hypothesis: valgus torque may not be the right way to measure ligament strain (how far it stretches compared with its length at rest) or stress (the amount of force being placed on it). Considering that decades of baseball research, including much of what has come out of ASMI, leaned on valgus torque, Buffi's findings had potentially significant implications, particularly if another researcher could replicate them or Buffi could show similar findings in a different study.

Now the public won't know, at least not in the immediate future. Buffi's knowledge goes directly into the Dodgers' information silo.

"I traded the opportunity to impact a ton of people, which I do want to do because I'm still only twenty-nine," Buffi said. "I just thought this opportunity to get in the ground floor—I had to make a choice. It feels like a selfish decision. But I did the best I could."

In a conversation with Buffi about spreading potential innovations to the masses, Friedman said all the right things about being open-minded. Buffi wasn't so naive as to think the Dodgers would simply give away proprietary information for the good of baseball. There are championships to be won, and the easiest way to do it is with a pitching staff full of healthy arms and the wisdom to flip those whose arms won't be.

When he called Boddy to tell him he took the Dodgers job, Buffi teared up. "I'm a sensitive guy," he later said. He was fond of Boddy, appreciative of the opportunity to write about his work, certain that Driveline would maintain its spirit of research and development without him.

"I was pretty pissed for about twenty minutes for the future of Driveline," Boddy said. "The company is going to go on. It just sucks. For all of baseball. It sucks that not everybody's going to know about his work, no matter what happens with the Dodgers. The worst-case scenario is he has a breakthrough with them. Because then the world won't see it." He sighed. "You can only learn you hate pro ball one way," Boddy said. "By working in it."

Boddy's own moral position was soon put to the test when the Indians wanted more information on his weighted-ball program and a better understanding of his command drills. They offered him a consulting deal to evaluate the deliveries of draft prospects. He jumped at it. "The short-term money in this business is lying to nine-year-olds about select and travel baseball," Boddy said. "The long-term money is becoming a cornerstone that pro teams rely on, which gives you implicit power, and dominating college baseball so you have a constant feeder system of high-level clients."

Over the winter, Boddy spoke to a captive audience at Vanderbilt that included its most distinguished baseball alum and Casey Weathers's college teammate David Price. When I asked Price in February 2015 what he thought of Boddy, he said: "I couldn't believe he had the knowledge he did about building arm strength. It all made sense. I got it." Maybe Price would work with him in the future. For now, though, he wasn't changing anything. Price was a free agent after the 2015 season, and he wouldn't risk deviating from what he knew. On December 1, 2015, Price signed a seven-year, $217 million contract with the Boston Red Sox. It was more than three times as much as their first offer to Jon Lester.

Maybe Boddy would've made Price better. Maybe he would've suffered a season-ending injury like Nick Hagadone, who trained with Boddy going into 2015 and underwent surgery a few months later. Knowledge in baseball was fluid as ever. Even Alex Anthopoulos, the Blue Jays' general manager, admitted that Toronto no longer treated pitchers of Noah Syndergaard's, Aaron Sanchez's, and Justin Nicolino's ilk with strict inning limits. Anthopoulos could have pointed to their clean arms—especially Syndergaard blasting 100-mph fastballs for the Mets as a World Series starter—as evidence that restrictions did work. He didn't. It would have been self-serving and intellectually dishonest.

"Over the last four or five years, there's more Tommy Johns, even from some guys who have been protected," Anthopoulos said. "They still got hurt. They still broke down. We owed it to ourselves to reevaluate things."

It's true everywhere, even on the cutting edge, where the rest of baseball must place itself sooner than later. If major league teams refuse to stop spending well over a billion dollars on free agent arms—with Price's $217 million deal and the Arizona Diamondbacks lavishing Zack Greinke with $206.5 million, teams guaranteed pitchers nearly $1.5 billion in the winter of 2015—perhaps it would behoove them to prioritize learning about what they don't know. Inside Major League Baseball's offices, this comprises two efforts. The first concerns kids. Over the next five years, MLB plans on extending its tentacles deep into baseball's youth network, not just to endear itself to a fading fan base but to strengthen control of its feeder system. By targeting Perfect Game—baseball could buy it out, force changes, or crush it—MLB would send a strong message to the youth baseball–industrial complex: join in the effort or go away. The blowback will be significant, not just from Perfect Game but from the year-round baseball racket. Equipment sales exceed $500 million annually. Year-round facilities exist to serve a game that now has a twelve-month season. The fear of a slain cash cow would set loose an army of lobbyists from across the industry on MLB. Ultimately, the power resides on Park Avenue.

And that's where part two factors in: Nobody will know whether the Inverted W really is sinister or how the ARPwave may actually heal UCL tears without scientific research, a world into which MLB has already dipped its toes without drowning. Baseball needs to dive in headlong. Considering the monetary cost of arm injuries—and the prospect of even more, at salaries climbing above $34 million per year, as the sport fills with players from the Perfect Game generation—baseball should look at this as a crucial investment in itself and its health rather than a loss leader.

MLB's epidemiologists need access to more data, from baseline and follow-up testing to nutritional profiles and sleep patterns. Doctors, trainers, managers, and coaches must agree that there is no one-size-fits-all solution for the arm and shift toward individualized programs, the kind Trevor Bauer espouses. Every body is different. Every arm is different. The idea of standardized throwing protocols is antiquated and nevertheless convention across the game. An expanded health staff—more athletic trainers, more strength coaches, more massage therapists—would help craft plans to address weaknesses while respecting limitations. Medical analyses would feed the HITS database with even more information for the researchers trying to snuff out injuries.

Patterns could emerge, and even if they don't, the league's open-mindedness toward third-party vendors like KinaTrax and Motus and other emerging technology companies could promote innovation. Baseball needs whatever it can muster. Average fastball velocity continues to rise toward 93 mph. Velocity exists because velocity works. And because velocity works, ridding the game of it will be far more difficult than the other deep-seated issues. So as noble as it is for ASMI to suggest young pitchers learn to throw at less than 100 percent, it is not realistic. Velocity is here to stay. The only sane option is to train pitchers' arms to handle it without harming them through overtraining.

The truest sign of MLB's long-term commitment—and the hardest to imagine because of baseball's institutional stubbornness—would include a think tank where the game houses its research, explores the novel training modalities championed at places like Driveline, and prepares the next generation of trainers and other medical personnel. This is the village's hub in Billy Beane's it-takes-a-village approach. This is where top amateur players come for pre-draft physicals, where athletic trainers and PTs and masseuses get specialized on-the-job educations, where curious, interested, or desperate players can go to participate in studies about weighted balls, electrical stimulation, and the technological advances that lie ahead. It finds minds like James Buffi and hires them for the good of the whole sport. It is baseball's chance to build a culture of knowledge and bury its culture of fear.

All of that knowledge eventually would wend its way throughout teams' systems and into the minor leagues, where today every team treats players in whom they've invested tens of millions of dollars—and on whom they'll spend hundreds of millions more—with all the solicitude of a goldfish getting a sprinkle of its daily flakes.

"We just have so far to go in this sport," Boddy said, and it's from the rec-league fields where my son plays to the festivals of nine- and ten-year-olds getting radar-gunned at Perfect Game events to the showcase circuit on steroids to colleges that major in moral hazard to behind-the-times pro ball and all the way to North Carolina, where Todd Coffey just wanted to prove he still belonged.

CHAPTER 16

Spring

January 7, 2015

Late at night, Todd Coffey sat in the dark with a flashlight and his fish. The LED display on the sixty-five-gallon tank automatically shut off at 11:00 p.m., at which point the blue hippo and clownfish retreated to the corners of the tank while the shrimp and crabs and snails came to life. They would dance around the coral and plants, regal and beautiful, seduced by the beam Coffey held. And when he finally tired around 3:00 a.m. and decided to pop his Ambien, Coffey clicked off the flashlight and the show was over.

January 8, 2015

Baseball's offseason calendar consists of two distinct periods: before and after Christmas. Almost every notable transaction takes place prior to the holiday, at which point the industry shuts down for a week. Come the New Year, those still unemployed find a job market that registers somewhere between unfriendly and hopeless.

Todd Coffey needed a team. "I thought I had him jobs back in December," said Rick Thurman, his agent, "and all the clubs went AWOL." Baltimore, Houston, Tampa Bay, Texas, Colorado, and Pittsburgh had shown slivers of interest. "I'd prefer it to be Pittsburgh," Coffey said. "I don't like American League–style baseball. And it's not because they hit better. So that cuts it to Colorado and Pittsburgh. And if I don't even like to play catch when I go to Colorado, why would I go there to play?"

He harbored no expectations of a major league contract, even though he still saw himself as a big leaguer. Coffey felt that his 1.83 ERA in the Pacific Coast League at least merited a minor league deal. "My arm feels freaking phenomenal," Coffey said. "Way better than it did last year."

Earlier in the week, a team from Japan called Thurman, whose contacts there go back decades, and asked for Coffey's medical records. The team never followed up.

January 30, 2015

With pitchers and catchers reporting to their teams in less than three weeks, an email popped into Coffey's AOL in-box at 10:10 a.m. on an otherwise uneventful Friday,

> Hi Todd—this is Terry Reynolds with the Reds. Will you be working out for teams? If so when and where? Good luck and thank you.
>
> Terry Reynolds

Reynolds was director of pro scouting for the Cincinnati Reds, the team that had drafted Coffey back in 1998. This was the perfect circle. Kismet. Coffey wrote back with his cell phone number and said he would love to chat. They connected, and Reynolds said he would reconnect with him Monday.

Hi Todd—We would like to have one of our scouts come over and see you this week. Can you give me the exact date, time and location of your next bullpen session? Are you throwing at 100% in your sessions?

Thanks for your help,

Terry

Coffey was throwing at about 90 percent, and he had a bull-pen later that week. The Reds were sending Cam Bonifay, the former Pittsburgh Pirates general manager who was now a special assistant to Reds GM Walt Jocketty.

"It tells me something that they reached out to me personally," Coffey said. "They know me. They know what I can do. That's why there's pressure on it. They just want to see what my arm looks like. I don't think they're worried about whether something is perfect. They know me."

Their bullpen coach, Mack Jenkins, had been the Triple-A pitching coach when Coffey was called to the big leagues for the first time. Jim Riggleman, the Reds' third-base coach, had managed Coffey in Washington. The last time they'd seen each other, Riggleman had shaken his hand and said: "If you ever need anything, give me a call."

Coffey didn't. His arm would take care of this.

February 6, 2015

On the poster she made for her father, fourteen-year-old Hannah Coffey wrote "Me and Daddy" above a drawing of Coffey in a red jersey and gray pants next to her. Both were smiling. The sun glistened. The sky was blue, the grass green. Next to the picture, Hannah wrote a message.

Dear Daddy

I wanted to say good luck today! And to take a deep breath. Just have fun! Please have the spark today.

Love,

Hannah Nicole Coffey

Hannah had moved in with Coffey during the early stages of his rehab because she and his ex-wife fought too much. Together, Hannah and Coffey watched history shows. He taught her that if a book is good enough, they'll make a movie or TV program out of it.

Around three p.m., Hannah showed up to the field at nearby Chase High in Forest City, North Carolina, along with Jennifer and Coffey's father. Coffey had arrived about a half hour earlier, carrying his gear in a Los Angeles Dodgers bag. The day didn't match Hannah's picture; it was partly cloudy, light wind, 45 degrees. Coffey stalled for a few minutes and chatted up Bonifay, telling him about signing with the Reds for a thousand bucks. It was a typical warm-up, darts delivered from progressively longer distances until his arm loosened up and he took to the mound. Bonifay used only his eyes. No radar gun. No notepad. Just the instincts of a scout who had seen enough thirtysomething pitchers trying to make it back to the big leagues to know which might succeed and which would struggle. Coffey spun his fastballs and sliders, finished strong, and bid Bonifay adieu, figuring he would hear from the Reds soon thereafter to formalize a deal.

"They said they wanted to see I was healthy," Coffey said. "Obviously, I showed I was healthy. I'm ready to roll. He didn't have a gun. He didn't care about velocity."

When the bullpen ended, Hannah ran into the dugout. She hadn't gotten a chance to give him one last piece of paper before he threw. It wished him good luck. To the right, she drew a baseball that said "MLB" in tiny letters.

February 7, 2015

Like every free agent in baseball desperate for a job, Todd Coffey clicked on MLBTradeRumors.com daily. Less than twenty-four hours after his showcase, he read the news: Cincinnati signed reliever Burke Badenhop and gave reliever Kevin Gregg a minor league deal. The circle wasn't perfect after all.

February 10, 2015

The Atlanta Braves called. It was John Coppolella, the assistant general manager in name but in reality the puppeteer for most of the Braves' offseason maneuvers. They'd dismantled the team, trading star outfielders Justin Upton and Jason Heyward, all with the expectation of rebuilding by the time they moved into a new stadium in 2017.

Coffey regretted not having signed with the Braves the previous season, and this was his opportunity to rectify the mistake. Coppolella was offering the opportunity, only with a catch: "He wants me to do a minor league deal with no invite," said Coffey, who couldn't remember a scenario in which a player with more than six years of service time did not receive an invitation to major league camp. Neither could Thurman. Coppolella explained to Coffey that the Braves had signed so many players their complex at ESPN Wide World of Sports near Disney World simply didn't have the locker space for him.

Coppolella promised Coffey that he could attend the late-

February minicamp for some of the Braves' top prospects, so he wouldn't need to report in early March with the rest of the minor leaguers. He would pitch in five to eight major league spring-training games, too. The short-term opportunity was no good, Coppolella admitted. This was a long-term play.

"I don't know," Coffey told me. "I really don't know. I'm trying to process it." He'd have to dress with the minor leaguers and practice with the minor leaguers. "Straight off the top of my head, I'm like, 'Hell no,' but I didn't have any time in the big leagues last year," Coffey said. "Part of me says to sign with 'em, but not being there in big league camp sucks. It really does. You don't really hear of too many people who get into the big leagues without being in big league camp. He says there's opportunity there, but is there?" If Coffey did agree, he wanted some guarantees. No roommate on the road. That was a deal breaker. And opt-outs. Lots of opt-outs. Like, one a month, or an immediate one if another team wants him in the big leagues.

The larger truth of his situation remained unspoken: there were no opportunities elsewhere, either.

Coffey told Coppolella he would sleep on it.

February 11, 2015

From the transaction wire:

> Atlanta Braves signed free agent RHP Todd Coffey to a minor league contract.

I'VE SEEN THE AGONY OF an elbow that won't get better. It's ugly on the body and the psyche and the soul. There will be more players like Daniel Hudson in the coming years, ones whose arms simply won't relent. It's why I can't say it surprised me when I received a text message from Hudson on March 14, 2015.

What's your take on my situation? You're an expert, and
I have zero clue what I want to do and what's best for me.

In the midst of trying to figure out whether he wanted to
be a starter or reliever, Hudson's arm started to hurt. I went to
Diamondbacks camp to see him. He pointed to the painful area:
above the elbow and down to the tip, on the back of his upper
arm. The weird part: It felt fine when he was throwing. Then he
picked up a sock and lofted it toward a laundry basket, like he was
shooting a free throw. That caused the discomfort. Extending his
arm at thousands of degrees per second didn't bother him, and
neither did internally rotating his shoulder even faster. Something
harmless made him wonder if it was betraying him again.

I wasn't sure what to say. I wasn't a doctor, a trainer, a physical therapist, a strength-and-conditioning guru, a biomechanist.
Like Hudson, I simply wanted to decipher as much of the arm's
mystery as I could. Of the little bit of anatomy I picked up, I
knew a tiny muscle called the anconeus wrapped around the back
of the elbow. Perhaps that was tugging? Far more likely was a
strained triceps or triceps tendinitis. And that was fine. Triceps
issues never corresponded with UCL troubles.

"Darvish?" Hudson said.

He was right. The Texas Rangers did suggest publicly that
Yu Darvish's injury during the spring of 2015 was to the triceps,
though privately the team understood he needed Tommy John
surgery. It still gave Hudson pause. His unsettled standing made
for an even odder spring than it already was. In September 2014,
Arizona fired manager Kirk Gibson and GM Kevin Towers,
Hudson's two greatest advocates. When the Diamondbacks traded
Miguel Montero to the Cubs in the offseason, Hudson became
the longest-tenured player on the roster. Most of his friends and
confidants were gone. The Diamondbacks wanted to start him.
Hudson feared his arm wouldn't hold up to it.

One day during batting practice, Hudson was shagging balls in the outfield and crossed paths with pitching coach Mike Harkey, a holdover from the previous season. The fourth overall pick in the 1987 draft, Harkey was the Chicago Cubs' ace-in-waiting. At twenty-four, after a fantastic rookie season, he underwent shoulder surgery. Harkey was never the same and threw his last pitch at thirty.

"I was like, 'Did you ever get to a point where you kind of just realize that you're never going to not feel something in your arm?'" Hudson said. "And he goes, 'Yeah, I did. I kind of realized that it wasn't going to feel a hundred percent every single day, so I just stopped worrying about it.'"

For the rest of his career, Daniel Hudson will live in fear. Every little twinge, every slight tingle, every tiny jolt, and he'll wonder: Again? And he'll take that thought, bury it, and throw another pitch, because the alternative is a worse fate.

"I've put in all the frickin' work that I can. I completely changed the way I throw, you know? What else can you do?" Hudson said. "If it goes again, it's gonna go again."

ON HIS FIRST DAY OF minicamp in the shadow of Disney World, Todd Coffey was told he needed to pull his pant legs up and get rid of his beard. He had spent half of his thirty-four years in professional baseball; he knew some organizations still believed clean-shaven cheeks and showing off socks instills some sort of lesson in players. The Atlanta Braves were one such team, though the rules applied only to players in minor league camp and not those on the major league side. Already the day felt odd enough for Coffey. He was the oldest player in the nine-pitcher minicamp by nearly a decade. Most of the other players knew one another and caught up on their offseasons. Coffey was thinking about his stupid pants.

"I don't know why it bothers me that much, but it does," he said. "It really, really bothers me. I think because I felt like I've earned the right to wear my uniform any way I want to." Because Coffey loved baseball and refused to disrespect it, the next morning he jogged onto the field with his pants pulled midcalf, his socks yanked high, and a vestigial red mustache adorning his then-Braves upper lip. It was the least he could do after the previous day, when then-Braves manager Fredi González walked up, introduced himself, and shook his hand.

"I saw him go by and I made a point to come say hi to him," González said later. "Just respect. He was a guy that pitched in the big leagues, I don't know how many years? Top of my head, seven? He signed a minor league deal. He wasn't even a nonroster invitee, and I think Coppy called him and said, 'Hey do you want to pitch?' And he didn't bitch or moan or anything. He goes, 'Yeah, I'd love to pitch.' And he's out here with the early camp with the young guys and is, 'Why not?' I respect that a lot. I just wanted for him to feel comfortable."

Now, on the second day—after a morning in which Braves trainers asked for Coffey's weight, only for him to say: "Nah, I'm good"—he threw a bullpen in front of Coppolella, Braves president of baseball operations John Hart, and the brains behind Atlanta's century-spanning run of dominance, team president John Schuerholz. Coffey fired fastballs and sliders for fifteen minutes, shook the hands of the brass, and headed to the boredom of pitchers' fielding practice and running drills. He made good time on his first sprint and asked a strength-and-conditioning coach how quickly he ran it.

"About thirty-two," the coach said. "But you can do it in thirty."

"If you say I can do it in thirty," Coffey said, "I'm-a do it in thirty."

He did it in thirty, and by the third sprint, Coffey sucked down breaths with ravenous thirst, his hogshead chest heaving. As he went for round four, another coach marveled at Coffey's toothpick legs somehow supporting his torso in defiance of the laws of physics.

On the way back to the minor league clubhouse, as Coffey walked by a truck for Ellie Lou's Brews & BBQ that said "We'll Rub You the Right Way," a fan asked him to autograph some old baseball cards. For the moment, Coffey felt like a big leaguer again. "You don't know what you miss 'til you're out. You really don't," Coffey said. "Does it suck? Yeah, it sucks ass. Can I do anything else about it? No. It is what it is right now. But I've always made my own opportunities."

On March 7, in the Braves' fourth game of the spring, Coffey was summoned from minor league camp for an inning. He struck out two. His fastball hit 94. For most of the game, Coffey hung on the bench with former Braves star Fred McGriff, who had retired the year before Coffey's debut. They talked about how players are too soft these days. "I am such a fucking old man," Coffey said.

Five days after the first outing, Coffey was summoned again in a more precarious situation: first inning, bases loaded, two outs. He allowed a two-run single, reloaded the bases with a walk, and escaped with a flyout. For the next ten days, Coffey waited for another shot with the big league team. He kept his arm fresh in minor league games until the Braves summoned him once more March 23. Coffey allowed two runs on three singles. "Was actually happy with it, even though I gave up two runs," he said. "They were the types of runs I like to give up. All ground-ball hits."

Concerned with the lack of major league action, Coffey asked coaches and others what they thought about his stuff. Coffey does this with such sincerity, such an earnest disposition, it's damn near impossible to tell him the unvarnished truth. It's almost as though Coffey's optimism is a contagion that causes white lies. While Braves officials assured Coffey that his stuff was good, the private reports differed. Neither the sinker nor the slider moved like it once did. "Flat," one scout said. And with the average fastball for a reliever approaching 93 miles per hour, whatever speed advantage Coffey once had, had been nullified by the velocity revolution.

He whiled away his days with a light morning workout, a minor league game in the afternoon, and trips with Jennifer and Declan to one of the four nearby Disney parks at night. Coffey stomached "It's a Small World" more times than he could count. Declan, now two, rode through the Haunted Mansion and started clapping at the sight of someone hanging by his neck. It was like every other day in the last two and a half years: the same thing, over and over, with one goal in mind. And even though Coffey hadn't spent a full day in the major league camp, when asked where he expected to start the year, he said: "I think a big league spot. There's no doubt in my mind that I'm going to Triple-A if I don't have a spot in the big leagues. I've been ninety-three to ninety-four. Just the way they've pitched me and treated me. I've gotten regular work."

By April 1, it had been more than a week since Coffey had pitched in a major league game, and his assignment was indeed a joke: the back fields in Lakeland, Florida, pitching against Double-A kids from the Detroit Tigers system. It was a strictly friends-and-family affair, fields with no seats and benches so uncomfortable Coffey preferred to stand. He wore number 99 on his back and a fuller mustache on his face. "I'd feel weird if it weren't there," Coffey said.

He trotted to the mound in the ninth inning. The first hitter chopped a 91-mph sinker off home plate for a single. The next grounded a 90-mph sinker into a double play. And after his velocity came back against the third hitter—Coffey said his arm finally loosened up, and he started with three straight pitches at 93—it took a slick catch by the Braves' top prospect, second baseman José Peráza, to end the game. Coffey didn't know if he got a save. He wasn't paying attention to the score and jogged off the field and out of the heat quickly.

"Want some water?" a coach asked.

"Nah," Coffey said. "I don't believe in it. Water's for the weak. Tequila. Real man's drink."

Both laughed as Coffey packed his bag. He hauled it over his shoulder and headed toward the bus. Parked adjacent to it were four car haulers stuffed with trucks and SUVs, Audis and Lexuses. The apogee of automotive excessiveness sat atop one of the eighteen-wheelers: Tigers starter Alfredo Simon's Mercedes-Benz S63 AMG, covered front to back in chrome. It shined like a beacon.

"Just another reminder," Coffey said. "It's where you want to be. Where I deserve to be right now. Get out there with no adrenaline and throw like that? Get me into the season, it's gonna be harder, better." He grew up loving the Braves, and even if the team looked like it was going to stink, he could make up for the time he missed last season, maybe even close a game or two if the Braves traded All-Star closer Craig Kimbrel, which they did within the week. Coffey was convinced everything was coming together, that this wouldn't be Seattle 2.0, that outings like the one on April Fools' Day would convince the Braves of his worthiness.

Before he got onto the bus, Coffey reached into his glove and flipped the game ball to me. "Your first save," he said.

I thanked him and made sure to keep it in a safe place. I figured he might want it someday.

WHEN THE PHONE IN THE bullpen rang, Daniel Hudson's body tensed up. Being a relief pitcher means being ready to throw at any moment, pushing the arm from zero to 60 in supercar time. On May 23, 2015, a day after he threw two perfect innings, the dugout summoned him once more.

"Get Huddy ready for the next hitter," the instructions went, and off went the training wheels once and for all. Two years of being babied, coddled, and nursed back to health disappeared with one phone call. It was like Hudson was just another pitcher: summoned for one out in the eighth inning of a tight game, throwing on back-to-back days, testing the fortitude of his arm. Following a pair of changeups to Chicago Cubs outfielder Chris Coghlan, Hudson reached back—far back, like he always would, bad habits so hard to break—and threw a baseball harder than he ever had thrown it.

The only time the radar gun lies is when it spits numbers onto stadium scoreboards. On occasion, they add a mile or two or three per hour, whether it's to oblige the psyche of the man on the mound or excite fans. And those guns once said Hudson was flirting with triple digits, which was all well and good, if not entirely truthful.

This pitch to Coghlan was tracked by three cameras—one behind home plate, one in center field, one down a baseline—that followed the ball from the moment it left his hand to when it crossed the plate. It drifted 5¼ inches away and spun 1,995 revolutions per minute and crossed the plate for a strike at 98 miles per hour. And for someone who long wondered whether he was supposed to throw a pitch again, he couldn't have asked for a more definitive answer.

Around baseball, people watched Hudson with great interest. Other Tommy John survivors' futures were tenuous. Stephen Strasburg couldn't seem to stay off the disabled list. Matt Harvey went through his innings drama. Jarrod Parker, a little more than a year removed from asking Hudson what it was like to come back from a second UCL reconstruction, collapsed to the ground during a rehab start. He suffered an avulsion fracture in the medial epicondyle, the same injury seen in the Japanese children visiting Naotaka Mamizuka's baseball clinic. Parker needed another surgery. No major league pitcher had ever returned from a pair of Tommy Johns and a broken elbow.

"You want to not feel anything in your elbow ever again?" Hudson said. "Just don't throw."

Hudson's arm scare during spring training turned out to be nothing more than triceps tendinitis. He was offered a chance to jump into an MRI tube to confirm the diagnosis. He declined. Hudson gobbled anti-inflammatories for five days, rested, and returned for one final spring start in which he threw seventy-two pitches. When he woke up the next morning his arm felt fine.

"Honestly, at this point, if I just sat there and thought about my elbow, it would start aching," Hudson said. "I swear to God. I feel like it would. I don't know if I'm just wired weird to where, once I get on the mound, I don't think about anything else except throwing the baseball. I don't know if I'm just wired differently than other people."

Mike Harkey assured him his future was in the rotation, and Hudson even made a spot start in May after a line drive brained rookie starter Archie Bradley and sidelined him for a week. Bullpen work suited Hudson well, though, the short, high-intensity bursts allowing him to better monitor his delivery, which too often got out of whack and started resembling his presurgery motion. His hand stayed on top of the ball better and his arm didn't wind up behind him quite as much, but the basics were too ingrained. He threw how he threw. He'd throw how he'd always thrown.

And when it blew—an elbow like Hudson's, it always is a matter of when, with the hope that it's a decade and not a year—he could call it a good career and not be lying to himself. Baseball was going to end at some point, and the two years away had given Hudson a far better sense of what life was going to look like when it did. He liked what he saw.

In Hudson's bedroom, two oversized nightstands abut his bed. Sara spent two years convincing her husband the room needed them. At five thousand dollars apiece, they were an extravagant purchase, ridiculous in Hudson's mind, but Sara was convinced they were important.

When Hudson goes to sleep, his right arm flexes into the air, almost like he's cocking it to throw a baseball. The second his eyes open, he focuses on his right arm and straightens it slowly. And when it's fully extended and no pain shoots through it, Daniel Hudson will roll over, hunt for the open wooden spot on the nightstand next to the mercury-glass lamps, ball up his fist, and knock twice, thankful for at least one more day his arm is still capable of wondrous things.

ON THE MORNING HE WAS released, Todd Coffey didn't even have time to change into his uniform. He showed up in the Atlanta Braves' minor league clubhouse, a space cramped with twenty-somethings that smelled like hangover and Axe body spray, and was summoned immediately to meet with Jonathan Schuerholz, the assistant farm director and the son of the Braves' president. He said Coffey did not make the Triple-A roster and that he wished him the best of luck wherever he ended up. It was quick and painful.

Coffey cleared his locker and bolted out. He wanted to go far away but ended up at Epcot instead because his kids were in town and they wanted to go. He didn't understand. This wasn't like Seattle, the difference between Triple-A and the major leagues. He couldn't even crack a minor league roster.

"I'm baffled beyond baffled," Coffey said. "If I'd have been sucking, I could read the writing on the wall. I'm pretty honest with myself."

Because every other team spent its spring paring down rosters in the same fashion as Atlanta, Coffey found no immediate suitors. He refused to consider the independent leagues, the standard home for MLB vagabonds seeking employment, or the Mexican League, where an old friend offered him a job. He would wait and find other things to occupy his days. "Guess I can get back to extreme couponing for a short time," Coffey said.

Back into the routine he went: up at 11:00 a.m., off to the gym, throw in the afternoon, home for dinner, play with Declan, help Hannah with her homework, and avoid baseball at night.

"It's almost physically painful to watch some of these guys throw shit up there and get their asses handed to them," Coffey said. "Like, in my chest. It's nausea. Honestly, I could pitch in the big leagues tonight."

And he believed it. He really, truly believed it, every word of it, and that was the essence of Todd Coffey. When I suggested it might be his age, he pointed to older pitchers. And when I hinted at his weight scaring off teams, he noted there were worse bodies in the big leagues. And when I alluded to the two full seasons since his last major league outing, he blamed Seattle.

When Coffey stared in the mirror, a major league pitcher stared back at him. "I know my arm is good," Coffey said. "I know I'm ready to pitch. That's what sucks. I was going to have a better year than I did last year. I know I was."

May rolled around. Jobs opened up. Nobody called Coffey. He spent his days going through the motions, his nights with his fish tank, waiting until the LED shut down at 11:00, shining his flashlight, watching the show, going to sleep, doing it all again. He thought about retiring. He thought more and realized he couldn't. Maybe if his sinker wasn't hitting 93 and 94 in bullpen sessions.

He so badly wanted to be in the 80 percent that made it back. For himself and Jennifer, for Hannah and Declan, for Rutherfordton and the donor's family, even if they never wrote him back. Coffey spent more time than Daniel Hudson trying to return to the major leagues, and he refused to say it was for nothing.

Coffey started to consider independent ball and Mexico. Jennifer wanted to know the history of pitchers coming back to the big leagues from Mexico. The closest comparable to Coffey was Seth McClung, another big, red-haired, right-handed reliever with six major league seasons. He spent one year in Mexico, pitched well, and never played again. Only two players in the previous five years had made it to the major leagues after pitching in Mexico: Jean Machi, the San Francisco Giants' mop-up reliever, and Rafael Martin, who debuted with the Washington Nationals five years after he last pitched in Mexico.

"Maybe Mexico doesn't have the biggest success rate of people going back into affiliated ball," Jennifer said, "but you don't know if you don't try. He could be the one percent of people who get back. You have to exhaust every option before you throw in the towel."

On May 31, 2015, Coffey agreed to a contract with Los Diablos Rojos del México, the best team in the Mexican League. It's where Machi impressed the Giants and where Coffey now vowed to do the same for all thirty teams. He didn't know much about Mexico City and didn't know enough Spanish to realize he was a perfect fit for a team called the Red Devils. It was baseball, though, real baseball. And he needed to play as a peace offering to those who didn't believe he would be back, to the baseball gods he would worship forever.

Earlier in the week, I had asked Coffey whether the game was telling him something. The Mariners fiasco. Then the Braves. Radio silence thereafter. The mound is an addiction, an artery into the pitcher's heart, and the thought of life after it scared Coffey. There is no sadder thing in baseball than a man who isn't done with the game when the game is done with him.

A few days before Coffey left for Mexico, he sent the longest text message I'd ever received.

After our conversation yesterday I have done a lot of thinking about what we talked about and how if this game is telling me it's over, it's always telling people it's over. If you ever fall into the trap of thinking you're not good enough or you think the game has passed you by you will never succeed, even in high school, because people are always telling you there's no chance, but we still push and strive and work hard. My whole career I have been told I wasn't good enough, not going to be able to do it. I never listened to them. Why should I start listening to them now? It's all about an opportunity. You make your own opportunities. If you're not playing you cant be seen, just like in high school. If you listened to the people in high school that tell you you're not good enough and quit then I would've never got the opportunity to get where I got. So now another chapter in my career is getting back.

My resolve is strong, my heart is true. I will never give up. I will push it every day until I get that opportunity and when I do get that opportunity I will prove once again to everyone that I can still play this game. If this is the end, which I don't think so, then I'm going to leave this game the way I came into it—fighting and kicking to stay in it.

The light remained on. The show was not over. I told him I didn't expect anything less.

EPILOGUE

On July 27, 2015, in Cooperstown, New York, nearly fifty thousand people heard John Smoltz speak at his induction into the National Baseball Hall of Fame. Toward the end of his thirty-minute speech, he did something no inductee before him had ever done.

He wanted to talk about pitching arms.

Smoltz underwent UCL replacement on March 23, 2000. He came back at thirty-four years old and thrived, the second half of his career good enough to make him the first pitcher in the Hall of Fame with a Tommy John scar.

"It's an epidemic," Smoltz said. "It's something that is affecting our game. It's something that I thought would cost me my career, but thanks to Dr. James Andrews and all those before him, performing the surgery with such precision has caused it to be almost a false read, like a Band-Aid you put on your arm.

"I want to encourage the families and parents that are out there to understand that this is not normal to have a surgery at fourteen and fifteen years old. That you have time. That baseball is not a year-round sport. That you have an opportunity to be athletic and play other sports. . . .

"So I want to encourage you, if nothing else, know that your children's passion and desire to play baseball is something that they can do without a competitive pitch. . . . Please, take care of those great future arms."

For Daniel Hudson and Todd Coffey, Jon Lester and Trevor Bauer, for anyone pitching in Major League Baseball today, it is too late. Maybe the game can save Riley Pint and Anthony Molina or the kids playing at a Perfect Game showcase this weekend or even my son. He starts kid-pitch baseball this year, and while I think I understand how to protect him, I don't know for certain. There might be a mechanical flaw I can't see with the naked eye or even the slow-motion video on my iPhone. Maybe something lurks in his elbow, biding its time. It's an awful feeling, surrendering to the unknown, and yet my son and millions of other kids love baseball enough that we no longer have a choice.

After I finished this book, the baseball world kept spinning— and the people in it continued their journeys. Shortly before it went to press, I caught up with some of those I had followed for more than three years.

DANIEL HUDSON Less than a year after his comeback, as he neared the end of his first full season since 2011, Hudson, who had been the Diamondbacks' eighth-inning guy, showed enough prowess to warrant the occasional save opportunity. He was regularly hitting 98 miles per hour, occasionally touching 99, and on September 1, when the radar gun flashed three digits—100—Hudson had achieved what only a couple of dozen others would in 2015, and maybe another hundred had ever done. That joke he made to Dr. Lewis Yocum before his first surgery—"If I don't wake up throwing one hundred," he had said, half anesthetized, "I want my money back"—was no longer wishful thinking.

His arm held up for the rest of the season, and he finished 2015 with an average fastball velocity of 96.2 miles per hour. By the end of the year, only sixteen pitchers threw as consistently hard as him. The velocity didn't always translate into success, as Hudson finished the season with a 3.86 ERA, dragged down by a few massive blowups. He saw room to improve, whether by taking yoga classes before the 2016 season to improve his flexibility or simplifying his footwork during the delivery to resemble that of David Price, Sonny Gray, and Jake Arrieta.

Over the winter, Hudson texted me and asked whether I think he should spend the 2016 season as a starter or reliever. The Diamondbacks bolstered their rotation with the $206.5 million investment in Zack Greinke and overpaid in talent to acquire twenty-five-year-old right-hander Shelby Miller from Atlanta. Winning a rotation spot wouldn't be easy. Then again, free agency beckons for Hudson after 2016, and his old friend and teammate Ian Kennedy—who had the worst on-base-plus-slugging-against of any starting pitcher in 2015—signed a five-year, $70 million contract in January 2016 with the Kansas City Royals, coming off a World Series championship.

Deep down, Hudson worried about starting, worried about what it might do to his arm. Sara wanted him to stick in the bullpen, to succeed where he'd found success, and maybe he could cash in like the dozen-plus relievers who fetched multiyear deals in the winter of 2015, topped by the $31 million for sidearmer Darren O'Day.

In the end, Hudson planned on going into spring training as a starter, which I thought was the right move. Nobody knows what his arm is or isn't capable of doing; erring on the safe side isn't realistic because there is no safe side. Pitching in the bullpen was a perfect fallback plan, and it ended up being his reality. And for the first three months of the season, he was one of the best relievers in baseball. Then came the worst five weeks of Hudson's career that didn't involve a scalpel or scar. He allowed an inconceivable 33 runs in 9⅔ innings. It was a combination of awful luck on balls in play and an inability to put hitters away.

Hudson finished the 2016 season with an ERA over 5.00. His fastball was still there, though, and his changeup darted as ever, and as free agency beckoned, his agent, Andrew Lowenthal, cast a wide net looking for suitors. Nearly twenty teams showed interest in Hudson. On December 19, 2016, he signed a two-year, $11 million deal with the Pittsburgh Pirates. It wasn't the $15 million he turned down. It didn't need to be. "It was just right," he said.

TODD COFFEY On July 3, 2015, in his eleventh outing for Los Diablos Rojos del México, Coffey heard a pop in his knee. He limped off the field, his ERA 4.66, his morale nonexistent, the major leagues a million miles away, and that was before the doctor tried to pump him with a shot of something he didn't want. "And to top it all off," Coffey said, "I ran out of gas on the way from the park to the hotel."

Thus ended Coffey's Mexican League experiment, a month that earned him a few thousand dollars and a torn meniscus. It was lonelier there than he had expected—just him and baseball and movies at the hotel. Ripping up cartilage in his knee was almost a relief; no major league team was calling on him, and now he had more time to consider his future. He said he wanted to pitch in winter ball, but that didn't happen. Coffey would gear up for spring training, maybe even minus a few pounds; he and Jennifer had talked about how impressed teams might be if he showed up looking like a new man and not the same guy who by then would have spent almost four years out of the big leagues.

Coffey wasn't quitting. Not like this. Nothing was ever enough to persuade him. Finally convinced his body might be scaring off teams, he started a high-intensity-interval-training program and dropped forty pounds. On December

8, 2015, Coffey drove from North Carolina to Nashville, where baseball held its Winter Meetings. For the next two days, he trawled the Gaylord Opryland Resort & Convention Center, a monstrosity of a hotel so ostentatious it boasts an indoor river, trying to reconnect with old friends and show them how good he looked. "Just need a chance," he said. That's all he ever wanted.

His opportunity arrived. Just not where he had hoped. The Long Island Ducks, often the last stop for former major leaguers on their way out of the game, imported him to close games in the independent Atlantic League. Coffey notched 27 saves. He said his fastball consistently sat in the mid-90s. Nobody from the major leagues called. And it left Coffey wondering what was next and whether he ever would get to fulfill his promise to himself.

Hidden in a closet in Rutherfordton were the cleats from his last game with the Dodgers, and he promised himself he would wear them again. Coffey won't unwrap the shoes for any game outside the big leagues. If his team doesn't wear blue, he'll dye the shoes. Just one more game, one day to validate everything.

JON LESTER As happened to him every spring, Lester endured a so-called dead arm period in March 2015 that spooked Chicagoans who feared their $155 million ace was a lemon draped in blue pinstripes. Though Lester's yips on throws to first base were exposed and exploited to the tune of a record 44 stolen bases against a left-handed pitcher, he turned in a classically strong first season with the Cubs: 205 innings, 207 strikeouts, 47 walks, a 3.34 ERA. Even better: his batting average is no longer .000, thanks to 4 hits in 62 at bats. While Lester's 11–12 record looked more like that of a starter on a poor team, the Cubs were anything but. Theo Epstein and Jed Hoyer's bet on the kids worked, and a lineup half filled with rookies led Chicago to 97 wins and an NLCS berth. The Cubs have the talent to be the best team in baseball for the next half-decade, though in 2016 they were merely content with breaking a one-hundred-eight-year curse. After the best season of his career, and after winning the NLCS MVP award, Lester experiences something even better: He helped lead the Chicago Cubs to a World Series title, pitching in the epic, extra-innings game seven that closed out one of the finest championship series in baseball history

TREVOR BAUER Over the first two months of the 2015 season, Bauer looked like he finally figured out the major leagues. His ERA sat at 3.22. He was striking out more than a batter an inning. The command remained iffy, though not killer. Then came a mess of a stretch, with some bad luck and bad execution and bad results that eventually got Bauer demoted to the bullpen. By the end of the season, his future in Cleveland's rotation was tenuous, in part because, of the seventy-eight pitchers who qualified for the ERA title, his walk rate of 4.04 per nine innings ranked last. Even if he believed in it, the command training didn't translate to better results. So at the end of the season, frustrated with baseball, Bauer boxed up his stuff and sent it to the Seattle area. He planned on buying a house there and readied for another winter of experimentation with Driveline Baseball. Bauer proved integral to the 2016 Indians, as injuries devastated their pitching staff, and achieved national recognition during the ALCS when a drone he was repairing malfunctioned and mangled the pinky finger on his pitching hand. Once it healed, Bauer matched up against Lester in game five of the World Series and finished out game seven for the Indians.

KYLE BODDY Before he started training at Driveline, a

teenager named Drew Rasmussen threw in the low 90s, topping out around 92 miles per hour. A year later, as a freshman at Oregon State, Rasmussen threw a perfect game in his fourth start, his fastball crackling at 97 mph. Scouts considered Rasmussen a surefire first-round pick in the 2017 draft—and then, in a cruel joke April 1, 2016, news broke that he needed Tommy John surgery.

Nevertheless, the gospel of Kyle Boddy spread not just through major college programs but the major leagues. Top prospects came to his new facility in Kent, Washington, with a $5,500 high-speed camera, an Emotiv EPOC headset that measures brainwaves, and no holes in the floor. Veterans seeking extra oomph on lost fastballs found their way to Boddy. Organizations sought his input. Eventually, not only did the Dodgers buy into Boddy's theories, they handed him ten wayward arms in their organization, allowed him to expose them to a weighted-ball-intensive regimen, and studied the results. They confirmed the suspicion: When it comes to velocity, there's no doubt the Driveline program works.

In the coming years, Boddy plans to expand to the Phoenix area, maybe even move there. For now, he sequesters himself in the Pacific Northwest, far away from the Indians and Astros and other teams that suddenly see the college dropout as their pitching Svengali. He's part of pro ball now, part of the machine he loathes. He just hopes, like so many before him, that the changes he yearns to make will last.

JAMES BUFFI Once he started working with the Los Angeles Dodgers as a senior analyst for research and development, the details of Buffi's experimentation were no longer for public consumption. He continued to toil away with Doug Fearing's team of quants in the Dodgers' think tank as they looked to get back to the World Series for the first time in nearly thirty years. The Dodgers won consecutive division titles in 2016 and '16.

CASEY WEATHERS Between Class A Lynchburg and Double-A Akron, Weathers threw 49⅓ innings—the most of his career. He held the 100-mph velocity on his peak fastball most of the season. Never did he get much closer to 105.8 miles per hour than that, nor did he control his walks enough to merit a serious major league sniff from Cleveland. That didn't come in 2016, either. A weightlifting injury hindered Weathers most of the year, and he topped out at Double-A.

HARLEY HARRINGTON In addition to baseball and soccer, Harley has added competitive paddleboarding to his busy schedule. His father, Martin, read a story about how a kid was recently drafted despite not pitching from ages eleven to fifteen, and he wondered whether Harley might benefit from a hiatus. No one will accuse the Harringtons of obsessing too much over sports. One October day in 2015, when Harley's baseball team had a doubleheader scrimmage and his soccer team a game in Los Angeles, Martin made a difficult choice easy: he took the family to Sea World. Harley turned twelve over the summer and entered sixth grade in the fall of 2016. His future in baseball is unclear.

RILEY PINT On the morning of August 7, 2015, scout Kiley McDaniel tweeted a picture of his radar gun reading 100 miles per hour. Pint, now eighteen, authored the pitch, and he continued to confound scouts who loved his stuff but blanched at his inconsistencies. This was the sort of Pint they wanted to see, one good enough to merit a cover story in the amateur-ball bible *Baseball America*. One hundred miles per hour before he was even a senior in high school was scary good—and also just scary, considering velocity's perils. Teams weren't that put off. Pint was taken with the fourth overall pick by the Colorado Rockies on June 9, 2016. He received a $4.8 million signing bonus.

ANTHONY MOLINA The charges against Molina were dropped in late June 2015, according to his father, Nelson. The incident still sent him tumbling down prospect lists and in search of another scholarship. His solution: to throw in more showcases. Molina went to seven Perfect Game events in 2015 as well as the East Coast Pro showcase in Tampa and the Under Armour game in Chicago. His fastball sat from 89 to 94. He was drafted by the Los Angeles Angels in the 13th round. He did not sign and planned to pitch for Northwest Florida State College, a junior college in a small town called Niceville, in the spring of 2017.

BRAEDYN WOBORNY After his visit to Dr. Kevin Witte, Woborny quit pitching. As a full-time, switch-hitting catcher, he batted over .380 as a sophomore and expects to graduate from high school in 2017. He still has not gone to a Perfect Game event.

PERFECT GAME Tired of the exclusive, pay-for-play paradigm of Perfect Game, Major League Baseball started a series of one-day showcases called the Prospect Development Pipeline designed to attract the best baseball players in 17 metropolitan areas across the country. The league hopes the PDP will encourage kids to stick with the sport while not hemming them in with days off school and expensive tournament costs. All PDP events will be free.

MATT HARVEY The New York Mets chose him to start game one of the 2015 World Series in his first year back from Tommy John surgery, a rousing success even as the Mets lost that game and Harvey's other start, the deciding game five, to eventual champion Kansas City. Harvey endured severe struggles in 2016 before undergoing surgery to remove a rib and relieve his thoracic outlet syndrome. All five of the Mets' young aces had arm trouble in 2016.

STEPHEN STRASBURG After returning from a strained oblique on August 8, 2015, Strasburg was arguably the second-best pitcher in baseball over the last two months, after NL Cy Young winner Jake Arrieta. In 66⅓ innings, he struck out 92, walked 8, and posted a 1.90 ERA. The Nationals signed him to a seven-year, $175 million contract during the 2016 season. He finished the year on the disabled list with an arm injury.

YU DARVISH He spent the entire 2015 season rehabbing from Tommy John surgery as the Texas Rangers won the AL West despite his absence. They did the same in 2016 with him back in the rotation and throwing as hard as ever.

TOMOHIRO ANRAKU While his fastball continues to sit in the high 80s and low 90s, Anraku pitched well enough in the minor leagues that the Tohoku Rakuten Golden Eagles summoned him to the major leagues for one start at the end of the 2015 season. Anraku threw six shutout innings, allowing two hits, striking out four, and walking five. He threw only ninety-four pitches.

SHOTA TATSUTA Sent to the Hokkaido Nippon Ham Fighters' minor league team in the Eastern League, Tatsuta threw 12⅔ innings, gave up fifteen hits, walked six, struck out seven, and had a 7.82 ERA. He told the *Wall Street Journal* that he likes to spend his downtime shopping at outlet malls.

KIRK GIBSON   About six months after the Arizona Diamondbacks fired Gibson, he was diagnosed with Parkinson's disease. He continues to work as a color analyst for Fox Sports Detroit's broadcasts of Tigers games.

STAN CONTE   Following 24 years as a major league trainer, Conte resigned from the Los Angeles Dodgers following the 2015 season to start a consulting business. He plans on advising teams on how to keep players healthy.

JEFFREY DUGAS His modified Tommy John surgery inspired enough faith from Dr. George Paletta, the St. Louis Cardinals' team surgeon, that he tried it on a pair of major league pitchers with partially torn UCLs. In June 2016, Mitch Harris, the first Navy graduate to pitch in the major leagues in nearly a century, underwent the procedure. Less than two months later, he performed it on Seth Maness, a four-year major leaguer. Both are expected back by the beginning of the 2017 season. Teams will be watching both with great intrigue.

JACK ZDURIENCIK   The Seattle Mariners' general manager was fired on August 28, 2015, after six and a half seasons. The team's record under his stewardship was 505–595.

BRAD ARNSBERG   "Same shit as ever," the Diamondbacks' rehab coordinator said.

ACKNOWLEDGMENTS

On MAY 26, 2012, I sent a terribly desperate text message to a twenty-three-year-old named Danny Duffy. He was a left-handed pitcher with the Kansas City Royals, and two weeks earlier he had blown out his elbow. I told him I wanted to follow him and write a book about it. He said he wasn't interested. A few days later, I inquired whether an Atlanta Braves right-hander named Brandon Beachy might be interested. Nope. Turns out young men facing the most harrowing moment of their lives aren't terribly keen on strangers shadowing them for a year.

I knew without a player—without a heart—this book was nothing. I tried twice more, hoping one might say yes, exulting when that happened, and then delighting at my fortune when the other did the same. Then one year turned into two and bled into three because nothing is linear about the arm, nothing easy, except perhaps dealing with the two people who could best tell its story.

And maybe it's proximity bias, but I feel like it's true: as compelling as the tale of a superstar's comeback might seem, Daniel Hudson and Todd Coffey imbued this book with a realness born of their honesty and forthrightness and willingness to expose themselves in a manner no active icon would dare. Never once did they shoo me away. No questions were off-limits. They wanted their experiences told right as much as I did. I sought one interesting subject. I got two perfect ones.

Right alongside them were Sara Hudson and Jennifer Coffey, embodiments of strength, not just in how they navigate their way through the peculiar world of baseball wifedom but how they managed their husbands' psyches as they plumbed the depths. Life with a sick spouse can turn necrotic quickly; Sara and Jennifer were professional psychologists without a diploma on the wall. Their husbands are lucky, and both know it.

Luck, it turns out, suffuses this book. Jay Mandel of William Morris Endeavor took me on only because I hung by a pinkie to Dan Wetzel's coattails. Now Jay is a sounding board, a trusted advisor, and my conduit to this world of books I didn't quite understand. When I had bad ideas, he let me figure out on my own how bad they were; when I stumbled upon a good one, he helped me find the right people to nurture it. Between Jay and his indefatigable assistant, Lauren Shonkoff, WME takes care of its writers.

David Hirshey and R. D. Rosen are the editors I've long desired, caring for every last word, calling bullshit on my verbosity, challenging me to be better. This is a new book because of them, a better one—and it exists, too, because of the tireless work of Kate Lyons, whose ability to troubleshoot every last problem was nothing short of heroic. All of them saw something good and wanted to make it great. I hope I delivered that.

My other dynamic duo is Blake Schuster and Mike Vernon, whom I met as juniors at the University of Kansas and who today are the kind of journalists I'd want to hire. Hundreds of hours of recorded interviews were uploaded into a Dropbox, and they transcribed all of it faithfully, accurately, and without complaint. They read chapters right after I finished them and told me what worked and what didn't. This book is theirs every bit as much as it's mine.

Maybe out of fear that I didn't want to screw up material so ripe, maybe on compliment-fishing expeditions, I sent chapters and manuscripts to far too many people whose lives were far too busy to read them. And Greg Bishop and Eli Saslow and Andy McCullough and Chico Harlan and Adam Kilgore and Mike Rothstein still did because however fantastic they are as writers, they're better people. Same goes for the others who offered advice and help: Kevin Kaduk, Nick Piecoro, Molly Knight, Wright Thompson, Chris Jones, Barry Svrluga, Marc Carig, Les Carpenter, Patrick Hruby, Wayne Drehs, Jonah Keri, Doug Miller, Ken Rosenthal, Mark Pesavento, Mike Vaccaro, Mike Fannin, Will Leitch, and the inimitable Jane Leavy, who made my year by asking to read it and my decade by going through it one line at a time.

I'm not sure any other employer would've tolerated a full-time baseball writer spending as much time on a side project as I did, though nothing about Yahoo Sports surprises me anymore. Working there excites me every bit as much as it did ten years ago when Dave Morgan took a chance on a kid who had no business in such a big-boy job. Now I spend every day writing alongside Wetzel, Adrian Wojnarowski, Charles Robinson, Eric Adelson, Pat Forde, Marc Spears, Kevin Iole, Mike Osegueda, and the best partner possible, Tim Brown, and it challenges me to do better. The backing of editors Bob Condor, Johnny Ludden, Joe Garza, Al Toby, Marcus Vanderberg, and Melissa Geisler, not to mention the rest of the Yahoo! hierarchy, allows us to pursue great journalism, a rarity these days.

So much help came from inside the baseball establishment. MLB and the MLBPA agreed to let me see the HITS system, and Chris Marinak's guidance was imperative. He and Rob Manfred, Patrick Courtney, John D'Angelo, and plenty of others show how MLB is starting to care about the arm. Same goes on the union side: the late Michael Weiner was a beacon, and Tony Clark, Rick Shapiro, Greg Bouris, and others were just as eager to answer hard questions.

On the club side, Josh Rawitch and Casey Wilcox with the

Diamondbacks were ever accommodating, and Joe Jareck and Steve Brener with the Dodgers made things happen I didn't think possible. On the writing side, the words of Joe Sheehan, Kiley McDaniel, Rob Neyer, Harry Pavlidis, Jason Parks, Kevin Goldstein, Jacob Pomrenke, and Max Thompson provided necessary reassurance. On the agent side, Andrew Lowenthal and Rick Thurman gave incredible insight and depth not just into Hudson and Coffey but the business of baseball and how it truly works.

This book doesn't work unless more than 220 people answer my questions. Neil Roach, Kyle Boddy, and Glenn Fleisig were particularly kind with their tolerance of my ignorance. Other parts simply don't happen without the cooperation of Jon Bartner, Neal ElAttrache, Orr Limpisvasti, Theo Epstein, Jed Hoyer, and Jon Lester, the hand-holding of Hiro Abe, Gaku Tashiro, George Nishiyama, Brad Lefton, and Meredith Wills, or the generosity of Tommy John, Sandy Koufax, and Frank Jobe.

And now it's here, finally, for Debbie and Rich Passan to show off like proud parents. Their support means everything, as does that of Nicole and Aaron Atlas, Joan and Sam Sharpe, Amy and Adam Rieke, Catherine and Jason Pettus, Mary and Tom Martz, Pam and Eric Sharpe, and the rest of my wonderful family. Even Otto Rieke, who thought The Arm was a terrible title and instead suggested 50 Shades of Elbow, because he was certain it would sell better.

How Sara Passan puts up with his nonsense, as well as mine and that of our sons, Jack and Luke, I'll never quite understand. As I sequestered myself inside a set of noise-canceling headphones and in front of a computer screen, she nurtured two exceptional boys, and for that I'll forever be in her debt. She's a superlative mother, wife, friend, person. Her unbending loyalty is rare, her unremitting patience rarer yet, her uncapped kindness rarest of all. Someone who embodies all three is a miracle. I hope she enjoys this when she finally reads it.

The recognition for Jack and Luke goes beyond the standard love-you trope. In mid-May 2012, when Luke was barely a month old, I was in his room at 3 a.m., watching him take down 4 ounces of milk in painfully slow fashion, the precipice of delirium fast approaching. My eyes struggled to peel open and my mind raced from thought to thought and I wondered about what the Blue Jays were doing and the Orioles and why they approached pitching in the manner they did and how retrograde it seemed and it branched out so quickly that by the final ounce I had the idea for this book, which was either the stupid product of middle-of-the-night fever dreams or something that could help a lot of people.

I hope it's the latter. Jack is eight now. He's starting to throw harder. He's starting to ask questions about how to keep his arm healthy, too. And that's the goal, the raison d'être of the last three and a half years: to use the power of two men's stories to humanize a limb and get kids and parents alike wondering the same thing as Jack. Thank you for letting me try.

JEFF PASSAN is a baseball columnist at Yahoo Sports, where he has worked for the past decade. He is the coauthor of the critically acclaimed *Death to the BCS*. He lives in Kansas with his wife and sons.